Principles and Practice of Intravenous

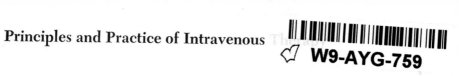

Principles and Practice of Intravenous Therapy

Second Edition

Ada Lawrence Plumer, R.N.

Supervisor and Instructor, Intravenous Department,
Massachusetts General Hospital, Boston

Member of the United States Pharmacopeia Advisory
Panel on Hospital Practices

Cofounder and Advisor of the National Intravenous
Therapy Association, Inc.

Little, Brown and Company   Boston

Library of Congress catalog card No. 75-14876

ISBN-0-316-71133-0(P)
ISBN-0-316-71132-3(C)

Printed in the United States of America

Preface

This book has been revised to meet the needs of the nurse, the medical student, the house officer, and all personnel who share the responsibility for intravenous therapy. It presents a source of practical information essential to safe and successful therapy.

In the past, intravenous therapy consisted chiefly of supplying necessary fluid to the fasting patient. Today it is much more complex and involved. Its use is extensive, and it is now an integral part of the daily treatment of medical and surgical patients. Frequently it is a lifesaving procedure; safe and successful therapy is essential and demands special knowledge and skill. Yet in spite of the increasing use and importance of parenteral therapy, little training is required of the average therapist to carry it out. It is considered sufficient by some that the therapist be able to perform a venipuncture. This modicum of knowledge does not contribute to the optimal care of the patient whose prognosis depends upon intravenous therapy, nor does it comply with legal requirements. The joint policy statements of most states require that the registered nurse be qualified by education and experience, but the majority of nurses have not been schooled in intravenous therapy in their basic or continuing education programs since most nursing schools do not include it in their curriculum. In order to perform intravenous therapy legally, nurses must seek this knowledge.

The medical staff also requires education and training. The medical student, on joining the hospital staff, is automatically expected to draw blood samples, insert intravenous cannulas, and start infusions. Techniques of venipuncture learned on a trial-and-error basis result in trauma to the veins; faulty handling of equipment and lack of aseptic technique contribute to serious complications. The house officer is required to insert catheters into the vena cava for central venous pressure monitoring and to perform therapeutic phlebotomies and many other related procedures.

Much has been published concerning cases of septicemia and fungemia which have been traced to in-use intravenous apparatus. Studies show that hospital personnel lack an understanding of asepsis and poorly carry out antiseptic practices.

Particulate matter infused through intravenous fluids may produce pathological changes that could adversely affect critically ill patients. For example, glass ampules may be the source of injection of thousands of glass particles into the circulation. Personnel directly involved in intravenous therapy remain ignorant of these dangers; yet it is their professional and moral responsibility to ensure that the patient receives fluids free from bacterial, fungal, and particulate contamination. This book provides information on these potential hazards and on the official recommendations for their prevention.

Our knowledge of fluid and electrolyte balance has increased; we now recognize an imbalance as a threat to life—a potential danger to the patient. This understanding has brought about an increase in the use of intravenous therapy and thus in the responsibility of the nurse. Knowledge of the fundamental concepts governing fluid and electrolyte balance contributes to safe therapy; knowledge of the endocrine response to stress assists the nurse in a better understanding of imbalances and problems associated with them. The nurse becomes alert to potential fluid and electrolyte disturbances, how they develop, and symptoms by which they are recognized.

Rapid and critical changes in fluid and electrolyte balance may be caused by the improper administration of intravenous fluids. Yet intravenous fluids, in spite of wide use, are the least understood of any vehicle used in the treatment of the hospitalized patient. Five percent dextrose in water, once considered a safe fluid, is now used more cautiously and recognized for the imbalances it may cause. The chapter titled *Parenteral Fluids and Related Fluid and Electrolyte Abnormalities* provides vital information for all personnel involved in the care of the patient receiving intravenous therapy.

Total parenteral nutrition has become a vital therapy in preventing starvation in many critically ill patients. Yet serious life-threatening complications may result from the care of these patients by untrained personnel.

Advances in drug therapy have further complicated intravenous therapy. The venous route offers pronounced benefits but is accompanied by problems and complications that are nonexistent in other forms of drug therapy. Very often the responsibility of compounding intravenous additives is left entirely to the nurse. With the continuous increase in drug products and parenteral fluids, the number of possible drug combinations is astronomical. This increases the likelihood of potential incompatibilities. Some basic knowledge should be available to those who share this responsibility.

Blood administration is an integral part of intravenous therapy.

Rapid advancement in transfusion therapy increases responsibility for administering this vital fluid. The therapist shares responsibility for safe administration. She must know the disadvantages as well as the advantages associated with blood and its components; she must be trained in the proper handling of blood and the basic principles of its safe administration. Knowledge of the fundamental principles of immunohematology provides a basis for understanding the problems associated with blood administration. It alerts the nurse to potential reactions, why they develop, and symptoms by which they are identified.

No matter what type of therapy is involved, an understanding of the basic principles of safe fluid administration is vital. With any infusion there is a certain element of risk. The therapist and the nurse involved in fluid maintenance must know the potential hazards and how to prevent their occurrence.

The patient's prognosis may depend upon his ability to receive a prolonged course of therapy. Preservation of the veins is important. Intravenous therapy may be given almost indefinitely if the therapist is skillful in (1) the choice of veins, (2) technique, and (3) the selection of proper equipment. The efficiency of the therapist may obviate the need of venous cut-downs and preclude the risk of adding the complication of thrombophlebitis to present illness.

With the increased use of intravenous therapy, there is a definite need for parenteral teams. More and more hospitals are establishing intravenous departments. In addition to the techniques and training essential to their function, this book also provides information on the organization of a team of intravenous nurses and the various duties that can be performed by this specialized group.

A. L. P.

Boston

Acknowledgments

I wish to express my deep appreciation to Grant V. Rodkey for reading the entire manuscript and offering valuable comments and suggestions, to Rita Colley for sharing her knowledge and expertise by contributing Chapter 13, *Total Parenteral Nutrition—Nursing Practice*, and to all the other individuals listed for their cooperation, help, and interest in reading and critiquing specific chapters or sections of chapters:

Grant V. Rodkey, M.D.

Associate Visiting Surgeon, Massachusetts General Hospital; Associate Clinical Professor of Surgery, Harvard Medical School

Mary Macdonald, R.N.

Director of Nursing, Massachusetts General Hospital

Legal Implications of Intravenous Therapy

Donald P. Todd, M.D.

Anesthesiologist, Massachusetts General Hospital; Associate Professor of Anesthesiology, Harvard Medical School

Technique of Intravenous Therapy
Venous Pressure

Benjamin A. Barnes, M.D.

Professor of Surgery and Chief of Transplantation Section, Tufts University School of Medicine–New England Medical Center Hospital

Fundamental Aspects of Fluid and Electrolyte Metabolism
Rationale of Fluid and Electrolyte Therapy
Parenteral Fluids and Related Fluid and Electrolyte Abnormalities

John F. Burke, M.D.

Visiting Surgeon and Chairman of Committee of Infection Control, Massachusetts General Hospital; Chief of Shriners Burn Institute; Associate Professor of Surgery, Harvard Medical School

Bacterial, Fungal, and Particulate Contamination
Parenteral Therapy for the Burned Patient

Joseph Fischer, M.D.
Associate Professor of Surgery, Harvard Medical School; Chief of Hyperalimentation Units, Massachusetts General Hospital

Total Parenteral Nutrition—Nursing Practice

Cyrus Hopkins, M.D.
Associate Professor of Medicine, Harvard Medical School; Epidemiologist, Massachusetts General Hospital

Total Parenteral Nutrition—Nursing Practice

Arlen Holter, M.D.
Resident, Department of Surgery, Massachusetts General Hospital

Total Parenteral Nutrition—Nursing Practice

Gellestrina T. DiMaggio, R.N.
Associate Director of Nursing, Massachusetts General Hospital

Total Parenteral Nutrition—Nursing Practice

Carole DeMille, R.N.
Infection Control Nurse, Massachusetts General Hospital

Total Parenteral Nutrition—Nursing Practice

John W. Webb, M.S.
Director of Pharmacy and Supplies, Massachusetts General Hospital; Clinical Professor of Pharmacy, Northeastern University School of Pharmacy and Allied Health Professions; Adjunct Professor of Hospital Pharmacy, Massachusetts College of Pharmacy

Intravenous Equipment
Intravenous Administration of Drugs

Sue Britten, B.S.
Former First Research Technician, Blood Bank, Massachusetts General Hospital

Basic Immunohematology

Morten Grove-Rasmussen, M.D.
Former Director of Blood Bank and Transfusion Service, Massachusetts General Hospital

Transfusion Therapy

Charles Huggins, M.D.
Director of Blood Bank and Transfusion Service, Massachusetts General Hospital; Associate Professor of Surgery, Harvard Medical School

Transfusion Therapy
The Therapeutic Phlebotomy

Sidney V. Rieder, Ph.D.

Chief of Clinical Chemistry Laboratories, Massachusetts General Hospital

Laboratory Tests

Mary Russell

Former Head Technician, Blood Bank, Massachusetts General Hospital

Blood Types

My appreciation is extended to the authors and publishers who have kindly allowed me the use of copyrighted material and to the manufacturing companies of intravenous equipment for their information and help. A special thanks to Paul Rosen, Medical Information, Abbott Laboratories, Hospital Products Division.

I am grateful to the Massachusetts General Hospital for giving me the opportunity to pioneer a program of intravenous therapy, one that has grown in thirty-five years from one nurse, myself, to the present thirty intravenous therapists.

Special thanks go to Cheryl Rust for her painstaking work in typing and assembling the manuscript, to Michael Seiler, Head Technician of the Blood Bank and Transfusion Service, for contributing the additional photographs for this second edition, and to Myra Ayer, Head Nurse, and Susan Pauley, Assistant Head Nurse, Intravenous Department, for their patience, helpful suggestions, and assistance in the development of this book. The artwork was done by Edith Tagrin of the Medical Arts Department, Massachusetts General Hospital.

Contents

Principles and Practice of Intravenous Therapy

1. History of Intravenous Therapy

The idea of injecting various substances, including blood, into the circulatory system is not new; it has been in the mind of man for centuries. In 1628 William Harvey's discovery of the circulation of the blood stimulated increased experimentation. In 1656 Sir Christopher Wren, with a quill and bladder, injected opium intravenously into dogs, and 6 years later, J. D. Major made the first successful injection in man [8].

In 1665 an animal near death from loss of blood was restored by infusion of blood from another animal. In 1667 a 15-year-old Parisian boy was the first human being to receive a transfusion successfully; lamb's blood was administered directly into the circulation by Jean Baptiste Denis, physician to Louis XIV [8]. The enthusiasm aroused by this success led to promiscuous transfusions of blood from animals to man with fatal results, and in 1687 by an edict of church and parliament animal-to-man transfusions were prohibited in Europe.

About 150 years passed before serious attempts were again made to inject blood into man. James Blundell, an English obstetrician, revived the idea. In 1834, saving the lives of many women threatened by hemorrhage during childbirth, he proved that animal blood was unfit to inject into man and that only human blood was safe. Nevertheless complications persisted; infections developed in donor and recipient. With the discovery of the principles of antisepsis by Pasteur and Lister, another obstacle was overcome, yet reactions and deaths continued.

In 1900 Karl Landsteiner proved that not all human blood is alike; classifications were made [8]. In 1914 a chemical, sodium citrate, was found to prevent blood from clotting [8]. From then on rapid advance has taken place.

Administration of parenteral fluids by the intravenous route has become widely used only during the past thirty-five years. The difficulty in accepting this procedure was due to lack of safe solutions. The solutions used contained substances called pyrogens, proteins which are foreign to the body and not destroyed by sterilization. These caused chills and fever when injected into the circulation. About 1923, with the discovery and elimination of these pyrogens, the administration of parenteral fluids intravenously became safer and more frequent.

Until 1925 the most frequently used parenteral solution was normal saline solution. Water, because of its hypotonicity, could not be administered intravenously and had to be made isotonic; sodium chloride achieved this effect [5]. After 1925 dextrose was used extensively to make isotonic solutions and to provide a source of calories [5].

In the early 1930s administration of an intravenous injection was a major procedure reserved for the critically ill patient. The doctor performed the venipuncture assisted by a nurse. The success of intravenous therapy and the great increase in its use led to the establishment of a department of specially trained personnel for infusion therapy. In 1940 the Massachusetts General Hospital became one of the first hospitals to assign a nurse as Intravenous Therapist. The services of the intravenous nurse consisted in administering intravenous solutions and transfusions, cleaning infusion sets, and cleaning and sharpening needles. Emphasis was placed on the technical responsibility of maintaining the infusion and keeping the needle patent. The sole requisite of the intravenous nurse was the ability to perform a venipuncture skillfully.

As knowledge of electrolyte and fluid therapy grew, more solutions became available, and further knowledge was needed to monitor the fluid and electrolyte status of the patient. Normal saline was no longer the only electrolyte solution. Today over 200 commercially prepared intravenous fluids are available to meet every need of the patient.

A whole new approach to intravenous therapy and a respite to the starving patient evolved in 1965 when members of the Harrison Department of Surgical Research at the University of Pennsylvania showed that sufficient nutrients could be given to juvenile beagle dogs to support normal growth and development [4]. This led to what is known today as total parenteral nutrition.

Improvements and innovations in equipment have reduced hazards; sets and needles are now disposable, reducing risks of pyrogenic reactions and hepatitis. Prior to the Second World War, the metal needle was used extensively for infusing parenteral fluids. Frequent infiltrations as well as difficulties with the metal needle led to the development in 1945 of the flexible plastic tubing known as the intravenous catheter [3]. This tubing was introduced into the circulation by means of either a cut-down or a needle. These procedures were cumbersome and required the same aseptic techniques as a small surgical procedure. In 1952 Aubaniac [1] first described the percutaneous approach to the subclavian vein, a procedure vital for monitoring the central venous pressure. Today this procedure has been applied to administering total parenteral nutrition. In 1958 the Intracath,* a plastic catheter lying within the lumen of the needle, was introduced in individual sterile packaging [2]. This type of catheter has reduced the need for the surgical procedure, the cut-down. At about the same time, a new innovation of the catheter, the Rochester needle,† was introduced by Emil Gauthier, Head of Rochester Products Company, and David John Massa, Anesthesiologist at the Mayo Clinic. This consists of a resinous catheter on the outside of a steel needle [7]; the catheter is slipped off the needle into the vein and the needle removed.

The catheter is invaluable in lifesaving procedures; nevertheless serious complications have been documented in the use of both the percutaneous and the surgically placed catheter. Intravenous therapy was fast changing from a purely technical responsibility to one that required a broad range of knowledge. The first change in the steel needle appeared in 1957 when McGaw Laboratories introduced the first grips made out of rubber and looking like an inverted T on a small needle. Shortly after this, small vein sets appeared with foldable wings replacing the metal hub. The traditional steel needle gave way to the winged infusion needle since the latter provided more comfort and was less apt to infiltrate.

In spite of all the advances in scientific and medical technology, complications have increased to alarming proportions. Our knowledge must now include the prevention of bacterial, fungal, and particulate contamination. Industry continues to provide equipment to increase the level of patient safety. Today filters are available which limit access of particulate matter, bacteria, and fungus to the bloodstream. Proper handling and use of this equipment are vital to the patient's safety.

Until recently the subcutaneous and the intramuscular routes were preferred for the parenteral administration of drugs. Today medications are commonly given intravenously, with 60 to 80 percent of infusion fluids containing additives.

Transfusion therapy has moved ahead by leaps and bounds. Not until 1940 did Karl Landsteiner and Alexander Wiener discover the Rhesus system. By 1968 RhoGAM had been manufactured and made available to the physician. RhoGAM relegates Rh hemolytic disease to a disease of the past [6].

Intravenous therapy has come a long way since the 1940s when the sole requisite of the intravenous nurse was the ability to perform a venipuncture skillfully. The value of the intravenous specialist is evidenced by the increasing numbers of parenteral teams and professional organizations throughout the United States. These organizations provide a forum for the interchange of ideas, information, experience, and

* Deseret Pharmaceutical Co., Inc., Sandy, Utah.
† Formerly, Rochester Products Co., now a Jelco Division of Johnson & Johnson.

knowledge, with the ultimate goal of raising standards and increasing the level of patient care.

We have reached a new, exciting era in intravenous therapy, one that has become complicated by great technical advances and spectacular medical and surgical achievements.

References

1. Aubaniac, L. L'injection intra veineuse sous-clariculaire: Advantages et technique. *Presse Medicale* 60:1456, 1952.
2. Burt, J. B. Personal communication, August 15, 1973.
3. Crossley, K., and Matsen, M. The scalp-vein needle. *Journal of the American Medical Association* 220:985, 1972.
4. Dudrick, S. J. Rational intravenous therapy. *American Journal of Hospital Pharmacy* 28:83, 1971.
5. Elman, R. Fluid balance from the nurse's point of view. *American Journal of Nursing* 49:222, 1949.
6. Queenam, J. T. Review of Rh Disease. In *RhoGAM One Year Later* (Proceeding of Symposium on RhoGAM Rho[D] Immune Globulin [Human], New York, April 17, 1969). Raritan, N.J.: Ortho Diagnostics, 1969.
7. Smith, S. S., Jr. Personal communication, July 26, 1973.
8. Williams, J. T., and Moravec, D. F. *Intravenous Therapy.* Hammond, Ind.: Clissold Publishing, 1967. Pp. 41–42.

2. Legal Implications of Intravenous Therapy

Because of the law and its interpretations, doubts and questions exist regarding the legal rights of nurses to administer intravenous therapy. Until the 1940s this function was performed solely by a physician and was considered a medical act. Violation of the Medical Practice Act is considered a criminal offense. In more and more hospitals the nurse is expected to administer intravenous infusions. She is asking, "Can I legally administer intravenous therapy on order of a physician?"

"Although the final decision whether or not the performance of venipuncture procedures are proper nursing practice cannot be made by the nurse, or the physician, or the hospital administration, individually or collectively, the court which may make final judgment has looked traditionally to the professions involved for assistance in such determinations" [4].

Professional and Government Regulations

To alleviate the nurse's fears regarding possible liability for claimed violation of the Medical Practice Act, the medical profession has issued joint policy statements with nursing associations on a number of procedures, including intravenous therapy. The American Nurses' Association defines a joint policy statement as "an authoritative document issued by a state nurses' association in conjunction with other significant health organizations and represent[ing] consensus on specific therapeutic measures in the area of nursing practice" [1].

Joint statements are written when questions arise regarding the nurse's professional responsibility or obligation to perform specific therapeutic measures and these questions are not answered in existing statutes (i.e., nursing practice acts and medical practice acts). This is considered the most useful way to deal with procedures that are carried out by members of both professions.

Sponsors of joint statements are the state nurses' association, which is concerned with the area of nursing practice, the state medical society, which is concerned with therapeutic measures that were formerly considered solely the practice of medicine and which legally must be prescribed by the physician, and the state hospital association, which is concerned with the issue of institutional liability for therapeutic measures performed in member health care facilities. "A joint statement should be issued by at least the State Nurses' Association and the State Medical Society in order to carry the full weight of professional opinion of the major disciplines concerned" [1].

A statement of this type regarding the role of nurses in intravenous therapy has been adopted in Massachusetts. Its text, which incorporates the rulings determined by the six organizations listed under Massachusetts in Table 1, is presented in Table 2. As Hargreaves [3] stated, however:

It is important for each nurse to note that this policy statement will not provide immunity if the practitioner is negligent. The nurse should realize and be aware that any policy statement made by the professional organizations or by the employing agency does not relieve him/her of responsibility for his/her acts.

Other ways of dealing with procedures are by rulings made by attorneys general, by state boards of nursing, and by the interpretation of the Nursing Practice Act. In some states the nurse practice acts relating to the definition of nursing are broad in wording and do not refer to specific procedures because it is believed that since practice changes rapidly it would be unfortunate if certain procedures had to be reviewed by state legislators before appropriate personnel could carry them out [6].

In 1972 I made a survey to determine the status of intravenous therapy in the country as it pertained to nursing. All fifty states and the District of Columbia were questioned and all responded. The results were as follows:

1. Thirty-four states (see Table 1) have issued joint policy statements.
2. One state has rulings by the attorney general.
3. Five states have rulings by the state nursing association.
4. Four states follow interpretation of the Nursing Practice Act.
5. Seven states have no statements.

All joint policy statements relate solely to the professional registered nurse, with the exception of two: One policy statement refers to registered professional nurses and other adequately trained health personnel, and one ruling by a state nursing association relates to nurse practitioners. As commonly defined in state nursing practice acts, the *professional nurse* carries out the administration of treatment and

Table 1 States Having Issued Joint Policy Statements as of 1972

State	Name of Statement	Participating Groups
Arizona	Intravenous Administration of Fluids Including Blood by Professional Registered Nurses (1962)	Arizona Medical Association Arizona Hospital Association Arizona State Nurses' Association
California	Intravenous Administration of Fluids, Including the Addition of Drugs, and the Starting and Administration of Blood by Registered Nurses (1957, amended 1967). Statement added on the use of intracatheters (1968)	California Medical Association California Hospital Association California Nurses' Association
Colorado	Intra-cath Intravenous (1964)	Colorado Nurses' Association Colorado Medical Society
	Intravenous Administration of Fluids and Medications (1965)	Colorado Nurses' Association Colorado Medical Society Colorado Hospital Association
District of Columbia	Venipuncture and the Administration of Intravenous Fluids for Registered Nurses of the District of Columbia (1969)	Medical Society of the District of Columbia Hospital Council of the National Capitol Area, Inc. District of Columbia Nurses' Association
Georgia	Intravenous Administration of Fluids, Blood and its Derivatives, and Drugs (1968). Policy refers to intravenous catheters	Georgia State Nurses Association Medical Association of Georgia
Hawaii	Statement on intravenous therapy duplicates that of California	
Illinois	Statement of Agreement refers to the administration of intravenous fluids by the registered professional nurse (1956)	Illinois Hospital Association Illinois State Medical Society Illinois Nurses' Association
	Written opinion (1962)	State of Illinois Department of Registration and Education
Iowa	Intravenous Administration of Fluids and Medications by Professional Nurses Practicing in Hospitals or Organized Agencies in Iowa (1968)	Iowa Nurses' Association Iowa Board of Nursing Iowa Medical Society
Louisiana	Administration of Intravenous Injections and Medications by Professional Nurses (1966)	Louisiana State Medical Society Louisiana State Nurses' Association
Maine	Venipuncture Procedure by Licensed Professional Nurses (1964)	Maine State Nurses' Association Maine League for Nursing Maine Medical Association Maine Hospital Association

Table 1 (*Continued*)

State	Name of Statement	Participating Groups
Maryland	Intravenous Administration of Fluids, Blood, and Medications by Professional Registered Nurses (1966)	Maryland State Nurses Association Maryland Medical Society
Massachusetts	Administration of Intravenous Fluids by Professional Registered Nurses (1965)	Massachusetts Nurses Association Massachusetts League for Nursing Massachusetts Heart Association Massachusetts Medical Society Massachusetts Hospital Association Massachusetts Board of Registration in Nursing
Michigan	Venipuncture and Intravenous Administration of a Foreign Substance (1965)	Michigan Nurses Association Michigan State Medical Society
Minnesota	Joint Statement on I.V. Administration of Fluids (1967). Relates to registered professional nurses and other adequately trained health personnel	Minnesota Nurses Association Minnesota State Medical Association Minnesota Hospital Association
Mississippi	Administration of Intravenous Solutions, Drugs, and Blood Transfusions when Performed by a Registered Nurse (1971)	Board of Directors of the Mississippi Nurses' Association Mississippi Board of Nursing Mississippi Hospital Association Mississippi State Medical Association
Missouri	The Registered Nurse and Administration of Intravenous Therapy (1972)	Primarily a joint effort of: Missouri State Medical Association Missouri Nurses' Association Vocal endorsement by: Missouri Hospital Association Missouri League for Nursing Missouri State Association of Licensed Practical Nurses, Inc. Missouri Pharmaceutical Association
Nebraska	Joint Statement on Guidelines for Nursing Practice (1970). Refers to administration of intravenous fluids and medications, including blood; a statement on intravenous catheters is included	Executive Committee of the Nebraska Hospital Association Board of Directors of the Nebraska Nurses' Association House of Delegates of the Nebraska State Medical Association
Nevada	Joint Statement on the Practice by the Professional Nurse to Administer Fluids Intravenously and Withdraw Venous Blood	Board of Directors of the Nevada State Nurses' Association (1965) Nevada Hospital Membership (1966)

Table 1 (*Continued*)

State	Name of Statement	Participating Groups
		Executive Committee of the Nevada State Medical Association (1966)
New Hampshire	Joint statement relative to the blood transfusion procedure and the administration of fluids and medications intravenously by the registered nurse (1966, revised 1970)	New Hampshire Nurses' Association New Hampshire Medical Society New Hampshire Hospital Association
New Mexico	Intravenous Administration of Fluids (Including Blood) by Professional Registered Nurses (1964)	New Mexico Nurses' Association New Mexico Hospital Association New Mexico Medical Society
New York	Insertion of Intravenous Catheters (1966)	Medical Society of the State of New York Hospital Association of New York State New York State Nurses' Association
North Dakota	Joint Statement on the Intravenous Administration of Fluids and Medications by Licensed Professional Nurses Practicing in North Dakota (1965)	North Dakota State Nurses Association North Dakota Medical Association North Dakota Hospital Association
Ohio	Intravenous Therapy (1962)	Ohio State Nurses Association Ohio State Board of Nursing Education and Nurse Registration Ohio Department of Health Ohio Department of Mental Hygiene and Correction Ohio Hospital Association Ohio League for Nursing Ohio State Medical Association Ohio State Medical Board
Oklahoma	Guidelines for Changes in the Area of Dependent Nursing Functions (1966). Relates to administration of intravenous fluids and blood by registered nurses	Oklahoma State Nurses Association Oklahoma State Medical Association Oklahoma Hospital Association
Oregon	The Role of the Professional Nurse in Parenteral Therapy (1963)	Oregon Nurses Association Oregon Association of Hospitals Oregon Medical Association
Pennsylvania	Statement on the Administration of Intravenous Fluids (1960)	Pennsylvania Nurses Association Pennsylvania League for Nursing Pennsylvania Medical Society

Table 1   (*Continued*)

State	Name of Statement	Participating Groups
		Pennsylvania Osteopathic Association Hospital Association of Pennsylvania
South Dakota	Venipuncture by Registered Nurses Practicing in South Dakota (1971)	South Dakota State Department of Health South Dakota State Medical Association South Dakota Hospital Association South Dakota Nurses' Association South Dakota Nursing Home Association South Dakota Board of Nursing
Tennessee	Joint statements on patient care includes policy on venipuncture for administering fluids by registered nurses (1968)	Tennessee Hospital Association Tennessee Medical Association Tennessee Nurses' Association
Utah	Joint statement of functions includes statement on the administration of intravenous fluids and insertion of intracatheters by registered professional nurses	Utah State Medical Association Utah State Hospital Association Utah State Nurses' Association
Vermont	Statement relates to venipuncture and the administration of fluids, blood, and medications intravenously (1968). Includes a statement on insertion of intravenous catheters	Vermont State Board of Medical Registration Vermont State Board of Nursing Vermont Hospital Association Vermont State Medical Society Vermont State Nurses' Association, Inc.
Virginia	Policy Statement on Intravenous Fluids and Blood Transfusions (1969)	Virginia Nurses' Association Virginia Hospital Association Medical Society of Virginia
West Virginia	A Policy on Intravenous Therapy for Registered Nurses (1963)	West Virginia Nurses Association West Virginia League for Nursing State Board of Examiners for Registered Nurses State Board of Examiners for Practical Nurses West Virginia State Hospital Association West Virginia State Medical Association West Virginia State Society of Osteopathic Medicine Medical Licensing Board

Table 1 (*Continued*)

State	Name of Statement	Participating Groups
Wisconsin	Responsibility of the Nurse in Maternal and Child Care (1965). Includes recommendations regarding intravenous fluids and blood transfusions by the registered nurse	State Medical Society of Wisconsin Wisconsin Nurses' Association Wisconsin Hospital Association
Wyoming	Statement on Intravenous Therapy (1969)	Wyoming Nurses' Association Wyoming State Medical Society Wyoming State Board of Nursing Attorney General's Office

Table 2. Massachusetts Joint Policy Statement

The Massachusetts Nurses Association and the Massachusetts League for Nursing in 1965 issued a Joint Statement Concerning Administration of Intravenous Fluids by Professional Registered Nurses. The following joint statement is set forth with the objective of providing for the health and welfare of the patient, and protecting the doctor, the nurse and the employing agency. The Massachusetts Nurses Association and the Massachusetts League for Nursing believe that it is a proper part of the practice of professional registered nurses to start and administer prescribed fluids intravenously (by needle) provided that:

1. The professional registered nurse, licensed to practice nursing in Massachusetts, should have had special, competent teaching in the technique;
2. Performance of the technique should be upon the order of a licensed doctor of medicine;
3. The order should be written for a specific patient;
4. Where the technique is to be performed in a hospital or any organized agency, the procedure should be performed within the framework of designated preparation and practice of the nurse established for the hospital or agency by a committee composed of representatives from the medical staff, the department of nursing and the administration; this framework of preparation and practice to be reproduced in writing and made available to every member of the medical and nursing staffs; and
5. It should be within the jurisdiction of that committee in a hospital or organized agency to:
   a. Decide if the nurses in the hospital or agency may perform the technique;
   b. Establish inservice teaching of the technique;
   c. Delineate the types of fluids that nurses may administer;
   d. Keep an approved list of medications that may be added to the fluid by the nurse and provide an inservice program that will acquaint the nurse with the reactions, contraindications, dosage and results of such drugs;
   e. Maintain a current list of qualified nurses on file.

medications as prescribed by a physician or dentist, the proper performance of which requires substantial specialized judgment and skill based on knowledge and application of the principles of biological, physical, and social sciences. Several states were asked whether they would include technicians, practical nurses, and nurses' aides, but they believed that these personnel are in violation of the Nursing Practice Act if they administer intravenous fluids and medications.

In the past, intravenous practice has been weighted on the technical side and emphasis so placed. Today, with rapid scientific, technological, and medical advances, intravenous therapy has become increasingly more complex and potentially more hazardous. Because intravenous therapy involves potential hazards and requires professional skill, knowledge, and judgment, joint policy statements assure maximal safety for the patient and protect the physician, the nurse, and the health care facility.

In order to answer the question "Can I legally administer intravenous therapy?" the nurse must ask herself:

1. Does the state law delegate this function to the registered nurse?
2. Does the particular institution's or agency's policy, with the approval of the medical staff, permit the registered nurse to perform this function?
3. Is the registered nurse limited in the types of fluids and medications she may administer by a list of fluids and drugs delineated by the hospital?
4. Is the order written by a licensed physician for a specific patient?
5. Is the registered nurse qualified by education and experience to administer intravenous therapy?

These requirements are common to the joint policy statements in most states.

The nurse may properly refuse to perform intravenous therapy if in her professional judgment she is not qualified and competent. It has been established by law that in a question of negligence, individuals are not protected because they have "carried out the physician's orders." They are held liable in relation to their knowledge, skill, and judgment [5].

In hospitals and states in which no written opinion relevant to intravenous therapy exists, what is the registered nurse's responsibility when ordered by a licensed staff physician to administer intravenous therapy? "A nurse is legally authorized and required to carry out any nursing or medical procedure she is directed to carry out by a duly licensed physician unless she has reason to believe harm will result to the patient from doing so" [2]. In order to meet her legal responsibility to the patient, the nurse must be qualified by knowledge and experience to execute the medical procedure, otherwise she may properly refuse to perform it. "Where there is no reason to question a physician's order, the nurse's failure to carry out such an order will subject her to liability for any consequent harm to the patient" [2].

States are recommending that schools of professional nursing include in their curriculum a course that will offer the student nurse clinical instruction and experience in intravenous therapy. The registered professional nurse would then be qualified to carry out the procedure when ordered by a licensed physician and determined as proper professional nursing practice of the employing health care facility.

Investigational Drugs

Today increasing numbers of investigational drugs are being administered intravenously. What is the responsibility of the nurse involved in the administration of these drugs? In 1957 the Board of Trustees of the American Hospital Association approved a statement of principles involved in the use of investigational drugs in hospitals, and in 1962 the Board of Directors of the American Nurses' Association endorsed it. It was reaffirmed by the American Hospital Association in 1973. Its text is presented in Table 3.

Investigational drugs, if approved by the appropriate hospital policy-making committee for intravenous administration by the nurse, should be added to any approved list of medications provided by the committee.

The Private-Duty Nurse

A private-duty nurse, who works under the direction, supervision, and control of a hospital and private physician, usually is subject to the rules and regulations of the hospital concerning all matters relating to nursing care. If the hospital policy-making committee has rules regarding who may and may not give intravenous therapy, the private-duty nurse is subject to the same rules that apply to the staff nurse. To prevent any misunderstanding on the part of the private-duty nurse, a specific sentence may be added to the hospital's joint policy statement noting that the private-duty nurse who has complied with the criteria applicable to the administration of intravenous therapy may give an intravenous infusion.

Legal Guidelines

The fear of the intravenous nurse of involvement in malpractice suits is increasing with the increase in the complexity of therapy and in the numbers of intravenous specialists. Many of the functions performed

Table 3. Statement of Principles Involved in the Use of Investigational Drugs in Hospitals[a]

Hospitals are the primary centers for clinical investigations on new drugs. By definition these are drugs which have not yet been released by the Federal Food and Drug Administration for general use.

Since investigational drugs have not been certified as being for general use and have not been cleared for sale in interstate commerce by the Federal Food and Drug Administration, hospitals and their medical staffs have an obligation to their patients to see that proper procedures for their use are established.

Procedures for the control of investigational drugs should be based upon the following principles:

1. Investigational drugs should be used only under the direct supervision of the principal investigator who should be a member of the medical staff and who should assume the burden of securing the necessary consent.
2. The hospital should do all in its power to foster research consistent with adequate safeguard for the patient.
3. When nurses are called upon to administer investigational drugs, they should have available to them basic information concerning such drugs—including dosage forms, strengths available, actions and uses, side effects, and symptoms of toxicity, etc.
4. The hospital should establish, preferably through the pharmacy and therapeutics committee, a central unit where essential information on investigational drugs is maintained and whence it may be made available to authorized personnel.
5. The pharmacy department is the appropriate area for the storage of investigational drugs, as it is for all other drugs. This will also provide for the proper labeling and dispensing in accord with the investigator's written orders.

a Approved by the Board of Trustees of the American Hospital Association, September 29, 1957, and the American Society of Hospital Pharmacists, 1957. Reaffirmed by the American Hospital Association, April 12–13, 1973.

Source: *American Journal of Hospital Pharmacy* 19:509 (Oct.), 1962. Copyright © 1962, American Society of Hospital Pharmacists, Inc. All rights reserved.

by the nurse have important legal consequences. An understanding of the legal principles and guidelines is necessary if daily professional actions are not to result in unwanted malpractice suits. It will be easier to arrive at a clearer understanding of these guidelines if a few of the legal terms involved are first defined.

Definitions

Criminal law relates to an offense against the general public because of its harmful effect on the welfare of society as a whole. Criminal actions are prosecuted by a government authority and punishment includes imprisonment or fine, or both. The administration of intravenous therapy, if performed in an unlawful manner, can involve the nurse in criminal conduct. Violation of the Nursing Practice Act or the Medical Practice Act by an unlicensed person is considered a criminal offense.

Civil law deals with conduct that affects the legal rights of the private person or corporation. When harm occurs the guilty party may be required to pay damages to the injured person.

A *tort* is a private wrong, by act or omission, which can result in a civil action by the harmed person. Common torts relevant to professional nursing practice include negligence, assault and battery, false imprisonment, slander and libel, and invasion of privacy. There are some defenses in civil actions, e.g., contributory negligence on the part of the plaintiff.

Coercion on a rational adult patient in order to insert a needle constitutes assault and battery. If the patient refuses treatment, and explanation and encouragement fail, the physician should be notified.

Malpractice is the negligent conduct of professional persons. Negligent conduct is not acting in a reasonable and prudent manner, with resultant damage to a person or his property. It is not synonymous with carelessness, although a person who is careless is negligent.

If a nurse with no previous training administers an intravenous infusion, performs an arterial puncture, or adds medications to intravenous fluids, and does it as carefully as possible but harm results, a civil court may rule her conduct as negligent; she should not have performed the act without previous training and experience. Such a negligent action is considered an act of malpractice because it involves a professional person. However, if the act of malpractice does not create harm, legal action cannot be initiated.

The rule of personal liability is "every person is liable for his own tortious conduct" [his own wrongdoing] [2]. No physician can protect the nurse from an act of negligence by bypassing this rule with verbal assurance. The nurse involved cannot avoid legal liability even though another person may be sued and held liable. The physician who orders an intracatheter cannot take responsibility for the nurse who is negligent in carrying out the procedure. If harm occurs, the nurse is liable for her own wrongdoing.

The rule of personal liability is relevant in medication errors. Medication errors are one of the most common causes of malpractice suits against nurses [2]. Negligence results from the administration of a drug to the wrong patient, at the wrong time, in an incorrect dosage, or in an improperly prescribed manner. If the physician writes an incomplete or partially illegible order and the nurse fails to clarify it before administration and harm results, the nurse is liable for negligence. The same applies to the administration of intravenous fluids. The nurse has a legal and professional responsibility to know the purpose and effect of the intravenous fluids and medications which she administers. She must take care to ensure that the patient receives the prescribed volume of fluid at the prescribed rate of flow. Fluid administered in an amount above or below that ordered constitutes an error that can result in fluid and electrolyte imbalances and lead to serious consequences for the patient and litigation for the nurse.

Approaches
The act of *observation* is the legal and professional responsibility of the nurse. Frequent observation is imperative for the early detection and prevention of complications. Complications that are not detected and are allowed to increase in severity because of failure to observe the patient constitute an act of negligence on the part of the nurse.

The rule of personal liability applies to a supervisor and a nurse under her supervision. A supervisor usually will not be held liable for the negligence of a nurse under her supervision, since every person is liable for his own wrongdoing. However, a supervisor is expected to know if the nurse is competent to perform duties assigned without supervision. A supervisor who is negligent in the assignment of an inexperienced nurse or a nurse who requires supervision may be held liable for the acts of the nurse [2]. The nurse herself is always held liable.

The nurse–patient relationship plays a significant role in influencing the patient in initiating legal liability against the nurse. The intravenous nurse must be particularly aware of and attentive to the emotional needs of the patient. Inserting needles and catheters can cause pain and apprehension in the patient. It is important for the specialist to develop an efficient interpersonal relationship. The nurse who is impersonal, aloof, and so busy with the technical process of starting an intravenous infusion that she has no time for establishing a kindly relationship with the patient is the suit-prone nurse whose personality may initiate resentment and later malpractice suits. The patient most likely to sue is the one who is resentful, frequently hostile, uncooperative, and dissatisfied with the nursing care. By demonstrating respect, care, and concern for the patient, as well as rendering skilled, efficient nursing care, the nurse may avoid malpractice claims.

Policies and procedures should be described in detail and all intravenous nurses required to know and review them periodically. This may be an important issue in civil court in determining whether or not the person involved in negligent conduct had adequate instruction in performing the act.

References
1. American Nurses' Association (Nursing Practice Department). *The Fundamentals of Joint Statements on Nursing Practice*. Kansas City, 1968.
2. Bernzweig, E. P. *Nurses' Liability for Malpractice*. New York: McGraw-Hill, 1969. Pp. 67, 71, 113, 125.

3. Hargreaves, A. Professional nurse practice committee. *Bulletin of the Massachusetts Nurses' Association*, September 1966. P. 21.
4. Maine State Nurses' Association. *Intravenous Procedure Manual*. Augusta, September 1965.
5. Minnesota Nurses Association. Joint statement on I.V. administration of fluids. *Minnesota Nursing Accent*, September 1967. P. 99.
6. Sward, K. M. Personal communication, June 1967.

3. Intravenous Equipment

Vast improvements and innovations in intravenous equipment have increased the safety of infusion therapy. Newer equipment affords greater accuracy both in regulating the rate of flow and in controlling the volume, vital considerations in drug and electrolyte therapy. Disposable equipment has replaced the permanent rubber tubing administration sets. Pyrogenic reactions were more frequent following blood and fluid infusions through reused sets; these reactions were associated with improperly cleansed and unsterile equipment. The reusable sets required meticulous care in cleansing, rinsing, packing, and sterilizing by autoclave. The disposable unit, delivered sterile to the hospital, has saved patients from needless reactions.

Specialized equipment is available to meet every need of the patient. An understanding of this equipment is vital to the staff nurse, who shares the responsibility for safe fluid administration, and to the intravenous therapist, whose knowledge ensures the use of proper equipment.

Fluid Containers

Sterile evacuated glass containers with premixed fluids first became available in 1929. Later, plastic containers became available for the storage and delivery of blood products. Recent years have found the plastic bag (Travenol Viaflex*) a popular container for parenteral fluids; it is easily transported with a minimal risk of damage and is easily disposed of. Since it contains no rubber bushing, coring is eliminated and particulate matter reduced. Air venting is not required, thereby reducing the risk of air embolism and airborne contamination. With glass containers, microporous filters serve to reduce these risks.

Plastic containers are susceptible to accidental puncture, which creates a port of entry for microorganisms. Since punctures may not be

* Travenol Laboratories, Inc., Morton Grove, Ill.

evident, the container should be squeezed prior to use. The Viaflex bag is sealed in a polyethylene overwrap to protect the bag and its contents.

Series connections are not recommended with the plastic container, and some manufacturers do not recommend them even with the glass bottles.

Because the plastic bag collapses as it empties, determination of the fluid level may be more difficult than with a rigid glass container.

Infusion Systems

There are basically three types of infusion systems currently available in the United States; the plastic bag, the closed system, and the open system (see Figure 1). The plastic bag contains no vacuum and needs no air to replace fluid flowing from the container since the container is flexible and collapses. All other systems employ glass bottles with a partial vacuum requiring air vents. The Cutter* and Abbott† systems are closed systems since only filtered air is admitted to the container; the air vent, containing the filter, is an integral part of the administration set. The open system is used by McGaw‡ and Baxter§; air enters through a plastic tube in the container and collects in the air space in the bottle.

Methods for adding medications to the fluid containers vary with each system. The plastic bag contains a resealable latex medication port through which the medication is injected. Since the plastic bag lacks a vacuum, medications must be added with a syringe and needle. A unit for creating a vacuum in the container is available to the pharmacist and provides speed and ease to the admixture program. When medications are added to the container during the infusion, special precaution must be taken to make certain the clamp on the administration set is completely closed and the flow interrupted before the medication is added. This prevents an undiluted, toxic dose of medication from entering the administration set and being infused. Medications and solutions should always be mixed thoroughly before administration, regardless of the system used.

In the closed system, medication may be added to the solution bottle during the infusion by using the air vent located in the administration set as a medication port. The filter is removed and the syringe is attached. An internal ball valve in the Abbott set and a one-way valve in the Cutter set permit injection of medication without leakage. Meticu-

---

* Cutter Laboratories, Berkeley, Calif.
† Abbott Laboratories, North Chicago, Ill.
‡ McGaw Laboratories, Glendale, Calif.; division of American Hospital Supply Corporation.
§ Baxter Laboratories, Morton Grove, Ill.; division of Travenol Laboratories, Inc.

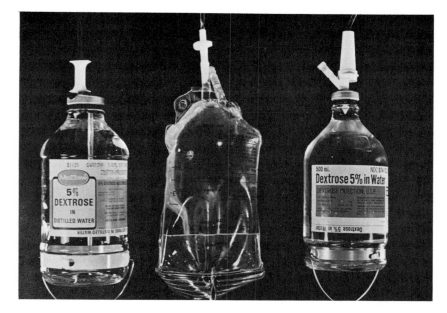

Fig. 1. Three types of infusion system. (*Left*) Closed system. (Abbott Laboratories, North Chicago, Ill.) (*Middle*) Plastic bag. (Viaflex, Travenol Laboratories, Inc., Morton Grove, Ill.) (*Right*) Open system. (McGaw Laboratories, Glendale, Calif.; division of American Hospital Supply Corporation.)

lous care must be observed to maintain sterility of the filter when removing the filter, adding the medication, and replacing the filter. The fluid bottle contains a solid rubber stopper through which medications may be added prior to infusion.

In the open system, bottles have a removable metal disk under which a sterile latex disk provides a closed method for aseptically adding a medication and a visible check for vacuum. The vacuum is noted by the depression in the seal and must be present to ensure sterility. Before the latex disk is removed, the medication is added through the outlet port with a syringe and needle; the vacuum draws the medication into the bottle. During infusion, the medication may be added through the designated area on the rubber bushing after the clamp on the administration set has been closed. The medication and solution must be mixed thoroughly by agitating the fluid before administration.

An important factor in the administration set is the rate of flow which the given set is gauged to produce; commercial sets vary—they may deliver from 10 to 25 drops per milliliter, depending upon the nature of the fluid. Increased viscosity causes the size of the drop to increase, so that a set that delivers 15 drops per milliliter will deliver 10 drops per milliliter when blood is administered. This information is of vital concern to the accurate control of the rate of infusion.

Pediatric Sets

It is frequently necessary to maintain the flow at a minimal rate. One method is to reduce the size of the drop by the use of special sets, originally designed for pediatric infusions. These sets are valuable for use in parenteral therapy for the adult patient, since by reducing the size of the drop it is possible to maintain a constant intravenous flow with a minimal amount of fluid. These sets deliver 50 to 60 drops per milliliter, depending upon the viscosity of the solution; at the rate of 60 drops per minute it would take 1 hour to infuse 60 ml. Adapters are available (see Figure 2) for changing the flow rate of the regular set to 50 drops per milliliter. The adapter can easily be removed when an increase in the flow is desired.

Sets for Monitoring Infusion Fluids

Sets are now available for measuring the amount of intravenous flow. Electronic meters allow a measured amount of solution to flow; the flow automatically stops when the required amount has been infused. A switch then triggers an alarm system which consists of a light at the nurses' station and a light and bell at the patient's bedside.

One set which monitors the patient's infusion fluids includes a small calibrated electrical switch attached to a hook from which the solution bottle hangs. When connected to a circuit containing a light or buzzer, this alert is calibrated to signal when the fluid level in the bottle drops to 50 ml. It can easily be calibrated to alarm at any desired level in order to give the nurse ample time to hang a new bottle before the intravenous container runs dry. This valuable device prevents patient discomfort and preserves veins by avoiding the necessity of restarting the infusion.

A valuable contribution to patient care has been provided by a unique monitor which accurately controls the rate of flow at a predetermined rate. A drop sensor is attached to the drip chamber and the intravenous tubing is placed in a slot on the front panel of the monitor. The prescribed rate of flow is dialed. Any change in the flow rate is automatically corrected by the clamp. Since this device eliminates the need to count drops and automatically adjusts the flow rate, valuable nursing time is saved and the risk of circulatory overload from a runaway clamp is reduced. Another feature of this monitor is the ability to detect infiltration. Whenever the needle is poorly positioned in the vein, the tubing is kinked, or an increase in back pressure develops owing to infiltration, an alarm sounds.

Medication Sites

Various devices are available for adding medications through the infusion needle or for setting up a secondary infusion. Some sets contain

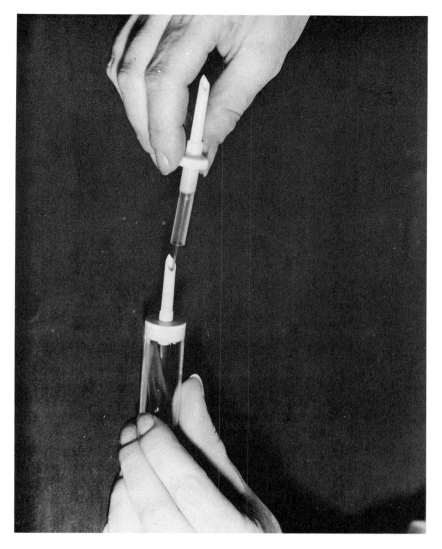

Fig. 2. Plexitron R38 M-50 administration set adapter for reducing drop size to $\frac{1}{50}$ ml inserted into drip chamber of administration set. This set will now deliver 50 drops per milliliter, enabling the patient to receive a slow infusion. (Travenol Laboratories, Inc., Morton Grove, Ill.)

Y-type injection sites which facilitate this procedure. Twin-site supplementary sets are available (see Figure 3) for attaching to regular sets lacking these injection sites. Three-way stopcocks provide another method of introducing drugs through the infusion needle. These are especially valuable for anesthesia and for the operating room when supplementary medications are required, and when transfusions and secondary infusions are necessary.

Any opening into the tubing may permit air to be sucked into the infusion, with the danger of resultant air embolism. If three-way stopcocks are used, caution must be exercised to see that the inlet which is not in use is completely shut off. The nurse should ever be on the alert for any faulty opening that allows air bubbles to escape into the flowing solution.

Series Hookup Sets

Series hookup sets serve a useful purpose in fluid therapy. They allow fluid to be added or solutions to be changed while the infusion continues and also reduce the risk of solution containers running empty. Although these sets vary with the type of container used, the principle is the same. The disposable unit connects the two containers. The air vent in the primary container is closed and the secondary bottle is vented. The second container will empty first, but there may be a certain amount of mixing of fluids: if the specific gravity is greater in the second bottle there will be no mixing; if the specific gravity is greater in the primary container there will be some mixing. This is a factor to be considered in the use of solutions containing drugs that are incompatible.

Another factor to be considered arises when a medication is added to the secondary bottle. If mixing of the fluids occurs, some of the drug will enter and remain in the primary bottle, resulting in a delay in its administration. The prescribed amount of drug will not be administered within the period of time ordered.

Since the series set, which is primarily a nursing aid, relieves the nurse of the necessity of checking the volume to prevent the bottle from emptying, periodic checks may be neglected. The rate of infusion is subject to change; if such a change goes undetected, it could result in the rapid infusion of large volumes of fluid, with the risk of circulatory overload.

Check-Valve Sets

Sets are available with an in-line check valve, which provides a more convenient and safer method for administering medications and fluids.

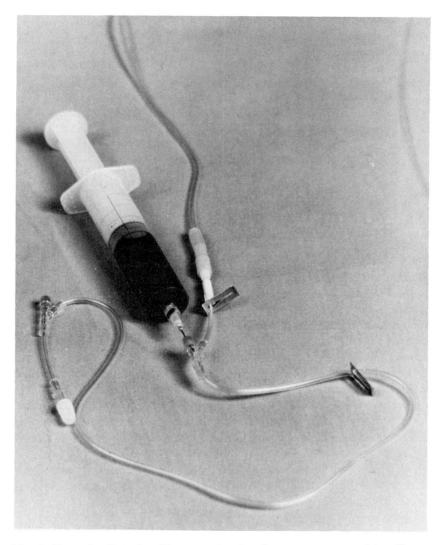

Fig. 3. Venotube Twin-Site Extension Set. Supplementary set containing Y-type injection sites. The needle is inserted directly through the medication site. (Dye added to facilitate photography.) (Abbott Laboratories, North Chicago, Ill.)

A secondary infusion or a single dose of medication can be administered "piggyback" into the injection site located below the check valve. The valve automatically shuts off the main-line infusion while the admixture is running and automatically allows the main infusion to start when the medication has run in. This valve prevents mixing of the two fluids, eliminates the risk of air entering the line when the secondary bottle empties, and prevents the cannula from becoming occluded by an interruption in the infusion. Since the rate of flow must be regulated by one clamp, the rate of administration remains the same for both fluids.

Controlled Volume Sets

With the increasing use and number of solutions containing drugs and electrolytes, greater accuracy in controlling the volume of intravenous fluids is necessary. There are several devices that permit accurate administration of measured volumes of fluids. One supplementary set, to be used in conjunction with an administration set, consists of five collapsible plastic chambers, each with a 10-ml capacity (see Figure 4). A clamp, depending upon its placement between the chambers, controls the volume from 10 to 50 ml. This controlled volume set is particularly valuable when used as a secondary intravenous set piggybacked through the medication site of the primary infusion; measured volumes of solution containing drugs may then be administered on an intermittent basis. Such a set, with the clamp applied, is ventless, thus avoiding the risk that air may be introduced into the flowing solution once the chambers have emptied, a potential danger in some Y-type administration sets.

Other sets containing vented calibrated buret chambers control the volume to 100 ml (see Figure 5). The buret chamber of some sets contains a rubber float which prevents air from entering the tubing once the infusion is completed.

Some calibrated buret chambers contain a microporous filter to block the passage of air when the chamber empties. The drip chamber, located directly below the filter, should not be squeezed, since back pressure may rupture the screen filter.

Y-Type Administration Sets

A variety of commercial sets are available for alternate or simultaneous infusion of two solutions. Some sets contain a filter and a pressure unit for blood infusions.

There may be a significant hazard of air embolism when the Y-type administration set is used ignorantly or carelessly. Constant vigilance is

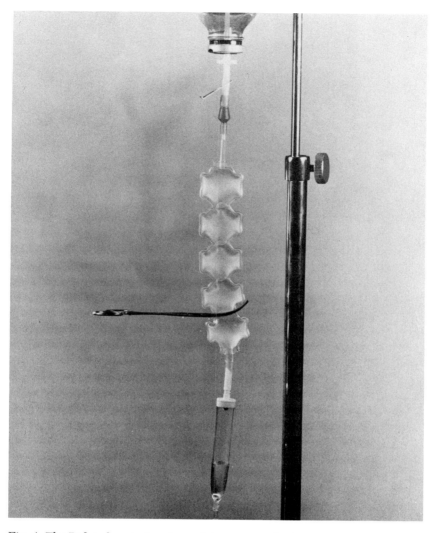

Fig. 4. The Pedatrol controls volume of intravenous fluids, permitting accurate administration of from 10 to 50 ml. (Travenol Laboratories, Inc., Morton Grove, Ill.)

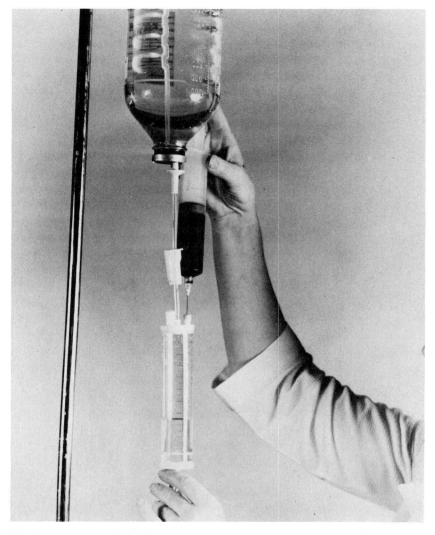

Fig. 5. Metriset. Calibrated chamber controls volume to 100 ml. Medications are added directly into the chamber through the medication plug. (McGaw Laboratories, Glendale, Calif.; division of American Hospital Supply Corporation.)

necessary if both solutions are administered simultaneously. If one container is allowed to empty, large quantities of air can be sucked into the tubing; the empty bottle becomes the vent owing to the greater atmospheric pressure in the empty bottle and tube over the pressure below the partially constricted clamp in the tubing of the flowing solution [3].

Positive Pressure Sets

Positive pressure sets (see Figure 6) are designed to increase the rapidity of infusions and are an asset when rapid replacement of fluid becomes necessary. They permit fluid to be administered by gravity, with a built-in pressure chamber available for rapid administration of blood should emergency arise. When used with the collapsible plastic blood unit, this system avoids the danger of air embolism; since the bag collapses, the need for air is eliminated. In contrast to the collapsible bag, the glass container must be vented to allow the fluid to flow; air pressure must be used when blood or fluid is forced into the bloodstream. As the last portion of blood from the container is forced into the bloodstream, the air under pressure may rapidly enter the vein before the clamp can be applied, resulting in a fatal embolus. According to Adriani [1], "Air pressure should not be used to force blood and other fluids into the blood stream."

The pump chamber must be filled at all times. The nurse should never apply positive pressure to infuse fluids; this is the responsibility of the physician.

The pressure cuff (see Figure 7) is another device which provides rapid infusion of blood. This cuff, with a pressure gauge calibrated in millimeters of mercury, fits over the plastic blood unit. Application of external pressure to the blood container permits rapid infusion of blood. This closed system avoids the inherent danger of air embolism.

Blood Warmers

Prewarmed blood may be indicated when conditions (such as massive hemorrhage) exist that warrant large and rapid transfusions; cold blood administered under such conditions may produce effects of cardiac and general hypothermia. Boyan [2] cited results of observations carried out in the operating rooms of Memorial (Sloan-Kettering Cancer Center) Hospital, New York, which showed that the incidence of cardiac arrest during massive blood replacement (3000 ml or more per hour) dropped from 58.3 percent to 6.8 percent when cold bank blood was warmed to body temperature during infusion. He stated: "To avoid the effects of cardiac and general hypothermia during massive hemor-

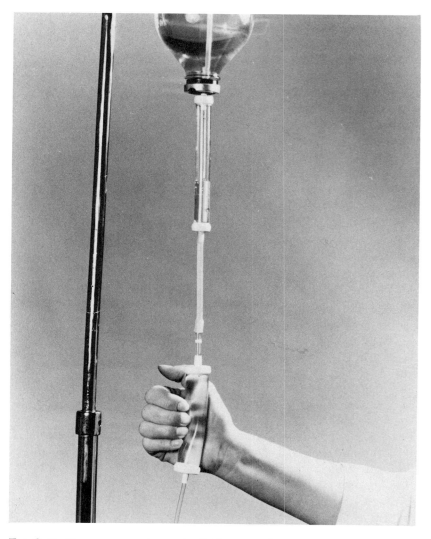

Fig. 6. Positive pressure set permits fluids to run by gravity, with pressure unit available for rapid infusion should emergency arise. (McGaw Laboratories, Glendale, Calif.; division of American Hospital Supply Corporation.)

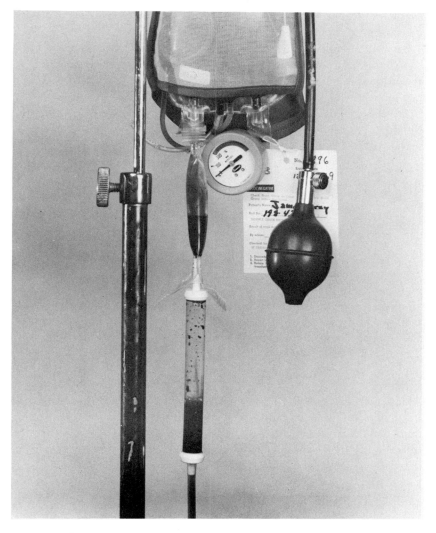

Fig. 7. Blood cuff, by means of external pressure, provides rapid infusion of blood. In-line filter is used. (Fenwal Laboratories, Morton Grove, Ill.; division of Travenol Laboratories, Inc.)

rhage, cold bank blood should be warmed to body temperature when administered rapidly and in large amounts."

Several manufacturing companies have devised units consisting of blood-warming coils that are placed in warm water baths (see Figure 8). In one unit the blood is warmed at an approximate rate of 150 ml per minute in the adult coil and at approximately 50 ml per minute in the pediatric coil. Some units contain a water bath automatically controlled to maintain a desired temperature of between 39° and 40° C, warming the blood to about 35° C.

Y-Type Blood Component Sets

Y-type blood component sets are available for the direct administration of platelets or cryoprecipitate (see Figure 9). One arm of the Y contains a spike for introducing into the component bag; the other arm, an adapter for attaching a 50-cc syringe. The blood component is aspirated into the syringe; the main clamp is then opened, the air expelled, and the main line filled. A small mesh filter is enclosed within the adapter. The venipuncture is made and the component administered by syringe. The necessity for starting an initial infusion is eliminated and loss of components in the tubing is avoided.

Filters

Administration sets with the standard clot filter of 170 microns are available for infusion of blood and blood components. The supplementary filter can be added to an in-use administration set, permitting infusion of blood; easy replacement of the filter, should clogging occur, allows multiple infusions of blood. Several manufacturers design blood filters with a pore size of 40 microns or less (see Figure 10) to trap microaggregates and protect the lung from this particulate matter. Recent evidence has demonstrated that cellular degradation develops with storage of banked blood. This debris has been implicated as a cause of respiratory insufficiency when large quantities of stored bank blood are infused (see Chapter 9). The small-pored filter is recommended for use when several units of stored bank blood are to be infused.

Final filters are available in a variety of forms, sizes, and material. Screen or membrane filters of 0.45 micron and 0.22 micron are bacterial particulate retention filters, and when wet block the passage of air (see Figure 11). Depth filters allow fluid to flow through a random path, absorbing and trapping the particles. They do not block the passage of air, and since the pore size is not uniform, they can not be given an absolute rating. See Chapter 9 for further information on the use of filters.

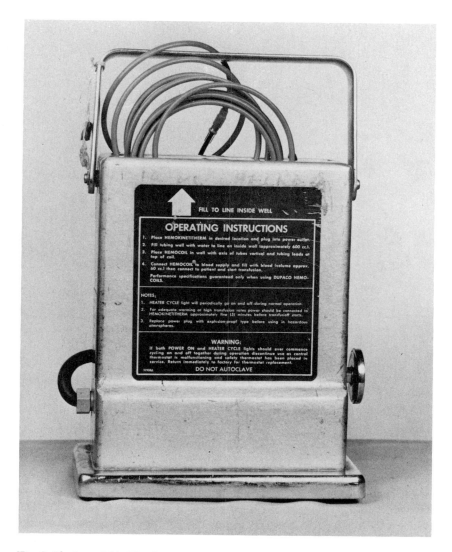

Fig. 8. Plexitron R66. Blood warmer with extension set. Extension coil with heating unit for administration of prewarmed blood. (Coil, Travenol Laboratories, Inc., Morton Grove, Ill.; heating unit, Hemokinetitherm Controlled Fluid Warmer, Dupaco Inc., Arcadia, Calif.)

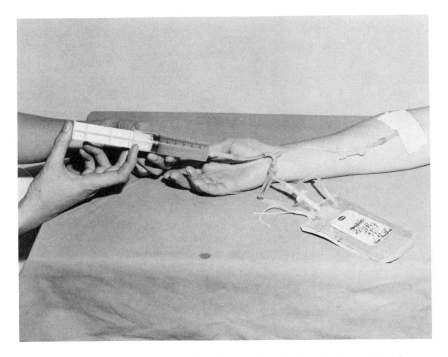

Fig. 9. Platelet recipient set. Platelets being infused through Y-type blood component set. (Fenwal Laboratories, Morton Grove, Ill.; division of Travenol Laboratories, Inc.)

Infusion Pumps

Infusion pumps have proved invaluable in neonatal, pediatric, and adult intensive care units, where critical infusions of small volumes of fluid or doses of high-potency drugs are indicated.

These pumps have increased the level of safety in parenteral therapy. In some models, the risk of air embolism is reduced by alarm systems and by the automatic interruption of the infusion when the container empties. A controlled rate of flow reduces the risk of circulatory overload.

Infusion pumps have saved valuable nursing time; the uniform control of fluid eliminates the need to count drops and adjust flow rates. Plugging of the needle, which occurs when blood backs into the needle owing to an increase in venous pressure due to coughing, crying, or strain, is eliminated; the pressure generated by the pump exceeds the maximum venous pressure.

Pumps are finding increasing uses in keep-open arterial lines and infusions of drugs, bloods, and viscous fluids such as hyperalimentation solutions.

There are many kinds and models of pumps, but most are based upon one of three principles—the roller, the peristaltic pump, and the syringe.

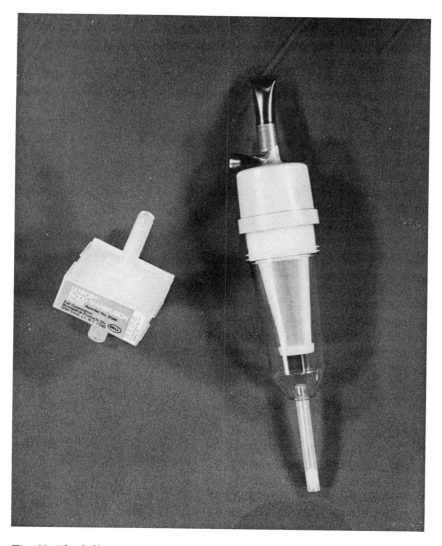

Fig. 10. Blood filters trap microaggregates in stored bank blood. (Ultipor Blood Transfusion Filter, Pall Corporation, Biomedical Products Division, Glen Cove, N.Y.)

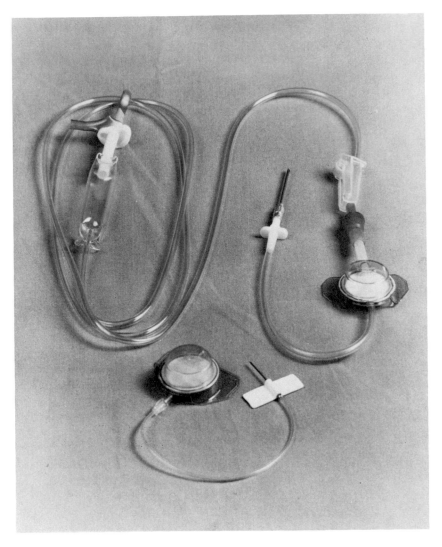

Fig. 11. Final filter administration set containing a 0.45-micron porosity filter which, when wet, prevents passage of air as well as particulate matter. (Travenol Laboratories, Inc., Morton Grove, Ill.)

Roller Pump

An example of the roller principle is found in the popular Holter* pump. A series of rollers on a revolving disk alternately stretch and relax the tubing, milking the fluid through the pumping chamber. The flow rate is dependent upon the diameter of the chambers and the speed of the roller disk. Four interchangeable pumping chambers, consisting of short lengths of suction tubing of different bore size, provide a wide range of flow rates in milliliters per hour, depending on the model used. Pumps with a flow rate of $\frac{1}{3}$ ml per hour (8 ml per day) are available for intensive care units. Microporous filters connected between the pump and the patient are recommended to prevent air from entering the bloodstream should the fluid container empty; the filter and the weld anchoring it to the chamber must be able to withstand the pressure of the pump. Tests indicate that the 0.45-micron filter will withstand the pressure exerted by the Holter Model 907 pump [4]. In order to block the passage of air, the filter must be wet.

Another popular roller pump, the Sigmamotor,† employs a series of cam-operated fingers controlled by a rotary pump shaft. The fingers press against the tubing in sequence, milking the fluid forward. The flow rate depends upon the revolutions per minute of the pump shaft; interchangeable heads provide flow rates from 0.50 to 1200 cc per hour. A supply monitor is available for use with the pump to prevent accidental air injection.

Peristaltic Pump

An example of the peristaltic pump is found in the IVAC‡ pump; the flow of fluid is controlled by a clamp which alternately pinches and releases the tubing of the administration set. Internal circuitry, working in conjunction with the drop sensor, automatically controls the rate of flow from 1 to 99 drops per minute, as dialed. The pump automatically stops at the last drop and sounds an alarm, preventing air from entering the infusion from an empty bottle.

Syringe Pump

The Harvard§ pump, a syringe-type pump, employs a filled syringe connected to an extension tube which leads to the cannula in the patient. The plunger is driven by a power source at a precisely controlled rate. The syringe, providing precise infusion by eliminating the variables of the drop rate, has proved valuable for critical infusions of small doses of high-potency drugs. A digital dial sets the rate in milliliters

* Extracorporeal Medical Specialties, Inc., King of Prussia, Pa.
† Sigmamotor, Inc., Middleport, N.Y.
‡ IVAC Corporation, San Diego, Calif.
§ Harvard Apparatus, Millis, Mass.

per minute or hour. As little as 0.06 ml per hour may be infused. A built-in alarm signals when 5 ml or less remains in the syringe, and the pump stops when the syringe empties.

The IMED* infusion pump provides constant infusion of a precise volume of fluid. A disposable cassette contains a sterile plastic syringe which repeatedly fills and empties, infusing fluid at a precise controlled rate from 1 to 299 cc per hour. An alarm sounds when the fluid container empties and automatically switches to a keep-open rate of 1 cc per hour preventing the needle from plugging. The volume administered can be noted by a glance at the volume control.

Catheters

One of the problems associated with the indwelling catheter (catheter inserted through the needle) is the risk of needle motion, with damage to the catheter and possible catheter embolism.

One unique device† permits removal of the needle after the silicone rubber catheter has been placed in the vein. A plastic sheath is stripped from the needle by pulling two tabs, exposing two needle halves which can then be removed from around the catheter.

Another device permits removal of the needle from within the catheter immediately upon entry of the catheter into the vein. A flexible self-sealing rubber tube connected to the hub of the introducer catheter allows a needle to be inserted into the introducer catheter (see Figure 12). The venipuncture is made, the needle is then removed, and the sterile catheter is slipped from its protective sleeve through the introducer catheter into the vein.

An over-the-needle catheter with extension wings has been designed to improve patient care (see Figure 13). The wings keep the hub flat and provide a means for taping and securely anchoring the needle, preventing irritating to-and-fro motion and reducing the potential risk of transport of bacteria into the puncture wound. Periodic inspection of the puncture site and daily dressing and tubing changes can be made without removing the tape; the catheter remains firmly anchored.

A radiopaque silicone central venous catheter has been devised for easy insertion through a Teflon introducer unit. This unique device eliminates catheter severance and provides the advantage of a soft, flexible inert silicone catheter. The catheter hub contains wings with eyelets which allow secure taping or suturing to the patient's skin. It is provided in a kit.‡

Still another central venous catheter makes use of an introducer

* IMED Corporation, La Jolla, Calif.
† Extracorporeal Medical Specialties, Inc., King of Prussia, Pa.
‡ Vicra Sterile, Inc., Dallas, Texas; division of Travenol Laboratories, Inc.

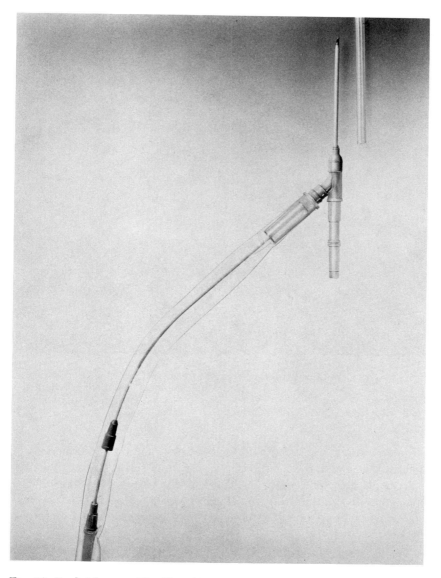

Fig. 12. Bard Advanset. Flexible self-sealing rubber tube allows insertion of the needle into the introducer catheter for venipuncture and its complete removal once the catheter has entered the vein. (Bard Hospital Division, C. R. Bard, Inc., Murray Hill, N.J.)

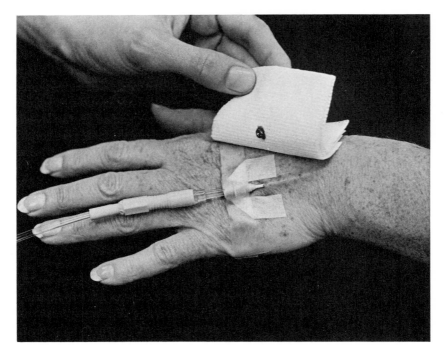

Fig. 13. Quik-Cath. Extension wings of the catheter allow unique methods of taping which prevents to-and-fro motion and permits periodic inspection and daily change of tubing without removal of the tape. (Vicra Sterile, Inc., Dallas, Texas; division of Travenol Laboratories, Inc.)

catheter.* After the venipuncture has been made and verified by a flashback of blood, the needle is removed from the catheter. The central venous catheter contains an anti-leak Luer-Lok connection that is then connected to the hub of the introducer catheter. The central venous catheter is threaded through the introducer catheter until the tip is properly placed.

References
1. Adriani, J.   Venipuncture. *American Journal of Nursing* 62:70, 1962.
2. Boyan, C. P.   Cold or warmed blood for massive transfusion. *Annals of Surgery* 160:282, 1964.
3. Tarail, R.   Practice of fluid therapy. *Journal of the American Medical Association* 171:45–49, 1950.
4. Webb, J. W., and Monahan, J. J.   Intravenous infusion pumps—An added dimension to parenteral therapy. *American Journal of Hospital Pharmacy* 29:54–59, 1972.

* Jelco Laboratories, Raritan, N.J.

4. Anatomy and Physiology Applied to Intravenous Therapy

Intravascular therapy consists of the introduction of fluids, blood, and drugs directly into the vascular system; that is, into arteries, into bone marrow, and into veins. The usual reason for using the *intra-arterial route* is to introduce radiopaque material for diagnostic purposes such as arteriograms for cerebral disorders. The dangers of arterial spasm and subsequent gangrene present problems which make this type of therapy hazardous for therapeutic use [2]. The *bone marrow*, because of its venous plexus, can be utilized for intravascular therapy. However, because infusions into the bone marrow can be dangerous, this route should be used only if other channels are unavailable. Repeated intramarrow injections could result in osteomyelitis. The *veins*, because of their abundance and location, present the most readily accessible route.

Applied to intravascular therapy, knowledge of the anatomy and physiology of veins and arteries is essential to the proficiency of the therapist and the welfare of the patient. Through a study of the superficial veins the therapist acquires a sense of discrimination in the choice of veins for intravenous use. Many factors must be considered in selecting a vein; the anatomical characteristics offer a basis for good judgment. The size, location, and resilience of the vein affect its desirability for infusion purposes.

Familiarity with the principles underlying venous physiology is also of prime value to the therapist. An understanding of the reaction of veins to the nervous stimulation of the vasoconstrictors and vasodilators enables the therapist to (1) increase the size and visibility of a vein before attempting venipuncture and (2) relieve venous spasm and thus assist in infusion maintenance.

With proficiency of the therapist, the primary goal of intravenous therapy is achieved: the welfare of the patient. Painless and effective therapy is desirable, promoting the patient's comfort and well-being, and often his complete recovery from disease or trauma as well. An integral part of this goal is the recognition and prevention of complications. The therapist, through her knowledge of anatomy and physiology, can reduce these risks.

Phlebitis and *thrombosis* are by far the commonest complications resulting from parenteral therapy. Although seemingly mild, they do present serious consequences: they (1) cause moderate to severe discomfort, often taking many days or weeks to subside, and (2) limit the veins available for further therapy. Injury to the endothelial lining of the vein contributes to these local complications. A thorough understanding of the peripheral veins alerts the therapist to observe precautions in technique in performing venipunctures. Proper technique in venipuncture minimizes the trauma to the vessel wall and provides an entry as painless and safe as possible. Examination of the superficial veins of the lower extremities alerts the therapist to the dangers resulting from their use. By avoiding venipunctures in veins prone to varicosities and sluggish circulation, the likelihood of phlebitis and thrombosis is decreased and the secondary risk of *pulmonary embolism* is reduced.

Awareness of the characteristics that differentiate veins from arteries assists the therapist in reducing the risk of *necrosis* and *gangrene;* these serious complications occur when a medication is inadvertently injected into an artery.

An understanding of the anatomy and physiology of the veins and arteries enables the therapist to recognize the existence of an *arteriovenous anastomosis;* failure to recognize this condition results in repeated and unsuccessful venipunctures performed in an attempt to initiate the infusion. These repeated punctures compound the trauma to the inner lining of the vein and increase the risk of the local complications already described, any of which limits the number of available veins, interrupts the course of therapy, and causes unnecessary pain and even dire consequences for the patient.

Vascular System

The circulatory system of the body is divided into two main systems, the pulmonary and the systemic, each with its own set of vessels. The *pulmonary system* consists of the blood flow from the right ventricle of the heart to the lungs, where it is oxygenated and returned to the left atrium. The *systemic system,* the larger of the two, is the one which concerns the intravenous therapist. It consists of the aorta, arteries, arterioles, capillaries, venules, and veins through which the blood must flow. The blood leaves the left ventricle, flows to all parts of the body, and returns to the right atrium of the heart via the vena cava. The *systemic veins* are divided into three classes: (1) superficial, (2) deep, and (3) venous sinuses [3].

Superficial Veins

The superficial or cutaneous veins are those used in venipuncture. They are located just beneath the skin in the superficial fascia. These veins and the deep veins sometimes unite; in the lower extremities they unite freely [4]. For example, the small saphenous vein, a superficial vein, drains the dorsum of the foot and the posterior section of the leg; it ascends the back of the leg and empties directly into the deep popliteal vein. Before the small saphenous vein terminates in the deep popliteal, it sends out a branch which, after joining the great saphenous vein, also terminates in a deep vein, the femoral vein. Because of these deep connections, great concern arises when it becomes necessary to use the veins in the lower extremities. Thrombosis may occur which could easily extend to the deep veins and cause pulmonary embolism [2]. Understanding this, the nurse should refrain from the use of these veins.

Varicosities occurring in the lower extremities, although readily available to venipuncture, are not a satisfactory route for parenteral administration. The relatively stagnant blood in such veins is prone to clot, resulting in a superficial phlebitis. Medication injected below a varicosity may result in another potential danger, a collection of the infused drug in the varicosity. This is caused by the stagnant blood flow. This "pocket" of infused medication may delay the effect of the drug when immediate action is desired; another concern is the danger of untoward reactions to the drug which may occur when this accumulation reaches the general circulation [1].

Arteriovenous Anastomosis

Deep veins are usually enclosed in the same sheath with the arteries. Occasionally an arteriovenous anastomosis may occur on a congenital basis or as the result of past penetrating injury of the vein and adjacent artery. When such trauma occurs, the blood flows directly from the artery into the vein; as a result, the veins draining an arteriovenous fistula are overburdened with high-pressure arterial blood. These veins appear large and tortuous. In these unusual circumstances the therapist's quick recognition of an arteriovenous fistula may prevent pain, complications, and loss of time due to repeated unsuccessful attempts to start the infusion.

Arteries and Veins

Knowledge of the characteristics differentiating veins from arteries and the position of each is important to the therapist so that she may avoid the complications of an inadvertent arterial puncture. Arteries and veins are similar in structure; both are composed of three layers of tissue. A close examination of these layers reveals their differing characteristics.

1. *Tunica intima,* or *inner layer,* consists of an inner elastic endothelial lining which also forms the valves in veins. These valves are absent in arteries. The endothelial lining is identical in the arteries and the veins, consisting of a smooth layer of flat cells. This smooth surface allows the cells and platelets to flow through the blood vessels without interruption under normal conditions. Care must be taken to avoid roughening this surface when performing a venipuncture or removing a needle from a vein. Any trauma that roughens the endothelial lining encourages the process of thrombosis whereby cells and platelets adhere to the vessel wall [2].

Many veins contain valves which are semilunar folds of the endothelium. These valves are found in the larger veins of the extremities; their function is to keep the blood flowing toward the heart. Where muscular pressure would cause a backing up of the blood supply, these valves play an important role. They occur at points of branching and often cause a noticeable bulge in the veins. Applying a tourniquet to the extremity impedes the venous flow. When suction is applied, as occurs in the process of drawing blood, the valves compress and close the lumen of the vein, preventing the backward flow of the blood. These valves thus interfere with the process of withdrawing blood. Recognizing the presence of a valve, the nurse may resolve the difficulty by slightly readjusting the needle.

These valves are absent in many of the small veins, which can therefore be utilized when, owing to obstruction from a thrombus in the ascending vein, they would otherwise prove useless. The needle may be inserted below the thrombosis, with its direction toward the distal end of the extremity; this results in a rerouting of the fluid and avoidance of the thrombosed portion.

2. *Tunica media,* or *middle layer,* consists of muscular and elastic tissue. The nerve fibers, both vasoconstrictors and vasodilators, are located in this middle layer. These fibers, constantly receiving impulses from the vasoconstrictor center in the medulla, keep the vessels in a state of tonus. They also stimulate both arteries and veins to contract or relax. The middle layer is not as strong and stiff in the veins as in the arteries, and therefore the veins tend to collapse or distend as the pressure within falls or rises. Arteries do not collapse.

Stimulation by a change in temperature or by mechanical or chemical irritation may produce spasms in the vein or artery. For instance, interrupting a continuous infusion to administer a pint of cold blood may produce vasoconstriction; this results in spasm, impedes the flow of blood, and causes pain. Application of heat to the vein promotes vasodilation, which will relieve the spasm, improve the flow of blood, and relieve the pain. The same results are obtained by heat when an irritating drug has caused vasoconstriction. In this situation, heat serves a twofold purpose: it (1) relieves the spasm and increases the blood flow and (2) protects the vessel wall from inflammation caused by the medication—with heat dilating the vein and increasing the flow of blood, the drug becomes more diluted and less irritating. The use of heat to achieve vasodilation is also an aid when it becomes necessary to use veins that are small and poorly filled.

Spasms produced by a chemical irritation in an artery may result in dire consequences. A single artery supplies circulation to a particular area. If this artery is damaged, the related area will suffer from impaired circulation and possibly from necrosis and gangrene. If a chemical agent is introduced into the artery, a spasm may result—a contraction that could shut off the blood supply completely. This problem is not as serious when veins are used, since many veins supply a particular area; if one is injured, others will maintain the circulation.

3. *Tunica adventitia*, or *outer layer*, consists of areolar connective tissue; it surrounds and supports the vessel. In arteries this layer is thicker than in veins because it is subjected to greater pressure from the force of blood within.

Arteries need more protection than veins and are so placed that injury is less likely to occur. Whereas veins are superficially located, most arteries lie deep in the tissues and are protected by muscle. Occasionally an artery is located superficially in an unusual place; this artery is then called an *aberrant artery*. An aberrant artery must not be mistaken for a vein. If a chemical which causes spasm is introduced into an aberrant artery, permanent damage may result [2].

Arteries pulsate and veins do not, a helpful differentiating characteristic.

Superficial Veins of the Upper Extremities

The superficial veins of the upper extremities are shown in Figures 14 and 15. They consist of the following: digital, metacarpal, cephalic, basilic, and median veins.

DIGITAL VEINS. The dorsal digital veins flow along the lateral portions of the fingers and are joined to each other by communicating branches [3]. At times these veins are available as a last resort for fluid administration. In some patients they are prominent enough to accommodate a 21-gauge scalp vein needle. With adequate taping the fingers can be completely immobilized, thereby preventing the needle from puncturing the posterior wall of the vein and causing extravasation of fluid.

METACARPAL VEINS. The three metacarpal veins are formed by the union of the digital veins [3]. The position of these veins makes them well adapted for intravenous use; the needle and adapter, in most

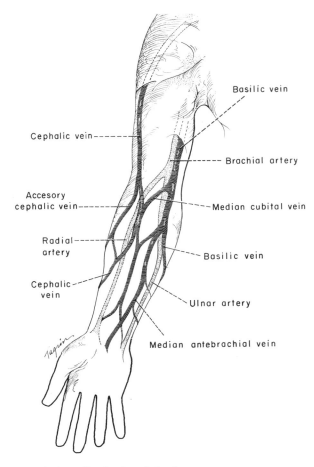

Fig. 14. Superficial veins of the forearm.

cases, lie flat between the joints and the metacarpal bones of the hand, the bones themselves providing a natural splint. The early use of the metacarpal veins is important in a course of parenteral therapy. Irritating fluid passing through a vein traumatized by previous puncture causes inflammation and pain. Therefore performing venipunctures for fluid administration at the distal end of the extremity, early in the course of therapy, is beneficial; it enables the nurse to initiate each successive venipuncture above the previous puncture site. Unnecessary inflammation and pain are avoided and opportunity for multiple venipunctures is provided.

Occasionally the use of the metacarpal veins in the elderly is contraindicated. Owing to inadequate tissue and thin skin in this area, extravasation of blood on venipuncture may readily occur.

CEPHALIC VEIN. The cephalic vein has its source in the radial part of the dorsal venous network formed by the metacarpal veins. Receiving trib-

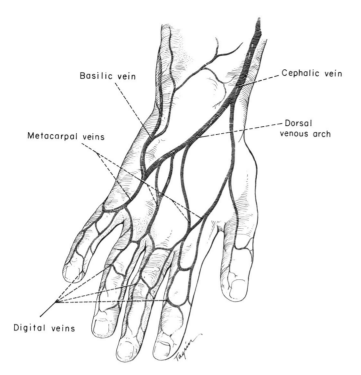

Fig. 15. Superficial veins of the dorsal aspect of the hand.

utaries from both surfaces of the forearm, it flows upward along the radial border of the forearm [3]. Because of its size and position, this vein provides an excellent route for transfusion administration. It readily accommodates a large needle and, by virtue of its position in the forearm, a natural splint is provided for the needle and adapter.

The *accessory cephalic vein* originates from either one of two sources: a plexus on the back of the forearm or the dorsal venous network. Ascending the arm, it joins the cephalic vein below the elbow. Occasionally it arises from that portion of the cephalic vein just above the wrist and flows back into the main cephalic vein at some higher point [3]. The accessory cephalic vein readily receives a large needle and is a very good choice for use in blood administration.

BASILIC VEIN. The basilic vein has its origin in the ulnar part of the dorsal venous network and ascends along the ulnar portion of the forearm. It diverges toward the anterior surface of the arm just below the elbow where it meets the median cubital vein. During a course of intravenous therapy this large vein is often overlooked because of its inconspicuous position on the ulnar border of the hand and forearm; when other veins have been exhausted; this vein may still be available. By flexing the elbow and bending the arm up, the basilic vein is brought into view.

MEDIAN VEINS. The *median antebrachial vein* arises from the venous plexus on the palm of the hand and extends upward along the ulnar side of the front of the forearm; it empties into the basilic vein or the median cubital vein. This vein, when prominent, affords a route for parenteral fluid administration. However, there are frequent variations of the superficial veins of the forearm, and this vein is not always present as a well-defined vessel.

The *median cephalic* and *median basilic veins* in the antecubital fossa are the veins most generally used for withdrawal of blood. Because of their size and superficial location, they are readily accessible for venipuncture. They receive a large-sized needle and, owing to the muscular and connective tissue supporting them, have little tendency to roll.

Since the median cephalic vein crosses in front of the brachial artery, care must be taken during venipuncture to avoid puncturing the artery. Accidental intra-arterial injection of a drug could result in permanent damage.

The basilic vein, outside the antecubital fossa on the ulnar curve of the arm, is the least desirable for venipuncture. On removal of the needle a hematoma may readily occur if the patient flexes his elbow to stop the bleeding rather than elevating the arm in the preferred manner.

The Skin

The skin is made up of two layers, the epidermis and the dermis. The *epidermis* is the uppermost layer which forms a protective covering for the dermis. Its degree of thickness varies in different parts of the body. It is thickest on the palms of the hands and the soles of the feet and thinnest on the inner surface of the limbs. Its degree of thickness also varies with age. In an elderly patient the skin on the dorsum of the hand may be so thin that it does not adequately support the vein for venipuncture when parenteral infusions are required.

The *dermis,* or underlayer, is highly sensitive and vascular. It contains many capillaries and thousands of nerve fibers. These nerve fibers are of different types and include those which react to temperature, touch, pressure, and pain. The number of nerve fibers varies in different areas of the body. Some areas of the body skin are highly sensitive; other areas are only mildly sensitive. The insertion of a needle in one area may cause a great deal of pain, while another area may be practically painless. In my experience the inner aspect of the wrist is a highly sensitive area. Venipunctures are performed here only when other veins have been exhausted.

Superficial Fascia

The superficial fascia, or subcutaneous areolar connective tissue, lies below the two layers of skin and is, in itself, another covering. It is in this fascia that the superficial veins are located. It varies in thickness. When a needle is inserted into this fascia, there is free movement of the skin above. Great care in aseptic technique must be observed, as an infection in this loose tissue spreads easily. Such an infection is called *cellulitis* [4].

References

1. Abbott Laboratories. Entering the Vein. In *Parenteral Administration*. North Chicago, Ill., 1965. P. 6.
2. Adriani, J. Venipuncture. *American Journal of Nursing* 62:66–69, 1962.
3. Warwick, R., and Williams, P. L. (Eds.). *Gray's Anatomy of the Human Body* (28th ed.). Philadelphia, Lea & Febiger, 1973. Pp. 700–703.
4. Kimber, D. C., Gray, C. E., and Stackpoles, C. E. *Textbook of Anatomy and Physiology* (15th ed.). New York: Macmillan, 1966. Pp. 69, 398, 423–431.

5. Technique of Intravenous Therapy

Approach to the Patient

The manner with which the nurse approaches the patient may have a direct bearing on his response to intravenous therapy. Since an undesirable response can affect his ability to accept treatment, emphasis must be placed on the significance of the nurse's manner and approach.

Intravenous therapy, though routine to the nurse, may be a new and frightening experience to the patient who is unfamiliar with the procedure. He may have heard rumors of fatalities associated with infusions or may misinterpret the treatment. By explaining the procedure to the patient, the nurse will alleviate his fears and help him to accept therapy.

The critically ill patient is particularly prone to fears which can at times become exaggerated, triggering an undesirable autonomic nervous system response usually known as a vasovagal reaction. Such a reaction may manifest itself in the form of syncope and can be prevented if the nurse appears confident and reassures the patient. Sympathetic reaction may follow syncope and result in vasoconstriction. Peripheral collapse then limits available veins, complicating the venipuncture. Repeated attempts at venipuncture can result in an experience so traumatic as to affect the further course of fluid therapy. Only a skilled person should perform a venipuncture on an anxious patient with limited and difficult veins.

Reactions to exaggerated fear may not only make therapy difficult, but may constitute a real threat to the patient with severe cardiac disease. Welt [6] has illustrated such a reaction in a case of pulmonary edema in a patient with renal insufficiency and hypertensive and arteriosclerotic heart disease with failure. No explanation of the infusion was made to the patient. When the needle was inserted, acute pulmonary edema occurred. The infusion was discontinued and in a few hours the patient recovered. Later that day, after the procedure was explained and the patient was sedated, 1000 ml of whole blood was tolerated. We can easily visualize such a reaction when we review the body's response to stress. Fear incites stimulation of the adrenal medulla to secrete the vasopressors which help maintain blood pressure and increase the work of the heart. Increased adrenal cortical secretions result in (1) sodium and chloride retention, which causes water retention, and (2) loss of cellular potassium, which draws water with it into the intravascular system. Increased antidiuretic hormone secretions cause a decreased urinary output, which results in retention of fluids and an increase in blood volume [4]. Such an increase may be sufficient to send a patient with an overburdened vascular system into pulmonary edema.

Selecting the Vein
The selection of the vein may be a deciding factor in the success of the infusion and in the preservation of veins for future therapy. The most prominent vein is not necessarily the most suitable for venipuncture: prominence may be due to a sclerosed condition which occludes the lumen and interferes with the flow of solution; or the prominent vein may be located in an area impractical for infusion purposes [2]. Scrutiny of the veins in both arms is desirable before a choice is made. The prime factors to be considered in selecting a vein are (1) suitable location, (2) condition of the vein, (3) purpose of the infusion, and (4) duration of therapy.

Location
Most superficial veins are accessible for venipuncture, but some of these veins, because of their location, are not practical. The *antecubital veins* are such veins, located over an area of joint flexion where any motion could dislodge the needle and cause infiltration or result in mechanical phlebitis. If these large veins are impaired or damaged, phlebothrombosis may occur which could limit the many available hand veins. The antecubital veins offer excellent sources for withdrawing blood and may be used numerous times without damage to the vein, provided good technique and sharp needles are used. But one infusion of long duration may traumatize the vein, limiting these vessels which most readily provide ample quantities of blood when large samples are needed.

Because of the close proximity of the arteries to the veins in the antecubital fossa, special care must be observed to prevent intra-arterial injection when medications are introduced. An artery can generally be detected by the thicker and tougher wall, the brighter red blood, and usually the presence of a pulse. *Aberrant arteries* in the antecubital area have been found to exist in one person out of ten. When a patient complains of severe pain in the hand or arm upon infusion, an arteriospasm due to an intra-arterial injection is to be suspected and the infusion must be stopped immediately.

Surgery often dictates which extremity is to be used. Veins should be avoided in the affected arm of an axillary dissection, such as a radical mastectomy; the circulation may be embarrassed, affecting the flow of the infusion and increasing the edema. When the patient is turned on his side during the operation the upper arm is used for the intravenous infusion; increased venous pressure in the lower arm may interfere with the free flow of the solution.

Objection is frequently expressed to the use of the veins in the lower extremities. As stated in Chapter 4, these objections arise from the danger of pulmonary embolism due to a thrombus extending into the deep veins. Complications may also arise from the stagnant blood in varicosities; pooling of infused medications can cause untoward reactions when a toxic concentration reaches the circulating blood. Varicosities, because of the stagnant blood, are prone to trauma. Phlebitis interferes with ambulation of the patient.

Condition of the Vein

Frequently the dorsal metacarpal veins provide points of entry that should be utilized first in order to preserve the proximal veins for further therapy. The use of these veins depends upon their condition. In some elderly patients, the dorsal metacarpal veins may be a poor choice; blood extravasation occurs more readily in small thin veins, and difficulty may be encountered in adequately securing the needle because of thin skin and lack of supportive tissue. At times these veins do not dilate sufficiently to allow for successful venipuncture; when hypovolemia occurs the peripheral veins collapse more quickly than do the large ones.

Palpation of the vein is an important step in determining the condition of the vein and in differentiating it from a pulsating artery. A thrombosed vein may be detected by its lack of resilience, by its hard, cord-like feeling, and by the ease with which it rolls. Use of such traumatized veins can only result in repeated venipunctures, pain, and undue stress.

Occasionally when thrombosis from multiple infusions interferes with the flow of solution and limits available veins, the venipuncture may be performed with the needle inserted in the direction of the distal end; lack of valves in these small peripheral veins permits rerouting of the solution and a bypassing of the involved vein.

Often large veins may be detected by palpation and offer advantage over the smaller but more readily discernible veins. Owing to the small blood volume, the more superficial veins may not be easily palpated and may not make a satisfactory choice for venipuncture.

Continual use by the nurse of the same fingers for palpation will increase their sensitivity. The thumb should never be used since it is not as sensitive as the fingers; also a pulse may be detected in the nurse's thumb, and this may be confused with an aberrant artery.

Although not apparent, edema may conceal an available vein; pressure for a few seconds with the fingers often helps to disperse the fluid and define the vein.

Purpose of the Infusion

The purpose of the infusion dictates the rate of flow and the solution to be infused—two factors which inherently affect the selection of the vein. When large quantities of fluid are to be rapidly infused, or when positive pressure is indicated, a large vein must be used. When fluids with a high viscosity such as packed cells are required, a vein with an adequate blood volume is necessary to ensure flow of the solution.

Large veins are used when hypertonic solutions or solutions containing irritating drugs are to be infused. Such solutions traumatize small veins; the supply of blood in these veins is not sufficient to dilute the infused fluid.

Duration of Therapy

A prolonged course of therapy requires multiple infusions which makes preservation of the veins essential. Performing the venipuncture distally with each subsequent puncture proximal to the previous one and alternating arms will contribute to this preservation.

The patient's comfort is also a factor that should be considered when infusions are required over an extended period of time; avoiding areas over joint flexion and performing venipunctures on veins located on the dorsal surface of the extremities will provide more freedom and comfort to the patient.

Selecting the Needle

Infusion may be administered through a catheter or metal needle.

Three types of catheter are available (see Figure 16):

1. *Plastic needle* (catheter mounted on a needle). Once the venipuncture is made, the catheter is slipped off the needle into the vein and the metal needle removed. Plastic stylets are available for insertion into the catheter to maintain patency for intermittent infusion.
2. *Intracatheter* (catheter inserted through the needle). The venipuncture is performed, the catheter is then pushed through the needle until the desired length is within the lumen of the vein, and the cut-

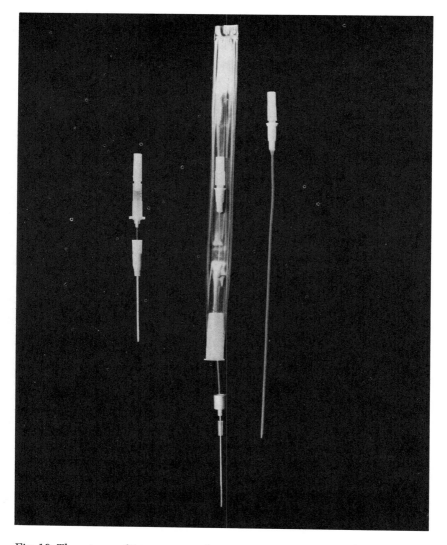

Fig. 16. Three types of intravenous catheter. (*Top*) Plastic needle. (Deseret Angiocath.) (*Center*) Intracatheter. (Deseret Intracath.) (*Bottom*) Inlying catheter inserted through a cut-down. (Deseret Cut-Down Catheter.) (Deseret Pharmaceutical Co., Sandy, Utah.)

ting edge is protected by a shield to prevent the catheter from being severed.

3. *Inlying catheter*. This catheter is inserted by means of a minor surgical procedure (cut-down) performed by the physician.

The choice of catheter depends upon the purpose of the infusion, and the condition and availability of the veins.

Plastic needles are used in the operating room to ensure a ready route for the administration of blood and fluid. In long-term therapy the plastic needle serves a purpose when difficulty arises in keeping the needle in the vein.

The intracatheter is used when a longer catheter is desired. It affords less risk of infiltration than the metal needle, often being used for administering drugs or hypertonic solutions which may cause necrosis if extravasation occurs.

An inlying catheter is required when (1) veins become exhausted from prolonged therapy, (2) obesity obscures the veins, and (3) peripheral veins have collapsed from shock.

Catheters are made of polyvinyl chloride, Teflon, and Silastic. For many years polyvinyl chloride was used almost exclusively. Ideally the catheter should be of a hemo-repellant material to reduce the risk of thrombi formation on the catheter. Silicone catheters are thought to be helpful in this respect. Most catheters are fully radiopaque for detection by x-ray in the event the catheter is severed and lost in the circulation.

Metal needles consist of the metal cannula and the scalp vein needle. The *metal cannula,* once the traditional intravenous needle, is made of a metal such as stainless steel that is noncorrosive and relatively inert in relation to the tissues. It is usually siliconized for ease of insertion and to minimize clot formation. It varies in length and gauge. The gauge refers to both the inside and the outside diameter of the lumen. The smaller the gauge, the larger is the lumen. Metal needles may be designed as *thin wall*. Because the wall of the needle is thinner than that of the standard needle, a larger lumen is obtained for the same external diameter, offering the advantage of higher flow rates. Today, the metal needle is used for short-term administration of blood and intravenous fluids. It is commonly used in the preparation and administration of medications.

In the past it was common hospital practice to infuse intravenous fluids once or twice a day over a 3- or 4-hour period. Because of this short duration, the incidence of phlebitis and infiltration was kept to a minimum. The metal needle provided a practical means of administering intravenous fluids with a minimum of complications. With the advent of intravenous antibiotics and other drugs, hospital practice changed, and intravenous fluids are now being administered on a keep-open or intermittent basis. The standard metal needle has given way to the scalp vein needle.

The *scalp vein needle* is similar to the metal cannula, with the hub replaced by two flexible wings. Originally designed for pediatric and geriatric use, it is now used in prolonged therapy for all ages. Two types of scalp vein needle are available, one with a short length of plastic tubing and a permanently attached resealable injection site, the other with a variable length of plastic tubing permanently attached to a female Luer adapter which accommodates an administration set. The scalp vein needle with the resealable injection site offers a method for the intermittent administration of medications or fluids. A dilute solution of heparin maintains patency of the needle when it is not in use (see Chapter 14).

The scalp vein needle is approximately ¾ inch long and ranges in size from a 23-gauge bore to a 16-gauge bore. It has definite advantages: the short bevel reduces the risk of infiltration from puncture to the wall of the vein, and the plastic wings provide a firm grip for inserting the needle and better control in performing the venipuncture. They fold flat against the skin, affording better anchoring power than the straight needle with a bulky hub.

The factors to be considered in selecting a metal needle are: length of bevel, gauge, and length of the needle.

A short *bevel* reduces the risk of (1) trauma to the endothelial wall, (2) infiltration from a puncture to the posterior wall, and (3) hematoma or extravasation occurring when the needle enters the vein. When a needle with a long bevel is inserted into the vessel, blood may leak into the tissues before the entire bevel is within the lumen of the vein.

Whenever possible the *gauge* of the needle should be appreciably smaller than the lumen of the vein to be entered; when the gauge of the needle approaches the size of the vein, trauma may occur. When a large needle occludes the flow of blood, irritating solutions flowing through the vein, with no dilution of blood, may cause chemical phlebitis. Mechanical phlebitis may result from motion and pressure exerted by the needle on the endothelial wall of the vein.

When large amounts of fluid are required, a needle of adequate size must be used; a small lumen interferes with the flow of solution. As Adriani [2] stated, "The flow of blood varies inversely as the fourth power of the radius of the lumen of the needle. Thus, a needle with an internal radius of 1 mm. delivering 1 cc. of blood with a fixed pressure on the plunger or in the infusion bottle delivers only $\frac{1}{16}$ of a cc. when the radius is reduced to $\frac{1}{2}$ mm." A large needle is also required with fluids of high viscosity. The rate of flow of the solution decreases in proportion to the viscosity of the fluid.

The flow of the solution varies inversely with the *length of the needle shaft*. If the length of the needle is increased, other conditions being equal, the volume flowing will be reduced [2]. Use of a short needle for infusions reduces the risk of infiltration. Because a short needle affords more play than a long needle, more motion is needed to puncture the vessel wall.

Securing Proper Lighting

The importance of proper lighting should not be overlooked. A few extra seconds spent in obtaining adequate light may actually save time and free the patient from unnecessary venipunctures. The ideal light is either an ample amount of daylight or a spotlight which does not shine directly on the vein, but which leaves enough shadow for clearly defining the vessel.

Applying the Tourniquet

Special care must be taken to distend the vein adequately. To achieve this, a soft rubber tourniquet is applied with enough pressure to impede the venous flow while the arterial flow is maintained; if the radial pulse cannot be felt, the tourniquet is too tight. In order to fill the veins to capacity, pressure is applied until radial pulsation ceases, and then released until pulsation begins. A blood pressure cuff may be used; inflate the cuff and then release it until the pressure drops to just below the diastolic pressure.

The tourniquet is applied to the mid-forearm if the selected vein is in the dorsum of the hand. If the selected vein is in the forearm, the tourniquet is applied to the upper arm.

Very little pressure is applied when performing venipunctures on patients with sclerosed veins. If the pressure is too great or the tourniquet is left on for an extended length of time the vein will become hard and tortuous, causing added difficulty when the needle is introduced. For some sclerosed veins a tourniquet is unnecessary and only makes the phlebotomy more difficult.

If pressure exerted by the tourniquet does not fill the veins sufficiently, the patient may be asked to open and close his fist. The action of the muscles will force the blood into the veins causing them to distend considerably more. Frequently a light tapping will help fill the vein. Occasionally these methods are inadequate to fill the vein sufficiently. In such cases application of heat is helpful. To be effective the heat must be applied to the entire extremity for 10 to 20 minutes and retained until the venipuncture is performed.

Preparation for Venipuncture

Check Solution and Container
Careful inspection must be made to ensure that the fluid is clear and free of particulate matter and that the container is intact—that there are no cracks in the glass bottle or holes in the plastic bag (see Chapter 9). The label must be checked to verify that the correct solution is being used and that the container is not outdated. Indicate the time and the date the bottle is opened; after 24 hours the fluid is outdated and should not be used.

Attach Administration Set to Fluid Container
The set is attached to the container by squeezing the drip chamber and entering the bottle with a thrust, not a twisting motion. The chamber is released, causing immediate function of the air vent and filling of the drip chamber on the suspension of the bottle. This prevents leakage of fluid through the air vent and expedites clearing the infusion set of air, thus preventing bubbles from entering the tubing.

Height of the Fluid Container
The fluid container is suspended at approximately three feet above the injection site. At this height adequate pressure is provided to achieve a maximum flow rate. The greater the height of the container, the greater the force with which the fluid will flow into the vein should the adjusting clamp release and the greater the risk of speed shock.

Preparing the Patient
The patient should be in a comfortable position with his arm on a flat surface. If necessary a strip of tape is used to secure the arm to an armboard and prevent an uncooperative or disoriented patient from jerking his arm while the needle is being inserted.

If the area selected for venipuncture is hairy, shaving will permit better cleansing of the skin and make removal of the needle less painful when the infusion is terminated.

Techniques in Venipuncture

Direct Method or Stab Technique
This method is performed with a thrust of the needle through the skin and into the vein with one quick motion. The needle enters the skin directly over the vein. This technique is excellent as long as large veins are available. However, owing to the many times one must resort to the use of small veins, this is not the preferred technique. Such an at-

tempt at entry into the small veins will result in hematomas. If the nurse chooses to use this technique she will never be adept at phlebotomies on tiny venules when the situation arises.

Indirect Method
This method consists of two complete motions:

1. Insertion of the needle through the skin. The needle enters the skin below the point where the vein is visible; entering the skin above the vein tends to depress the vein, obscuring its position.
2. Relocation of the vein and entry into the vein.

Basic Venipuncture
The basic venipuncture is performed as follows (see Figure 17):

1. Thoroughly wash and dry hands.
2. Apply tourniquet and select vein.
3. Prepare skin with an accepted antiseptic—70 percent isopropyl alcohol is usually used. Do not repalpate or touch skin.
4. After establishing a minimum rate of flow by adjusting the clamp, kink the infusion tubing between the third and little fingers of the right hand. When the kinked tubing is released, the minimum rate of flow will prevent a rapid infusion of fluid and drugs with the potential danger of speed shock. Obstructing the flow of solution manually expedites the procedure and leaves the hands free for anchoring the needle and caring for any collected blood samples.
5. Hold the patient's hand or arm with the left hand, using the thumb to keep the skin taut and to anchor the vein to prevent rolling.
6. Place the needle in line with the vein, about ½ inch below the proposed site of entry. The bevel-up position of the needle facilitates venipuncture and produces less trauma to the skin and the vein on puncture.

   In small veins it is often necessary to enter the vein with the bevel down to prevent extravasation; any readjustment of the needle should be made before releasing the tourniquet to prevent puncturing the vein and producing a hematoma [1].
7. Insert the needle through skin and tissue at a 45-degree angle.
8. Relocate the vein and decrease the needle angle slightly.
9. Slowly, with a downward motion followed immediately by a raising of the point, pick up the vein, leveling the needle until it is almost flush with the skin.
10. On entering the vein there may be a backflow of blood, which indicates successful entry. There may be no blood return if the vein

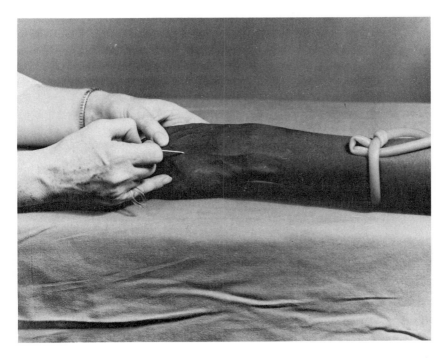

Fig. 17. Basic venipuncture. Infusion tubing is kinked between third and little fingers. Left thumb keeps skin taut and anchors vein. The needle is held in line with the vein at 45-degree angle.

is small. Usually pinching the rubber tube just above the needle adapter and then releasing it will back the blood into the plastic tubing. If doubtful of the needle's position in the vein, check by this method. With experience the fingers will become sensitive to the needle's entering the vein—the resistance encountered as the needle meets the wall of the vein and the snap felt at the loss of resistance as the needle enters the lumen. This is more difficult to discern on thin-walled veins with small blood volume. To prevent a through puncture, move the needle slowly, checking at each movement for a backflow of blood.

11. Once the vein is entered, move the needle cautiously up the lumen for about ¾ inch.
12. Release the tourniquet.
13. Release the pressure exerted by the little finger, unkinking the tube and allowing the solution to flow.
14. Check carefully for any signs of swelling.

If the vein has sustained a through puncture (evidenced by a developing hematoma) and the venipuncture is unsuccessful, the needle

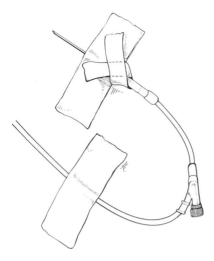

Fig. 18. Note that tape, securing tubing, is independent of needle; an accidental pull will not dislodge the needle.

should be immediately removed and pressure applied to the site. Never reapply a tourniquet to the extremity immediately after a venipuncture; a hematoma will occur, limiting veins and providing an excellent culture medium for bacteria.

Anchoring Needle and Securing Armboard

Needle
To anchor the needle, carry out the following steps (see Figure 18):

1. Use 1-inch wide tape over the hub and shaft of the needle. Tape the needle flush with the skin—no elevation of the hub is necessary and it would only increase the risk of a through puncture from the point of the needle.
2. Place a ½-inch strip of tape—adhesive up—under the hub of the needle. Place one end tightly and diagonally over the needle. Repeat with the other end, crossing over the first. This secures the needle firmly and prevents any sideward movement.
3. Loop the tubing and secure it with tape independently of the needle. This eliminates dislodging the needle by an accidental pull on the tubing.
4. Indicate the size of the needle and the date on the tape. This will help ensure removal of the needle within a safe period of time.

Armboard
The use of an armboard is helpful in immobilizing the extremity when undue motion could result in infiltration or phlebitis. It is a valuable

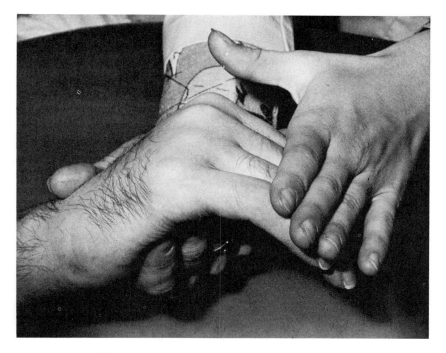

Fig. 19. Maximal flexion of the hand of a patient who has developed contracture from positioning the hand in a flat position. The patient cannot make a fist.

aid in restraining the arm when infusions are initiated on uncooperative, disoriented, or elderly patients or children, or when the needle is inserted on the dorsum of the hand or in an area of joint flexion. When the metacarpal veins are used the fingers should be immobilized to prevent any movement of the needle that could result in phlebitis.

The function of the hand may be endangered and even permanently impaired by the widespread hospital practice of flattening it on an armboard during intravenous therapy. This complication results from failure to recognize that the hand has both transverse and longitudinal arches and that if the knuckle joints (metacarpophalangeal) are immobilized in a straight position, they will develop contracture that will prevent motion (see Figure 19). Patients on long-term therapy with edema or muscular weakness are particularly vulnerable. Intensive physical therapy, splinting, and even surgery may be required to restore mobility.

To preserve maximal function, the hand should be immobilized in a functional position on the armboard. Robert Leffert* recommends 20 degrees of dorsiflexion of the wrist, 45 to 60 degrees of flexion of the metacarpophalangeal joints, with the palm slightly cupped and the

* Chief of the Surgical Upper Extremity Rehabilitation Unit and Department of Rehabilitation Medicine, Massachusetts General Hospital, Boston, Mass.

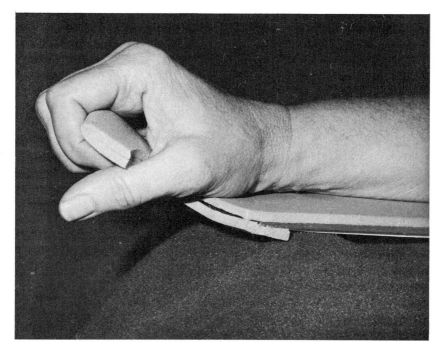

Fig. 20. The hand is immobilized in a functional position on the armboard to prevent contracture, which may endanger or permanently impair the function of the hand.

flexion increasing from index to little finger. The thumb should be in opposition so that it is away from the palm in the posture it would assume in pinch (see Figure 20).

If a plastic armboard is used, cover it with absorbent paper or bandage to prevent the arm from perspiring and sticking to the board. Make certain that any tape placed on the needle is independent of the board so that a motion of the arm on the board will not cause a pull on the needle. If restraint of the arm is necessary, the restraint is secured to the board, not to the patient's arm above the puncture area; such restraint might act as a tourniquet, causing a backflow of blood into the needle, resulting in clotting and obstruction of the flow.

Insertion of the Intracatheter

As the intracatheter is associated with a higher incidence of serious complications, only the experienced therapist, alert to the risks involved, should attempt venipuncture by this method. The inherent danger of infection from bacteria invading the vein through the cutaneous opening and being carried along the plastic cannula makes thorough skin preparation necessary. Trauma caused by the insertion of a large intracatheter is increased when performed by an inexperienced operator.

A catheter severed by the cutting edge of the needle can result in a serious complication when lost in the bloodstream. An intracatheter introduced into a vein over joint flexion increases the risk of complication if the extremity is not immobilized.

A catheter facilitates prolonged therapy but increases the risk of thrombophlebitis. Limiting the length of time the intracatheter is in use reduces the incidence of phlebitis; a time limit is sometimes difficult to enforce, however, since veins may be exhausted in critically ill patients whose life depends upon infusion therapy.

To minimize the danger of infection, the Center for Disease Control has recommended the use of plastic gloves after the hands have been thoroughly washed, the use of iodine-containing disinfectants as an excellent prepping solution, daily change of dressings with consideration given to a topical antiseptic iodophor ointment, and change of the cannula after 72 hours, preferably after 48 hours (see Chapter 9).

Local anesthesia is often employed to prevent discomfort when a large catheter is used; more nerve endings are traumatized by the large catheter than by a small needle. Since the subcutaneous tissue is comparatively insensitive, most of the pain occurs as the needle penetrates the skin [2]. Usually 0.5 or 1 percent procaine is used. Because of a possible sensitivity to procaine the patient should be questioned as to allergies. A minimal amount of procaine is injected intradermally with a 25-gauge hypodermic needle to raise a wheal through which the intravenous needle is passed. Care must be observed to prevent an inadvertent intravascular injection.

Technique for Venipuncture and Installation of Plastic Catheter
Steps to follow in placing a catheter mounted on a metal needle are as follows:

1. Thoroughly wash and dry hands. Optimal technique requires the use of sterile gloves and drapes.
2. Apply tourniquet and select vein.
3. Shave the skin if necessary and prepare with iodine and alcohol or an accepted antiseptic. Do not repalpate the vein or touch the skin.
4. Inject a local anesthetic intradermally if required.
5. Perform the venipuncture in the usual manner. When the needle has punctured the venous wall, introduce the needle ½ inch farther to ensure entry of the catheter into the lumen of the vein.
6. Hold the needle in place and slowly slide catheter hub until desired length is in the vein (see Figure 21). If the venipuncture is unsuccessful *do not reinsert the needle into the catheter;* to do so could sever the catheter.

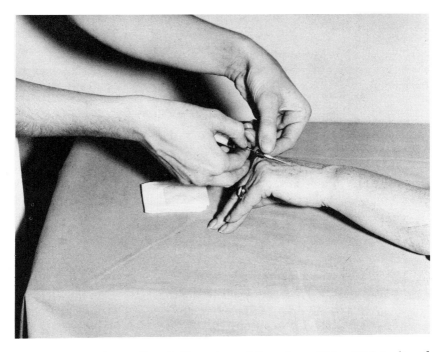

Fig. 21. Hub of the needle is held in place while catheter (Jelco I.V.) is slipped off the shaft until desired length is in the vein. (Jelco Laboratories, Raritan, N.J.)

7. Remove the needle by holding catheter hub in place. To minimize leakage of blood while removing the needle and connecting the infusion set, apply pressure on the vein beyond the catheter with the little finger (see Figure 22).

8. Attach the administration set which has been previously cleared of air and regulate the rate of flow.

9. Apply iodophor ointment.

10. Tape the catheter securely to prevent any motion which could contribute to phlebitis. Avoid taping over the injection site if antibiotic ointment is to be applied daily. Cover the injection site with a sterile sponge.

11. Loop tubing and tape independent of the catheter to prevent an accidental pull from withdrawing the catheter.

12. Indicate the date of insertion and size and type of the catheter on the tape.

Catheter Inserted Through the Needle

Although certain precautions must be observed, the same principles just listed are employed when the longer catheter is threaded through the needle.

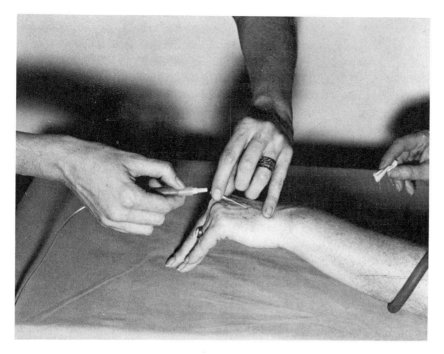

Fig. 22. Pressure on vein reduces leakage of blood which occurs when the needle is withdrawn from the catheter (Jelco I.V.) and the catheter is connected to the infusion set. (Jelco Laboratories, Raritan, N.J.)

1. Thoroughly wash and dry hands. Optimal technique requires the use of sterile gloves and drapes.
2. Apply tourniquet and select vein.
3. Shave the skin if necessary and apply an accepted antiseptic. Do not repalpate the vein or touch the skin.
4. Make the venipuncture.
5. Gently thread the catheter through the lumen of the needle into the vein until the desired length has been introduced.
6. Apply digital pressure on the vein to hold the catheter in place; withdraw the needle.
7. Apply pressure with a sterile sponge for 30 seconds to minimize bleeding through the puncture site.
8. Attach the needle to the infusion set and regulate the flow rate.
9. Slip the shield from the base of the needle over the bevel and tape; the shield must be kept in place to protect the cutting edge of the needle and prevent its severing the catheter. A tongue depressor is frequently used to secure the needle and catheter to further guard against kinking and breaking of the catheter at the junction of the needle.

10. Tape the catheter to prevent motion.
11. Indicate the date of insertion and type and size of the catheter on the tape.
12. Apply iodophor ointment.
13. A sterile pressure dressing over the venipuncture may be required for a short time; the puncture made by the needle is larger than the inlying catheter and seepage of fluid may occur.
14. An armboard should be used if the catheter lies over a point of flexion—motion contributes to phlebitis. The arm must not be fastened tightly to the armboard; vascular occlusion results in a plugged catheter and stasis edema may occur.

If the venipuncture is unsuccessful the needle and catheter must be removed *together;* to pull the catheter through the needle may sever the catheter and result in its loss in the circulation.

Intravenous Catheterization by Surgical Procedure

When lack of superficial veins prevents venipuncture, a surgical procedure for exposure and cannulation of the vein is performed by the physician. The commonest technique is insertion of the cannula or catheter into the exposed vein through the incision. This makes skin approximation difficult and may lead to a delay in healing and an increased risk of bacterial invasion in the vein through the incision.

Dudley [3] described a modified technique in which the incision is made in the usual manner to expose the vein. The cannula is then inserted slightly distal to the incision through a nick in the skin made by a small scalpel. The cannula is then introduced into the exposed vein in the usual manner. Later removal of the cannula does not disturb the incision.

References

1. Abbott Laboratories. *Parenteral Administration*. North Chicago, Ill., 1965. P. 10.
2. Adriani, J. Venipuncture. *American Journal of Nursing* 62:66, 1962.
3. Dudley, H. A. F. Modified technique for intravenous cannulation. *Surgery, Gynecology & Obstetrics* 111:513, 1960.
4. Metheny, N. M., and Snively, W. D., Jr. *Nurses' Handbook of Fluid Balance*. Philadelphia: Lippincott, 1967. Pp. 110–115, 147.
5. Pfizer Laboratories. Intravenous techniques. *Spectrum* 9:2–5, 1965.
6. Welt, L. *Clinical Disorders of Hydration and Acid-Base Equilibrium* (2d ed.). Boston: Little, Brown, 1959. P. 131.

6. The Staff Nurse's Responsibility in Maintenance of Infusions

Safe, successful fluid therapy depends not only upon the knowledge and skill of the intravenous nurse, but also upon the role the staff nurse plays in maintaining the infusion. The proper rate must be maintained, medications must be infused at their allotted time, and potential hazards prevented.

Sterile Technique

There is a great risk of infection if sterile technique is not observed. Solutions, once opened, must be used within 24 hours or discarded. Glucose is a culture medium and when exposed to air for an extended length of time becomes a potential vehicle for bacteria.

Prolonged intravenous therapy presents a hazard. To minimize the risk of deep phlebitis during a constant infusion, the tubing should be changed every 24 hours, using rigid sterile technique and making sure all air is expelled from the tubing before it is attached to the inlying needle.

Ambulating Patients with Infusions

Special precautions must be taken when ambulating patients with infusions. The fluid flask must be kept sufficiently high at all times to maintain a constant flow. Any cessation in the rate must be detected immediately and remedied before a clot is allowed to plug the needle.

Frequent Observation

Fluid maintenance requires frequent observation of patients receiving infusions. The attending nurse should visit the patient every hour, checking the rate of flow, the amount of solution remaining, and the site of infusion, as described in the following sections.

Rate of Flow

Since the rate of flow, once established, is often difficult to maintain, the staff nurse should check and readjust the flow whenever necessary. When an infusion stops, the cause must be immediately investigated and remedied.

When Infusion Stops

The following procedure is to be used when the infusion stops:

1. Check for infiltration.
2. Check the fluid level in the bottle.
3. Check for kinking of the tubing.
4. Open the clamp.
5. Check air vent (has it been inserted if required and is it patent?).
6. Check the needle for patency by kinking the tubing a few inches from the needle while pinching and releasing the tubing between the needle and the kinked tubing. Resistance if encountered should be treated with caution as a clot may have plugged the needle. If a patient complains of pain, a sclerosed vein may be the cause of the cessation of flow. In either case the needle must be removed.
7. Is the needle in line with the vein or up against the wall of the vein? A slight adjustment, by moving the needle, may remedy the problem.
8. If the intravenous solution is cold, as in the case of blood, venous spasm may result. Heat placed directly on the vein will relieve the spasm and increase the flow of the infusion.
9. If the infusion is blood, check the filter; heavy sediment may be slowing the flow. Replace the filter if necessary.
10. Increase the height of the bottle to increase gravity.
11. If unable to restart the flow after these procedures have been followed, restart the infusion.

Amount of Solution in Flask

Air embolism and *blood embolism* are significant hazards of infusion therapy and may be associated with delay in changing solution bottles. A fresh bottle of solution should be added before the level of fluid falls in the drip chamber. Failure to do this results in the following problems:

1. *Plugged needle.* Intravenous solutions flow into the vein by means of gravity. Once the fluid level has dropped in the tubing to about the level of the patient's chest, the blood will be forced back into the needle, occluding the lumen of the needle. Occluded needles should be removed, not irrigated. Fibrinous material injected into the vein

could propagate a thrombus, possibly resulting in an infarction. Irrigation may embolize small infected needle thrombi, which could result in septicemia. Aspiration aimed at dislodging the fibrin may cause the vein to collapse around the needle point traumatizing the vessel wall.

2. *Trapped air.* If the bottle is changed after the level of fluid drops in the tubing and before the needle plugs, the air is trapped in the tubing and forced into the patient by pressure of the fresh solution. Fatal air embolism can result. According to Mollison [2], when a blood container is allowed to run empty, and there is a negative pressure in the vein being used for the infusion, air may be drawn into the bloodstream. He stated, "It is easy to introduce air into the patient's veins at the beginning or when changing from one bottle to another." Infusions through a central venous catheter carry an even greater risk of air embolism than those through a peripheral vein. Since the central venous pressure is lower than the peripheral pressure there is a greater chance of a negative pressure causing air to be sucked into the patient's circulation when the bottle runs dry. According to Metheny and Snively [1], "Small amounts of air are not always harmful, yet as little as 10 ml may be fatal in some patients."

Before the flow ceases and the bottle empties, replace the empty bottle with fresh solution using the following procedure:

1. Vent fresh bottle if vent is required.
2. Kink tubing to prevent air from being introduced into the flowing solution.
3. Change flask. Hang solution bottle before unkinking tubing.
4. Readjust rate if necessary.

Nonfunctioning sets (leaking or plugged) should be removed.

Infiltration or Inflammation at Injection Site
Failure to recognize an infiltration before the swelling has increased to a sizable degree may:

1. Cause damage to the tissues.
2. Prevent the patient from receiving necessary and urgent medication.
3. Limit veins available for future therapy.

If the question of infiltration exists, compare the questionable extremity with the normal extremity. An infusion has infiltrated if

1. There is swelling about the site of the needle.
2. A tourniquet applied above the needle does not stop the flow of fluid.

Checking for an infiltration by a backflow of blood into the adapter is not a reliable method for the following reasons:

1. In small veins the needle may approach the size of the vein, occluding the lumen and obstructing the flow of blood; the solution flows undiluted so that no backflow of blood is obtained.
2. The needle may have punctured the vein, causing an infiltration, and at the same time be within the lumen of the vein, or the bevel may be only partially within the lumen of the vein, causing a swelling and still producing a backflow of blood on test.

Inspect the injection site for erythema, induration, or tenderness by palpation of the venous cord. If any of these signs occur, remove the needle or catheter. When replacing it, sterile equipment should be used and the site changed, preferably to the opposite arm. Should infection be noted, the catheter and the infusion fluid should be cultured and lot numbers of sets and infusions recorded (see Chapter 9).

Outdated Sets and Needles
The Center for Disease Control (C.D.C.) recommends changing intravenous tubing daily and needles and catheters every 72 hours, preferably every 48 hours (see Chapter 9).

Dressings
The C.D.C. recommends daily change of catheter dressings with consideration given to application of an antiseptic iodophor ointment.

Intermittent Infusions and Heparin Locks
For recommended procedures, see Chapter 14.

Termination of Infusion
To terminate the infusion follow this procedure:

1. Stop flow by clamping off tubing.
2. Remove all tape from needle.
3. With a dry sterile sponge held over the injection site, remove needle. The needle must be removed nearly flush with the skin. This prevents the point from damaging the posterior wall of the vein, thus encouraging the process of thrombosis.
4. Apply pressure instantly and firmly. Do not rub. Hematomas occur from needles carelessly removed and render veins useless for future use.

Small adhesive bandages, such as Band-Aids, should not be used unless specifically ordered. It must be emphasized that such a bandage is not used to stop bleeding and does not take the place of pressure. If ordered, it should be applied only after pressure has been applied and the bleeding stopped.

References

1. Metheny, N. M., and Snively, W. D., Jr. *Nurses' Handbook of Fluid Balance.* Philadelphia: Lippincott, 1967. P. 138.
2. Mollison, P. L. *Blood Transfusion in Clinical Medicine* (3d ed.). Springfield, Ill.: Thomas, 1961. Pp. 574-575.

7. Rate of Administration of Parenteral Infusions

One of the prime considerations in the administration of parenteral solutions is the rate of flow. Ideally the physician orders the rate of flow since in determining the rate he must consider the solution, the patient's condition, and the effect he wishes to produce. The nurse who initiates the infusion or who cares for its maintenance is responsible for regulating and maintaining the proper rate of administration. Occasionally when the rate has not been ordered the nurse must assume this responsibility.

Determining Factors for Infusion Rate

To determine the flow rate intelligently, the nurse must have a knowledge of parenteral solutions, their effect, and rate of administration. She must also understand other factors that influence the speed of the infusion. These factors include (1) surface area of the body, (2) condition of the patient, (3) age of the patient, (4) composition of the fluid, and (5) the patient's tolerance to the infusion.

Surface Area of the Body

The body surface area is proportionate to many essential physiological processes (organ size, blood volume, respiration, and heat loss) and therefore to the total metabolic activity. It provides a helpful guide for determining the amount of fluids and electrolytes and for computing the rate of infusions. The larger an individual, the more fluid and nutrients he requires and the faster he can utilize them. The usual infusion rate is 3 ml per square meter of body surface per minute (see nomograms for determining surface area, Chapter 11, Figure 29). This rate applies to maintenance and replacement fluids [5]. However, the speed must be carefully adjusted to each individual.

Condition of Patient

Since the heart and the kidneys play a vital role in the utilization of infused solutions, the cardiac and renal status of the patient affects the desired rate of administration. An expanded blood volume may occur when fluids, rapidly infused, overtax an impaired heart and renal damage causes retention of fluid. Patients suffering from hypovolemia must receive plasma and blood rapidly, but the desired speed of the infusion may be affected by impairment of the homeostatic controls. Therefore the rate should be specified by the physician. Vital signs must be carefully observed and the speed of the infusion decreased as the blood pressure rises.

Age of Patient

Because there is usually some degree of cardiac and renal damage in the elderly, fluids are administered slowly to prevent an increase in venous pressure which could result in pulmonary edema and cardiovascular disturbances [5]. Infants and small children are particularly prone to pulmonary edema when excessive quantities of fluid or rapidly infused fluids expand the vascular system [5]. The rate of administration must be determined by the physician and all precautions observed to ensure steady maintenance at the required rate of flow. If difficulty is encountered in controlling a constant rate, it should be reported and corrected at once.

The special pediatric infusion sets which deliver a smaller size drop (50 to 60 drops per milliliter) provide precision control of the rate of flow. The infusion pumps, such as the Holter pump,* are valuable in maintaining the exact rate of flow regardless of difficulties.

Composition of Fluid

The composition of the fluid affects the rate of flow. When the solution is used as a vehicle for administering drugs, the speed of the infusion depends upon the drug and the effect the physician wishes to produce. Potassium, because of its deleterious effect on the heart when infused at a rapid rate, should be administered with caution. "About 40 mEq. of potassium over an eight-hour period is an average rate for administering potassium parenterally. In emergencies, the rate of administration may be up to four times as fast" [4].

Concentration of solutions must be considered since the flow rate may alter the desired effect. When dextrose is administered for caloric benefits it is infused at a rate that will ensure complete utilization. Dextrose can be administered at a maximum speed of 0.5 gm per kilogram of body weight per hour [5, 7] without producing glycosuria in a normal individual. At this rate it would take approximately 1½ hours to administer a liter of 5 percent dextrose to an individual weighing 70 kg or twice as long for a liter of 10 percent dextrose [7]. This maxi-

* Extracorporeal Medical Specialties, Inc., King of Prussia, Pa.

mum rate is faster than usual and not customarily used except in an emergency.

When a diuretic effect is desired a more rapid infusion is necessary. If the solution is too rapidly infused for complete metabolism, the glucose accumulates in the bloodstream, increases the osmolality, and acts as a diuretic.

When oliguria or anuria occurs, the status of the kidneys must be determined before solutions containing potassium can be administered. Urinary suppression may be due to a blood volume deficit or to kidney damage. An initial hydrating solution, to test kidney function, is usually administered at a rate of 8 ml per square meter of body surface per minute for 45 minutes [2]. If urinary flow is not accomplished the rate is slowed to about 2 ml per square meter of body surface per minute for another hour. If urinary output has not occurred after this period, it is presumed that kidney damage is present [2, 5].

Tolerance

Tolerance to solutions varies with individuals and influences the rate of infusion. A 5 percent solution of alcohol can be administered at the rate of 200 to 300 ml per hour to sedate without intoxication in the average adult [5]. However, the rate must be adjusted to the individual.

When protein hydrolysates are infused, a slower rate of administration, 2 ml per minute, is necessary to test the patient's sensitivity to the protein [7]. Nausea and a feeling of warmth may occur from excessively rapid administration; if these symptoms do not subside when the rate of administration is decreased, the infusion should be stopped [5].

Computation of Flow Rate

Frequently the physician orders a total volume of fluid to be infused over a 24-hour period. If the nurse knows the volume and the flow rate of the administration set in use, she can easily compute the required rate of flow. A quick, easy formula for computing flow rate in drops (gtt) per minute is

$$\frac{\text{gtt/ml of given set}}{60 \ (\text{min in hour})} \times \text{total hourly volume} = \text{gtt/min}$$

If a set delivers 15 drops per milliliter and 240 ml are to be infused in 1 hour,

$$\frac{15}{60} \times 240 = \frac{1}{4} \times 240 = 60 \text{ gtt/min}$$

Whenever a set is used that delivers 15 drops per milliliter, merely divide the hourly volume to be infused by 4 and the number of drops per minute will be obtained.

If the set delivers 10 drops per milliliter, divide the number of milliliters to be infused by 6 for drops per minute:

$$\frac{10}{60} \times \text{hourly volume} = \frac{1}{6} \times \text{hourly volume} = \text{gtt/min}$$

Manufacturers of parenteral solutions have devised convenient calculators to assist the nurse in accurate rate determinations (see Figure 23). The Normosol Calculator by Abbott Laboratories is a concise, excellent device for calculating both rate determinations and surface area in square meters. The rate determinator is devised for use with Abbott sets or sets calculated as follows:

Fluid administration sets approximately	15 gtt = 1 ml
Blood administration sets approximately	10 gtt = 1 ml
Pediatric administration sets approximately	60 gtt = 1 ml

The calculator consists of a rotary dial containing three sectors, representing each of the three sets. To determine the flow rate, the dial is rotated until the set in use is aligned with the amount of fluid required for 1, 2, 3, or 4 hours. Drops per minute will be visible in the window contained in the represented sector.

On the opposite side a dial provides a nomogram for calculating surface area of the body in square meters. The weight in kilograms or pounds on the rotary wheel is aligned with the height in centimeters or inches. An indicator then points to the surface area in square meters.

The Minislide by Baxter Laboratories, Inc., provides the nurse with a handy, quick device for computing fluid rates. It consists of a slide rule containing four scales:

Top, scale A: total milliliters to be infused
Bottom, scale D: flow rate in drops per minute

The insert slides between scales A and D and contains

Scale B: number of drops per milliliter (10 to 60) a given set delivers
Scale C: time in hours for infusion

The flow rate or the infusion time at the prescribed rate may be determined by sliding the insert until the number of drops that the set delivers is aligned with total milliliters to be infused. Opposite the time (hours) for infusion, see drops required per minute; opposite the prescribed flow rate, see the infusion time (hours).

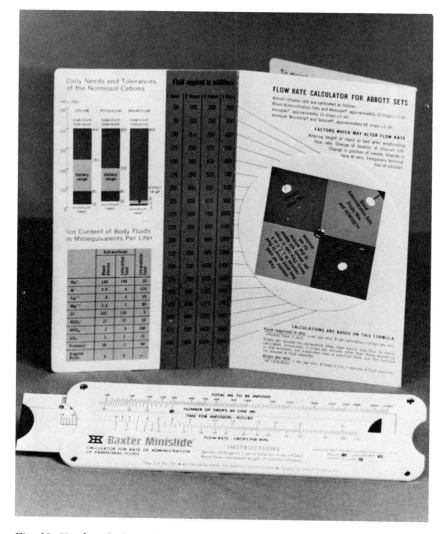

Fig. 23. Handy calculators for determining rate of flow of a given volume of fluid over a set period of time. (Normosol Calculator, Abbott Laboratories, North Chicago, Ill.; Minislide, Baxter Laboratories, Morton Grove, Ill.; division of Travenol Laboratories, Inc.)

Factors Affecting the Flow Rate

The infusion should be checked frequently to maintain the required rate of flow. Because of certain factors, the rate is subject to change.

Height of the Solution Bottle

Intravenous fluids run by gravity. Any change in gravity by raising or lowering the infusion bottle will change the rate of flow. When patients receiving infusions are ambulated or transported to x-ray, the solution bottle should be retained at the same height, or the speed of the infusion readjusted to maintain the prescribed rate of flow.

Clot in the Needle

Any temporary stoppage of the infusion, such as a delay in changing infusion bottles, may cause a clot to form in the lumen of the needle, partially or completely obstructing it. Clot formation may also occur when an increase in venous pressure in the infusion arm forces blood back into the needle. This results from restriction of the venous circulation and is most commonly caused by (1) the blood pressure cuff on the infusion arm, (2) restraints placed on or above the infusion needle, and (3) the patient's lying on the arm receiving the infusion [3].

Change in Position of the Needle

A change in the needle's position may push the bevel of the needle against or away from the wall of the vein [6]. Special precautions should be taken to prevent speed shock or overloading of the vascular system by making sure the solution is flowing freely before adjusting the rate.

Change in Temperature or Composition of the Solution

Stimulation of the vasoconstrictors from any infusion of cold blood or irritating solution may cause venous spasm, impeding the rate of flow [6]. A warm pack placed on the vein proximal to the infusion needle will offset this reaction.

Trauma to the Vein

Any injury such as phlebitis or thrombosis which reduces the lumen of the vein will decrease the flow of the solution.

Plugged Vent

A plugged vent in the solution bottle will cause the infusion to stop [1]. Check the vent needle for patency.

If there is any question as to the rate of administration, the therapist should check with the physician. This applies to intravenous administration of drugs in solution. The rates should also be established on patients receiving two or more infusions simultaneously. Any change in the rate from that normally used should be ordered by the attending physician.

The nurse should never exert positive pressure (manual pressure) to infuse solutions or blood. This should be the responsibility of the physician.

References

1. Abbott Laboratories. *Parenteral Administration.* North Chicago, Ill., 1969. P. 19.
2. Abbott Laboratories. *Fluid and Electrolytes.* North Chicago, Ill., 1960. P. 32.
3. Bard, C. R., Inc. *An Outline for the Use of IV Placement Units.* Murray Hill, N.J., 1970. P. 8.
4. Crowell, C. E., and Staff of Educational Design, Inc., N.Y. Potassium imbalance. *American Journal of Nursing* 67:358, 1967.
5. Metheny, N. M., and Snively, W. D., Jr. *Nurses' Handbook of Fluid Balance.* Philadelphia: Lippincott, 1967. Pp. 118–124, 256.
6. Pfizer Laboratories. Intravenous techniques. *Spectrum* 9:2, 1965.
7. Williams, J. T., and Moravec, D. F. *Intravenous Therapy.* Hammond, Ind.: Clissold Publishing, 1967. P. 49.

8. Hazards and Complications of Intravenous Therapy

Intravenous therapy subjects the patient to numerous hazards, many of which can be avoided if the nurse understands the risks involved and uses all available measures to prevent their occurrence. The *local complications* occur most frequently and include thrombophlebitis and infiltrations. The *systemic complications* are the most serious and consist of the following:

1. Pyrogenic reactions
2. Pulmonary embolism resulting from
   a. Blood emboli—"clots"
   b. Air emboli—"bubbles"
3. Pulmonary edema
4. Speed shock

Local Complications

Occasionally local complications are not recognized until considerable damage is done. Early recognition may prevent (1) extensive edema depriving the patient of urgently needed fluid and medications, (2) necrosis, and (3) thrombophlebitis with the subsequent danger of embolism. The local complications occur as the result of trauma to the wall of the vein.

Thrombosis

Any injury that roughens the endothelial cells of the venous wall allows platelets to adhere and a thrombus to form. Because the point of the needle traumatizes the wall of the vein where it touches, thrombi form on the vein and at the tip of the needle [11]. Thrombosis occurs when a local thrombus obstructs the circulation of blood. It must be remembered that thrombi form an excellent trap for bacteria, whether carried by the bloodstream from an infection in a remote part of the body or introduced through the subcutaneous orifice [3].

Thrombophlebitis
Thrombophlebitis is the term used to denote a twofold injury: thrombosis plus inflammation. The development of thrombophlebitis is easily recognized. A painful inflammation develops along the length of the vein. If the infusion is allowed to continue, the vein progressively thromboses, becoming hard, tortuous, tender, and painful [7]. Early detection may prevent an obstructive thrombophlebitis which causes the infusion to slow and finally stop. This condition is most painful, persisting indefinitely, incapacitating the patient, and limiting valuable veins for future therapy.

Usually a sterile inflammation develops from a chemical or mechanical irritation. When the inflammation is the result of sepsis it is much more serious and carries with it the potential danger of septicemia and acute bacterial endocarditis.

There is always the inherent danger of embolism when thrombosis occurs. The more pronounced the inflammation and the more intense the pain, the more organized the thrombus is apt to become. It has been frequently stated that embolism is less likely to occur from the well-attached clot of thrombophlebitis than from phlebothrombosis [6].

Phlebothrombosis
Phlebothrombosis denotes thrombosis and usually indicates that the inflammation is relatively inconspicuous. It is thought to give rise to embolism since the thrombus is poorly attached to the wall of the vein [6]. Both thrombophlebitis and phlebothrombosis have a degree of inflammation and are associated with potential embolism.

CONTRIBUTING FACTORS. Any irritation involving the wall of the vein predisposes the patient to thrombophlebitis. Inflammation to the vein will occur from any foreign body and is mediated by the following: (1) duration of the infusion, (2) composition of the solution, (3) site of the infusion, (4) technique, and (5) method employed [2].

Duration of the infusion is a significant factor in the development of thrombophlebitis. As the duration of time is lengthened, the incidence and degree of inflammation increase. Infusions left in place over 24 hours are prime offenders [2, 4].

The *composition of the solution* may play a role. Venous irritation and inflammation may result from the infusion of hypertonic glucose solutions, certain drug additives, or solutions with a pH significantly different from that of the plasma. Solutions of dextrose are known to be irritating to the vein [4, 5]. The United States Pharmacopeia specifications for pH of dextrose solutions range from 3.5 to 6.5; acidity is necessary to prevent "caramelization" of the dextrose during autoclaving and to preserve the stability of the solution during storage. Studies have been performed which show a significant reduction in thrombophlebitis when buffered glucose solutions have been infused [5]. Abbott Laboratories, recognizing this problem, identifies the pH of each solution and provides Neut, a sodium bicarbonate 1 percent additive solution, to increase the pH of acid intravenous solutions. This additive, however, poses a problem of incompatibility when added to solutions containing drugs. Abbott's circular on Neut calls attention to the precaution that "When Neut is added to solutions, the compatibility of these solutions with other drugs may be altered." According to Williams and Moravec [14], "It is quite likely that changes in pH produce the largest number of incompatibilities." As an example, tetracycline hydrochloride, with a pH of 2.5 to 3.0, is unstable in an alkaline environment.

The *site of infusion* can be a factor contributing to thrombophlebitis. The veins in areas over joint flexion undergo injury when motion of the needle irritates the venous wall. The veins in the lower extremities are especially prone to trauma, enhanced by the stagnant blood in varicosities and the stasis in the peripheral venous circulation.

Small veins are subject to inflammation when used to infuse an irritating solution. The infusion needle may occlude the entire lumen of the vein, obstructing the flow of circulating blood; the solution then flows undiluted, irritating the wall of the vein.

Technique can mean the difference between a successful infusion and the complication of thrombophlebitis. Only minimal trauma results from a skillfully executed venipuncture, whereas a carelessly performed venipuncture may seriously traumatize the venous wall.

Phlebitis associated with sepsis may be related to the technique of the operator. There is always the risk of infection if sterile technique is not zealously observed. Thorough cleansing of the skin is important in preventing infections. Maintenance of asepsis is essential during long-term therapy, particularly in the use of the intracatheter [10].

Methods employed to infuse parenteral solutions may foster septic thrombophlebitis. This complication is most often associated with the intracatheter. The intracatheter threaded through the needle remains sterile, does not come in contact with the skin, but provides a large subcutaneous orifice facilitating entry of bacteria around the catheter and seepage of fluid.

The catheter mounted on the needle is not without fault as it comes in direct contact with the skin before being introduced into the vein. However, the tight fit through the skin may bar further bacterial entry.

PREVENTIVE MEASURES. In performing venipunctures, the therapist should exercise every caution to avoid injuring the wall of the vein needlessly. Multiple punctures, through-and-through punctures, and damage to the posterior wall of the vein with the point of the needle can cause thrombosis. The risk of phlebitis may be minimized if the nurse

1. Refrains from using veins in the lower extremities.
2. Selects veins with ample blood volume when infusing irritating substances.
3. Avoids veins in areas over joint flexion.
4. Anchors needles securely to prevent motion.

To prevent septic phlebitis, thorough preparation of the skin, together with aseptic technique and maintenance of asepsis during infusion, is imperative.

Periodic inspection of the injection site will detect developing complications before serious damage occurs. Complaints of a painful infusion make it necessary to differentiate between early phlebitis and venospasm from an irritating solution. If the latter is present, slowing the solution and applying heat to the vein will dilate the vessel and increase the blood flow, diluting the solution and relieving the pain. Following hypertonic solutions with isotonic fluids will flush the vein of irritating substances.

If inflammation accompanies the pain, a change in the injection site should be considered. To continue the infusion will only bring progressive trauma and limit available veins. An enforced time limit for removal of the needle reduces the incidence of phlebitis [2, 4].

During removal of the infusion needle, care must be taken to prevent injury to the wall of the vein; the needle should be removed at an angle nearly flush with the skin. Pressure should be applied for a reasonable length of time to prevent extravasation of blood.

Infiltration

Dislodgment of the needle with consequent infiltration of fluid is not uncommon and is too frequently considered of minor significance. With the increasing numbers of irritating solutions and the frequency with which potent drugs are infused via intravenous solutions, serious problems may occur when the fluid invades the surrounding tissues. Hypertonic, acid, and alkaline solutions are contraindicated for hypodermoclysis and are not intended for other than venous infusions. If they are allowed to infiltrate, necrosis may occur (see Figures 24 and 25).

If necrosis is avoided, edema may nevertheless

1. Deprive the patient of fluid and drug absorption at the rate essential for successful therapy.
2. Limit veins available for venipuncture, complicating therapy.
3. Predispose the patient to infection.

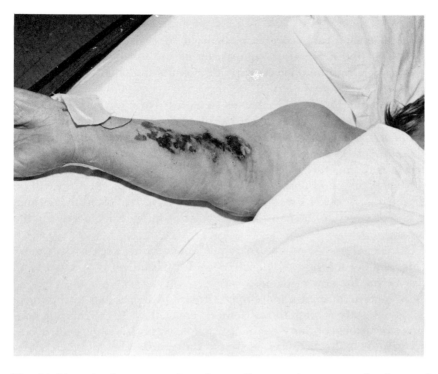

Fig. 24. Necrosis of tissues resulting from infiltration of concentrated solution of potassium chloride.

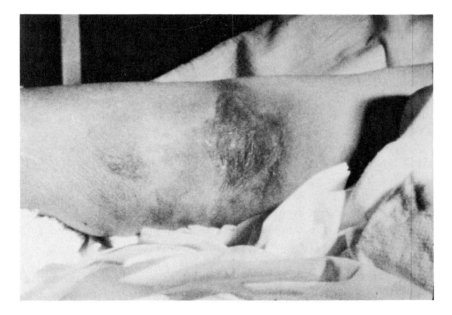

Fig. 25. Necrosis from infiltration of hypertonic solution.

Extravasation can easily be recognized by the increasing edema at the site of the infusion. A comparison of the infusion area with the identical area in the opposite extremity assists in determining whether there is a swelling.

Frequently the edema is allowed to increase to great proportions because of a misconception that a backflow of blood into the adapter is significant proof that the infusion is entering the vein. This is not a reliable method for checking a possible infiltration. The point of the needle may puncture the posterior wall of the vein, leaving the greater portion of the bevel within the lumen of the vein. Blood return will be obtained on negative pressure, but if the infusion is allowed to continue fluid will seep into the tissues at the point of the needle, increasing the edema.

Occasionally a blood return is not obtained on negative pressure. This may occur when the needle occludes the lumen of a small vein, obstructing the flow of blood.

To confirm an infiltration, apply a tourniquet proximal to the injection site tightly enough to restrict the venous flow. If the infusion continues regardless of this venous obstruction, extravasation is evident.

Once an infiltration has occurred, the needle should be removed immediately.

Systemic Complications

Pyrogenic Reactions

Pyrogenic reactions occur when pyrogens (proteins foreign to the blood) are introduced into the bloodstream, producing a febrile reaction. This sudden occurrence of chills and fever may be accompanied by general malaise, headache, and, depending upon the severity of the reaction, backache, nausea, and vomiting. If the infusion is allowed to continue, the increased absorption of pyrogens may induce the more serious symptoms of vascular collapse and shock.

A pyrogenic reaction calls for immediate termination of the infusion. Vital signs should be observed, the physician notified, and the solution saved for any necessary cultures.

Improvement in equipment (disposable plastic infusion sets) and the use of commercially prepared solutions have greatly reduced the number of pyrogenic reactions. Still, reactions do occur. Special precautions can reduce the incidence of pyrogenic reactions.

USE OF PYROGEN-FREE SOLUTIONS. The solution should be carefully inspected for abnormal cloudiness or for the presence of extraneous particulate matter which may represent fungi.

Methods of sterilization of parenteral fluids vary with manufacturing companies. If the method used produces a vacuum in solution bottles, presence of a vacuum should be noted; lack of vacuum indicates possible loss of sterility and contamination.

USE OF FRESHLY OPENED SOLUTIONS. Protein solutions, such as albumin and protein hydrolysates, must be used as soon as the seal is broken. To refrigerate these opened solutions for future use can result in serious consequence.

Other solutions should be used within 24 hours. The wise practice of indicating on the bottle the time and date that the seal is broken safeguards patients from possible contaminated infusions, especially patients on keep-open infusions for intermittent drug therapy.

PROTECTION OF SOLUTION FROM CONTAMINATION. In the drug-additive program, sterile technique is essential to prevent organisms from being introduced into the solution. All drugs must be reconstituted with a sterile diluent. Once opened, any unused diluent should be discarded.

Keep-open solutions, terminated temporarily for blood infusion or drug therapy, must be protected from contamination. Sterile caps are available for some containers; sterile sponges may provide protection.

Pulmonary Embolism

Pulmonary embolism occurs when a substance, usually a blood clot, becomes free floating and is propelled by the venous circulation to the right side of the heart and on into the pulmonary artery [6]. Emboli may obstruct the main pulmonary artery or the arteries to the lobes, occluding arterial apertures at major bifurcations [6]. Obstruction of the main artery results in circulatory and cardiac disturbances. Recurrent small emboli may eventually result in pulmonary hypertension and right heart failure [8].

PREVENTIVE MEASURES. Certain precautions must be taken to prevent this serious complication from occurring.

1. Blood or plasma must be infused through an adequate filter to remove any particulate matter which could result in small emboli.
2. Veins on the lower extremities should be avoided when venipunctures are performed. These veins are particularly prone to trauma, predisposing the patient to thrombophlebitis. Although superficial veins rarely seem to be the source of emboli of consequence [6], a thrombus may extend into the deep veins, resulting in a potentially viable clot; superficial and deep veins unite freely in the lower extremities.
3. Positive pressure should not be employed to relieve clot formation. To check for patency of the lumen of the needle, kink the infusion

tubing about 8 inches from the needle. Then kink and release the tubing between the needle and the pinched tubing—if the tubing becomes hard and meets with resistance, obstruction is evident, necessitating removal and reinstatement of the infusion.

4. Special precautions should be observed in the drug-additive program. Reconstituted drugs must be completely dissolved before being added to parenteral solutions; it is the inherent nature of red cells to adhere to particles, adding to the danger of clot formation.

5. Solutions should be examined to detect any particulate matter.

AIR EMBOLISM. Air embolism is a significant possible complication of every infusion, although its occurrence is usually associated with blood infused under pressure. Fatal embolism may occur when small bubbles accumulate dangerously and form tenacious bubbles that block the pulmonary capillaries [1]. Recognition of the circumstances which contribute to this hazard and measures taken to prevent their occurrence are imperative for safe fluid therapy.

Infusions run by gravity. If the container is allowed to run dry, air enters the tubing and the fluid level drops to the proximity of the patient's chest. The pressure exerted by the blood on the walls of the veins controls the level to which the air drops in the tubing. A negative pressure in the vein may allow air to enter the bloodstream. A negative pressure occurs when the extremity receiving the infusion is elevated above the heart [9]. Infusions flowing through a central venous catheter carry an even greater risk of air embolism when the flask empties than those flowing through a peripheral vein; since the central venous pressure is less than the peripheral venous pressure, there is more apt to be a negative pressure which could suck air into the circulation.

If the fluid bottle on a continuous infusion should empty, fresh solution will force the trapped air into the circulation. To remove the air from the administration set (see Figure 26):

1. Place a hemostat close to the infusion needle.
2. Hang the fresh solution.
3. With an antiseptic, clean the rubber section of the tubing proximal to the hemostat and below the air level in the tubing.
4. Insert a sterile needle to allow the air to escape.
5. Remove clamp and readjust flow.

The Y-type infusion set (see Figure 27) is a less obvious source but one by which great quantities of air can be drawn into the bloodstream. Running solutions simultaneously is the contributing factor. If one vented container empties, it becomes the source of air for the flowing

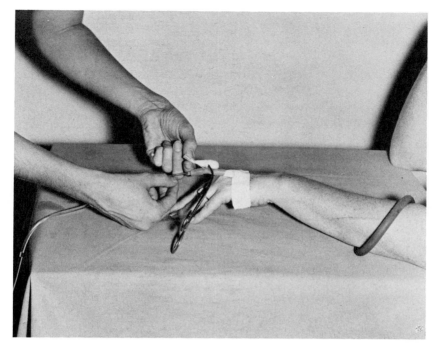

Fig. 26. Removing air from infusion set. The hemostat prevents air from entering the vein while a sterile needle allows air to escape from administration set.

solution. This is explained by the fact that the atmospheric pressure is greater in the open tubing to the empty bottle than below the partially restricted clamp on the infusion side. Recurrent small air bubbles are constantly aspirated into the flowing solution and on into the venous system. The introduction of air may be prevented by running one solution at a time. Vigilance is imperative if vented solutions are ordered to run simultaneously. The tubing must be clamped completely off before the solution bottle is allowed to empty [12].

This same principle is involved in the piggyback setup for secondary infusions. The potential danger of air embolism exists whenever solutions from two vented sets run simultaneously through a common needle.

All connections of an infusion set must be tight. Any faulty opening or defective hole in the set allows air to be emitted into the flowing solution. If a stopcock is used, the outlets not in use must be completely shut off.

The regulating clamp on the infusion set should be located no higher than the chest level of the patient. Since the pressure exerted by the blood on the venous wall will normally raise a column of water from 4 to 11 cm above the heart, a restricting clamp placed above this point

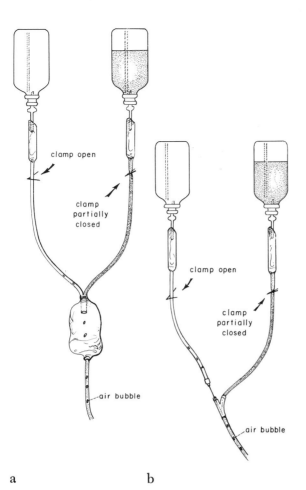

clamp open

clamp
partially
closed

clamp open

clamp
partially
closed

air bubble

air bubble

a   b

Fig. 27. (a) Bottle runs dry during simultaneous infusion of fluids through Y-type administration set. Pressure below the partially constricted clamp is less than atmospheric, allowing air from the empty bottle (atmospheric) to enter infusion.
(b) Secondary infusion "piggybacked" through injection site of a primary intravenous set. Lacking an automatic shut-off valve, air from the empty container will enter the circulation. The same principle is involved as in the Y-type set.

will result in a negative pressure in the tubing [9]. If great enough, the pressure can suck air into the flowing solution should a loose connection or a faulty opening exist between the clamp and the needle [9]. The lower the clamp, the greater is the chance of any defects occurring above the clamp, where positive pressure could force the solution to leak out [12].

An infusion set long enough to drop below the extremity gives added protection against air's being drawn into the vein should the infusion bottle empty. Inlying pressure pumps on administration sets should be kept filled at all times. Manual compression of an empty chamber will force air into the bloodstream.

OCCURRENCE OF AN AIR EMBOLISM. The nurse should be familiar with the symptoms associated with air embolism which arise from sudden vascular collapse: cyanosis, drop in blood pressure, weak rapid pulse, rise in venous pressure, and loss of consciousness. If air embolism occurs the patient should be turned on his left side with his head down [9]. This causes the air to rise in the right atrium, preventing it from entering the pulmonary artery. Oxygen is then administered and the physician notified.

Pulmonary Edema

Overloading the circulation is a real hazard to the elderly patient and to those with impaired renal and cardiac function. Fluids too rapidly infused increase the venous pressure, with the possibility of cardiac dilatation and subsequent pulmonary edema.

PREVENTIVE MEASURES. Measures should be taken to prevent pulmonary edema.

1. Infusions should be maintained at the flow rate prescribed.
2. Positive pressure should never be applied by the nurse to infuse solutions. If the patient requires fluids at such rapidity that positive pressure is required, it then becomes the physician's responsibility.
3. Solutions not infused within the 24-hour period ordered should be discarded and not infused with the following day's solutions.
4. Fluids administered in excess of the quantity ordered can overtax the homeostatic controls, increasing the danger of pulmonary edema. The attending nurse must be alert to any signs or symptoms suggestive of circulatory overloading. Venous dilatation, with engorged neck veins, increased blood pressure, and a rise in venous pressure, should alert the nurse to the danger of pulmonary edema. Rapid respiration and shortness of breath may occur. The infusion should

be slowed to a minimal rate and the physician notified. Raising the patient to a sitting position may facilitate breathing.

Speed Shock

Speed shock is the term used to denote the systemic reaction which occurs when a substance foreign to the body is rapidly introduced into the circulation. The rapid injection of a drug permits its concentration in the plasma to reach toxic proportions, flooding the organs rich in blood, the heart and the brain. As a result, syncope, shock, and cardiac arrest may occur [1].

PREVENTIVE MEASURES. Certain precautions can minimize the potential danger of speed shock.

1. Controlled volume infusion sets give added protection by preventing large quantities of fluid from being accidentally infused. These sets control the volume from 10 to 100 ml.
2. The pediatric-type infusion sets, by reducing the size of the drop, provide greater accuracy, thereby reducing the risk of rapid administration. They are valuable when solutions containing potent drugs must be maintained at a minimal rate of flow.
3. An extra clamp ensures greater safety should the initial clamp on the infusion set let go.
4. Upon initiating the infusion, ascertain that the solution is flowing freely before adjusting the rate; movement of a needle in which the aperture is partially obstructed by the wall of the vein could cause an increase in the flow, contributing to the danger of speed shock.

References

1. Adriani, J. Venipuncture. *American Journal of Nursing* 62:66–70, 1962.
2. Bard, C. R., Inc. *An Outline for the Use of IV Placement Units.* Murray Hill, N.J., 1970. Pp. 8, 9.
3. Druskin, M. S., and Siegel, P. D. Bacterial contamination of indwelling intravenous polyethylene catheters. *Journal of the American Medical Association* 185:966–968, 1963.
4. Editorial. Thrombophlebitis following intravenous infusions. *Lancet* 1:907–909, 1960.
5. Fonkalsrud, E. W., Pederson, B. M., Murphy, J., and Beckerman, J. H. Reduction of infusion thrombophlebitis with buffered glucose solutions. *Surgery* 63:280–284, 1968.
6. Hickan, J. B., and Sieker, H. O. Pulmonary embolism and infarction. *Disease-A-Month,* Jan. 1959.
7. McNair, T. J., and Dudley, H. A. F. The local complications of intravenous therapy. *Lancet* 2:365–368, 1959.

8. Mavor, G. E., and Galloway, J. M. D. The ileofemoral venous segment as a source of pulmonary emboli. *Lancet* 1:873, 1967.
9. Metheny, N. M., and Snively, W. D., Jr. *Nurses' Handbook of Fluid Balance*. Philadelphia: Lippincott, 1967. Pp. 137–140.
10. Moran, J. M., Atwood, R. P., and Rowe, M. I. A clinical and bacteriologic study of infections associated with venous cutdown. *New England Journal of Medicine* 272:554–556, 1965.
11. Pfizer Laboratories. Intravenous technique. *Spectrum* 9:2–5, 1965.
12. Tarail, R. Practice of fluid therapy. *Journal of the American Medical Association* 171:45–49, 1950.
13. Vere, D. W., Sykes, C. H., and Armitage, P. Venous thrombosis during dextrose infusion. *Lancet* 2:627–630, 1960.
14. Williams, J. T., and Moravec, D. F. *Intravenous Therapy*. Hammond, Ind.: Clissold Publishing, 1967. P. 59.

9. Bacterial, Fungal, and Particulate Contamination

Scientific, technological, and medical advances have extended the life-saving capabilities of intravenous therapy. However, in spite of these advances, intravenous-associated morbidity and mortality continue to increase.

The literature is full of warnings regarding intravenous fluids and administration sets as potential vehicles for transmission of infection in hospitals. Cases of septicemia and fungemia have been directly traced to contamination of in-use intravenous apparatus and solutions [8, 11]. In 1969, 33 patients with fungal septicemia had been seen over an 18-month period in one university hospital. This complication was the primary cause of death in 13 patients. A correlation with prolonged intravenous catheterization was found [8].

From 1970 to 1971, 150 cases of bacteremia associated with intravenous therapy occurred in eight United States hospitals. These were associated with intravenous fluids of a major manufacturer; gram-negative bacteria were found contaminating sterile equipment. As a result, the Center for Disease Control (C.D.C.) performed a study of all commercial intravenous systems in use in hospitals. The study showed a minimum of 6 percent prevalence of contamination within tubing and bottles after infusion equipment had been in use [4]. Conditions were shown to exist that potentially contributed to contamination: the characteristics of the apparatus itself and the manipulation of sets and solutions by hospital personnel. Hospital staffs were found to lack an understanding of asepsis, and therefore to practice poor antiseptic technique.

Much has been published concerning the alarming escalation of intravenous therapy complications, but owing to a lack of communication hospital personnel remain ignorant of the potential dangers. In hospitals utilizing intravenous teams, communication is better and personnel are more cognizant of complications and their warning symptoms. Infusion-associated infections "can be minimized if physicians, nurses, and other hospital personnel adhere to established infection control procedures when administering intravenous fluids" [17]. As long as intravenous therapy is taken for granted and the staff remain uninformed, intravenous-associated infection will continue to plague the recovery of the ill patient. About 8 million Americans (at least one-fourth of all hospitalized patients in the United States) receive intravenous therapy each year [26]. These patients must be protected from the hazards complicating intravenous infusions.

To this end, official government organizations are developing improvements in their requirements, guidelines, and standards for hospital practice. Learning the technical maneuvers of venipuncture is often accomplished by trial and error; the trauma resulting from such an approach contributes to complications. To overcome this and other problems, hospitals should require periodic reassessment of therapeutic measures and training procedures. The principles of asepsis relevant to intravenous therapy should be taught to all personnel involved in the preparation, administration, and maintenance of the intravenous infusions.

A background knowledge of the epidemiology of nosocomial infections helps to instill in the therapist a greater awareness of the importance of aseptic and antiseptic technique in the prevention of infection. Epidemiology has been defined as "the division of medical science concerned with defining and explaining the interrelationship of the host, the agent and environment in causing disease" [36]. The host is the organism or patient from which a parasite obtains its nourishment. Bacteria which cause disease are said to be agents of the specific disease they cause [36].

Sources of Bacteria

There are three main sources of bacteria responsible for intravenous-associated infection: the air, the skin, and the blood. Microorganisms (flora and fauna) characteristic of a given location are referred to accordingly, thus the terms *skin flora, intestinal flora,* and so on.

The Air

The number of microbes per cubic foot of air varies, depending upon the particular area involved. Where infection is present, bacteria escape in body discharges, contaminating clothing, bedding, and dressings. Activity, such as bed making, sends bacteria flying into the air on particles of lint, pus, and dried epithelium [21]. Increased activity causes a rise in the number of airborne particles and provides an environment that interferes with aseptic technique and potentially contributes to contamination. Patient areas and utility rooms are places where airborne microorganisms may be plentiful. These contaminants find easy access to unprotected intravenous fluids.

The Skin

The skin is the main source of bacteria responsible for intravenous-associated infection. The bacteria found on the skin are referred to as *resident* or *transient*. Resident bacteria are those normally present, and they are relatively constant in a given individual. They adhere tightly to the skin, and usually include *Staphylococcus albus* as well as diphtheroids and *Bacillus* species [21]. Since not all bacteria are removed by scrubbing, meticulous care must be observed to avoid touching sterile equipment.

"The 'transient' flora is loosely attached to the skin and is composed of bacteria which have been picked up by the individual from his environment, and it varies from day to day in quality and quantity. . . . It is scant on clean protected skin, and profuse on dirty, greasy, exposed areas of the body" [21]. The transient bacteria are responsible for infection carried from one person to another. Touch contamination is a potential hazard of infection since hospital personnel move about frequently, touching patients and objects. Frequent hand washing is imperative.

The skin of the patient offers fertile soil for bacteria growth. "It has been estimated that a minimum of 10,000 organisms are present per square centimeter of normal skin" [42]. A square centimeter is equal to 0.155 square inches. Organisms such as *S. epidermidis, S. aureus,* gram-negative bacilli (especially *Klebsiella, Enterobacter,* and *Serratia*), and enterococci are ubiquitous on the skin of hospital patients [26].

The Blood

The blood may harbor potentially dangerous microorganisms. Therefore care must be taken to prevent bacterial contamination from blood spills when drawing samples and performing venipuncture. However, more likely to be a problem in blood is the hepatitis virus. The hepatitis virus is easily transmitted and can be destroyed only by heat or gas sterilization. Proper care of contaminated needles, syringes, and intravenous sets is imperative. Adequate precaution and warning on blood samples possibly contaminated with hepatitis virus are necessary to prevent spread of infection among hospital employees.

Factors Influencing the Survival of Bacteria

Infection depends upon the ability of bacteria to survive and proliferate. The factors that influence their survival are: (1) the specific organisms present, (2) the number of such organisms, (3) the resistance of the host, and (4) the environmental conditions [29].

The Specific Organisms

Bacteria are referred to as *pathogenic* or *nonpathogenic*. Pathogenic bacteria are capable of producing disease. All bacteria should be considered pathogenic. Reports show that bacteria previously considered nonpathogenic may produce infection. In one study, *Serratia* was implicated in 35 percent of cases of gram-negative septicemia resulting from intravenous therapy [1]. "Evidence is piling up that we can no longer ignore culture reports showing that patients or equipment are positive for organisms supposedly 'non-pathogenic for men'" [28].

Bacteria are classified as *gram-positive* and *gram-negative*. In recent years gram-negative bacteria have replaced gram-positive bacteria as the leading cause of death from septicemia [32]. "The single most important reason for the seriousness of the problem is probably the increased usage of antibiotics highly effective against gram-positive organisms but only selectively effective against gram-negative organisms. With the competitive inhibition of gram-positive bacteria eliminated, the more resistant gram-negative organisms have proliferated in the hospital environment" [25].

Number of Organisms

The number of contaminants present influences the probability of production of an infection. The power of bacteria to proliferate must not be underestimated. It is simply not true that a small amount of bacteria from touch contamination is harmless. Contamination of intravenous fluids and bottles with even a few organisms is extremely dangerous since some fungi and many bacteria can proliferate at room temperature in a variety of intravenous solutions to more than 10^5 organisms per milliliter within 24 hours [14].

Host Resistance

The resistance of the host influences the development and course of septicemia. Underlying conditions such as diabetes mellitus, chronic uremia, cirrhosis, cancer, and leukemia may adversely affect the patient's capacity to resist infection. Various forms of treatment such as immunosuppressive drugs, corticosteroids, anticancer agents, and extensive radiation therapy may depress immunological response and permit the invasion of infection. Therapy may mask infection so that septicemia may be unrecognized until autopsy [1].

Environmental Factors

Environmental factors that affect the survival and propagation of bacteria in intravenous fluids are (1) the pH, (2) the temperature, and (3) the presence of essential nutrients in the infusion.

Some organisms grow rapidly in a neutral solution and are less likely to grow in an acid medium. Buffering of acidic dextrose solutions has been recommended for prevention of phlebitis [15], but at the same time, the neutral environment provided by the buffer may enhance the survival and proliferation of bacteria.

The temperature of the fluid may affect the ability of bacteria to multiply. At room temperatures, strains of *E. cloacae, E. agglomerans,* and other members of the tribe Klebsiellae have been found to proliferate rapidly in commercial solutions of 5 percent dextrose in water [4, 26]. Total parenteral nutrition fluids should be used as soon as possible after preparation, and when it becomes necessary to store them temporarily they should be refrigerated at 4° C; at this temperature growth of *Candida albicans* is suppressed [26].

The presence of certain nutrients is essential to the growth of bacteria. Blood and crystalloid solutions provide nutrients that broaden the spectrum of pathogens capable of proliferation. Maki and associates [26] stated that the administration of blood or reflux of blood into the infusion system may provide sufficient nutrients to broaden this spectrum. The American Association of Blood Banks requires blood to be stored at a constant controlled refrigeration of 1° to 6° C.

It has been reported [30] that saline solutions are likely to contain enough biologically available carbon, nitrogen, sulphur and phosphate together with traces of other material to support, under favorable conditions, the survival and multiplication of any gram-negative bacillus introduced to as many as a million organisms per milliliter.

Factors Contributing to Contamination and Infection

Local complications of phlebitis and sepsis, as well as systemic complications, pyrogenic reactions, and septicemia, are hazards of prolonged intravenous therapy which complicate recovery. Contamination may occur via the administration sets, the medication sites, and supplementary apparatus such as extension tubes, containers of fluid, and cannulas. Each time a medication is added, a bottle is changed, or supplementary equipment is added, the likelihood of contamination increases. Dudrick [12] pointed out that "each violation of the system's integrity geometrically increases the chances for contamination of the tubing, the bottle, or the catheter."

Breaks in aseptic technique contribute to contamination. Too much reliance on antibiotics has fostered a decline in aseptic technique. "Instead of overcoming contamination, antibiotic therapy has simply changed the spectrum of organisms from gram-positive to gram-negative" [28]. "Experience has suggested that antibiotic therapy, particularly with large and prolonged dosage, may have contributed to the development and increasing incidence of gram-negative septicemia.

In some instances, toxemia and shock seemed to be temporarily intensified, presumably by the sudden destruction and lysis of gram-negative bacteria and the liberation of endotoxin" [1].

Faulty Handling

Faulty handling and procedures contribute to contamination. Containers of parenteral fluid are accepted as being sterile and nonpyrogenic on arrival from the manufacturer. The potential risk of contamination occurring in transit or in use is frequently overlooked by hospital personnel. However, through faulty handling or carelessness bottles may become cracked or damaged. Bacteria and fungi may penetrate a hairline crack in an intravenous bottle, even though the crack is so fine that fluid is not lost from the bottle (see Figure 28). Robertson [34] reported two cases in which fluid contaminated with fungi was inadvertently administered; the bottles were cracked. These two patients were treated with an effective drug (amphotericin B), and recovery was complete.

Intravenous solutions of dextrose, as well as providing carbon and an energy source, include the extra nutrients needed to support the growth of 10 million organisms per milliliter. If the fluid is not examined closely, its opalescence may be overlooked, and subsequent infusion of a few hundred milliliters of such contaminated fluid will result in deep shock or possibly death [30].

Prior to use containers of fluid should be examined, preferably against a light and dark background, for cracks, defects, turbidity, and particulate matter; plastic containers should be squeezed to detect any puncture hole. Accidental puncture may occur without being evident and provide a point of entry for microorganisms [26, 41]. Any bottle with a crack or defect must be regarded as suspect and not used. Any glass bottle lacking a vacuum when opened should not be used.

Airborne Contamination

Studies by Hansen and Hepler [20] showed that intravenous fluids in an open intravenous stream (without an air filter) may become contaminated by airborne microbes when the container vacuum is replaced by unsterile air. When a 1-liter glass container is opened, approximately 100 ml of air rushes in to replace the vacuum. In areas with a high concentration of airborne particles, contamination of unprotected fluids is a potential risk. Many hospitals, recognizing this risk, are having intravenous bottles opened and the appropriate set added in the pharmacy under the sterile environment of a laminar flow hood. An alternative to this method is the use of the filter needle to break the vacuum and allow sterile air to enter the container.

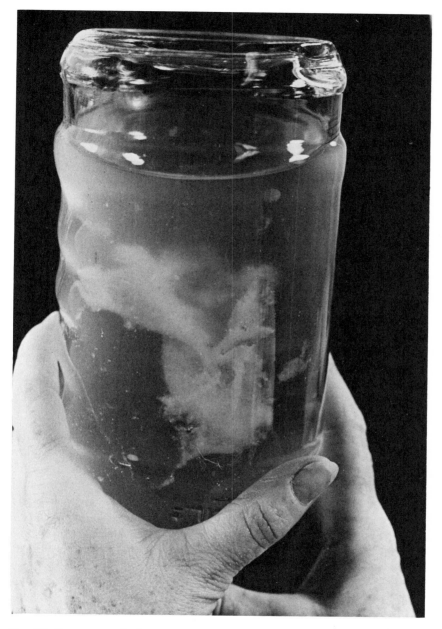

Fig. 28. Intravenous fluid contaminated with fungi which penetrated a hairline crack in the container.

Discarding Outdated Intravenous Solutions

Several studies [4, 8, 11] have demonstrated that intravenous fluids and sets often become contaminated while in use. The longer the container is in use, the greater the proliferation of bacteria and the greater the infection should contamination inadvertently occur. The use of 250-cc containers for keep-open infusions and central venous pressure monitoring reduces the length of time the container is in use and the risk of infusing outdated fluids. Every container should be labeled with the time the bottle is opened. The C.D.C. recommends that intravenous fluid containers and sets be changed at least every 24 hours [5].

Studies [5, 27] have shown that once microorganisms capable of growing in infusion fluid are introduced into an in-use system, they may continue to multiply in the tubing of the infusion apparatus if the same set is retained, despite frequent bottle changes. Studies have further revealed that "routine once-daily complete change of all I.V. administration apparatus, especially at the time of replacement of infusion devices (polyethylene catheters, needles, etc.), can greatly decrease the hazard of extrinsic contamination by preventing introduced organisms from propagating to dangerous levels" [14].

Strict asepsis must be maintained during bottle and tubing changes. Should the spike or the adapter of the set become contaminated by inadvertent contact with unsterile objects, the set must be discarded. A sterile sponge placed under the hub of the cannula during the attachment of a sterile set will reduce the risk of touch contamination.

Admixtures

Allowing untrained hospital personnel to add drugs to intravenous containers potentially contributes to the risk of contamination. This risk is reduced when admixtures are prepared under laminar flow hoods by trained personnel adhering to strict aseptic technique such as is regulated by a pharmacy additive program. Such a program may not be practical or possible in all hospitals, and even where it exists, the necessity for nurses and physicians to prepare admixtures in an emergency does arise. All personnel involved in the preparation and administration of intravenous drugs should receive special training in the preparation of admixtures and the handling of intravenous fluids and equipment. Adherence to strict aseptic methods is vital. It must be understood that touch contamination is the primary source of infection and that although laminar flow hoods prevent airborne contamination, they do not ensure sterility when a break in aseptic technique occurs.

Manipulation of In-use Intravenous Equipment

Intravenous fluids can be inadvertently contaminated by faulty techniques in the manipulation of equipment. In open systems, where solutions are not protected by air filters, the simple procedure of hanging the bottle may be taken for granted and the risk of contamination overlooked. When an administration set is inserted into the bottle and the bottle is inverted, the fluid tends to leak out the vent onto the unsterile surface of the container. Regurgitation of the contaminated fluid into the bottle occurs when the bottle vents. Instructions in the use of the equipment often go unread and unheeded. Squeezing the drip chamber of the administration set before inserting it into the container and releasing it when the bottle is inverted will prevent regurgitation of fluid and minimize the risk of contamination.

Injection Sites

Meticulous care, both aseptic and antiseptic, must be observed in the use of injection sites since they are a potential source of contamination when used to "piggyback" infusions. The location of the injection site, at the distal end of the tubing, exposes it to patient excreta and drainage which enhance the growth of microorganisms and contribute to contamination. The injection site must be *scrubbed* with an accepted antiseptic; 70 percent isoproply alcohol is commonly used. The needle inserted into the injection site should be securely taped to prevent an in-and-out motion of the needle from introducing bacteria into the infusion.

Three-way Stopcocks

Three-way stopcocks are potential mechanisms for transmission of bacteria to the host since their ports, unprotected by sterile covering, are open to moisture and contaminants. Connected to central venous catheters and arterial lines, they are frequently used for drawing blood samples. Aseptic practices are vital in preventing the introduction of bacteria into the line. A sterile catheter plug attached at the time the stopcock is added and changed after each use will reduce the risk of contamination.

Whenever fluid leakage is discovered at injection sites, connections, or vents, the intravenous set should be replaced. McDonough [28] stated that "many of the gram-negative organisms, including *Serratia*, have been found contaminating intravenous solutions and equipment. Their entry from 'standing water' about loose or defective caps or other ports is simple and swift; and their resultant sepsis in the patient is equally swift."

Scalp Vein Needles

Scalp vein needles are recommended for parenteral infusions since studies show that the use of this device results in very low rates of infection or serious local reactions [37]. Because the insertion of a scalp vein needle is relatively atraumatic and phlebitis is not a common complication, the same vein may be used repeatedly. Phlebitis and thrombophlebitis occur frequently with plastic catheters, often preventing reuse of the same vein and necessitating the placement of catheters by surgical cut-down. The low morbidity associated with the scalp vein needle suggests that except in carefully selected cases it ought to be the needle of choice for parenteral therapy [7].

Plastic Catheters

Plastic catheters are associated with a high incidence of complications in comparison with the steel needle. "Venous complications from plastic catheters were found to be approximately 2½ times more prevalent than with steel needles" [37].

The traumatic insertion of a catheter often results in the formation of local thrombi which can support bacterial or fungal proliferation. The trauma is increased when a large catheter is used or when the venipuncture is performed by inexperienced personnel.

Characteristics inherent with the catheter encourage the introduction of bacteria through the cutaneous opening. In the over-the-needle catheter, the catheter is larger than the cutaneous puncture wound made by the inlying needle. The result is a definite drag through the skin as the catheter is slipped off the needle, with the potential risk of transporting cutaneous bacteria into the puncture wound. Skin flora has been implicated as an important source of organisms responsible for catheter-associated infection. In the through-the-needle catheter, the sterility of the catheter is maintained by its sterile protective sleeve and the sterile needle through which the catheter is slipped into the vein. Once the catheter is within the lumen of the vein, the needle is withdrawn, leaving a puncture wound larger than the catheter and one through which fluid can seep and bacteria can gain entrance.

Skin Preparation

Microbes on the hands of hospital personnel contribute to hospital-associated infection. Too often breaks in sterile technique occur from failure to wash hands before changing bottles or sets or preparing admixtures. Besides the usual skin flora, antibiotic-resistant gram-negative organisms frequently contaminate the hands of hospital personnel [26].

To maintain asepsis, the C.D.C. recommends that hands be thoroughly washed and that sterile gloves be worn during insertion of the intravenous cannula [5].

Adequate and reliable preparation of the patient's skin and maintenance of asepsis is imperative when a catheter is used for intravenous therapy. The skin, the first defense barrier of the body, is broken, providing a vulnerable port for the migration of bacteria. Skin flora has been implicated as a source of contamination of catheters. In a study made of 118 patients receiving intravenous therapy via an indwelling polyvinyl catheter, 53 catheters were found to be contaminated with bacteria; in 28 of these the organisms were comparable to those cultured from the skin of the patient before the skin was cleaned with iodine [3].

Frequently the question arises of whether or not to shave the skin. The need to remove the hair is not substantiated by scientific evidence; antiseptics used to clean the skin also clean the hair. Shaving facilitates removal of the tape, but may produce microabrasions which enhance the proliferation of bacteria [26].

Seventy percent alcohol is frequently used to prepare the skin site for venipuncture. How reliable is alcohol? Studies show that ethyl alcohol, 70 percent by weight, is an effective germicide for the skin when *applied with friction for 1 minute*. It is as effective as 12 minutes of scrubbing and reduces the bacterial count by 75 percent [42]. Since a minimum of 10,000 organisms per square centimeter are present on normal skin, the count would be reduced to 2500. Too frequently the use of alcohol consists of a quick wipe which fails to reduce the bacterial count significantly.

Iodine and iodine-containing disinfectants are still the most reliable agents for preparing the skin for venipuncture since they provide bactericidal, fungicidal, and sporicidal activity. Because of occasional patient allergy to iodine, the possibility of sensitivity should be investigated before its use.

Quaternary ammonium compounds such as aqueous benzalkonium chloride are inactivated by organic debris and are ineffective against gram-negative organisms, and so should not be used for skin disinfection [26].

The tourniquet itself may very well provide a source of cross-infection and contamination since it is used repeatedly from patient to patient and handled just prior to venipuncture. This possibility should be kept in mind and the tourniquet disinfected periodically.

Once the venipuncture is completed and the cannula is within the lumen of the vein, it must be securely anchored; to-and-fro motions of the catheter in the puncture wound may irritate the intima of the vein and introduce cutaneous bacteria. Thought should be given to the possible contamination of the adhesive tape that is used to secure the cannula. Rolls of tape last indefinitely and may be a source of contamination; they are transported from room to room, placed on patients' beds and tables, and frequently roll to the floor. Furthermore, before venipuncture, strips of tape often are torn off the roll and placed in convenient locations on the bed, table, and uniform. These facts should be borne in mind when adhesive tape is applied about the catheter and over the puncture wound. The puncture wound must be considered an open wound and asepsis must be maintained.

Care of the Catheter

Use of topical antiseptic iodophor ointment should be considered, and the wound should be protected by a sterile dressing. The dressing should be changed daily using aseptic technique and the ointment re-applied. Occlusive dressings create a moist, warm environment which may alter the cutaneous flora and enhance the proliferation of bacteria [26].

Recommendations [17] require that indwelling cannulas be left in place no longer than 72 hours and preferably for only 48 hours. The date and time of insertion written on a piece of tape and placed in the vicinity of the dressing will alert the nurse and assist in ensuring removal within a safe period of time.

Frequent observations should be made for signs of malfunction of the cannula, infiltration, and phlebitis characterized by erythema, induration, or tenderness. Such signs require immediate removal of the cannula. Fuchs [16] has noted that the major factor influencing the frequency of catheter colonization is the presence of other catheter complications such as subcutaneous infiltration and phlebitis. He defined *colonization* as positive culture of the catheter tip without evidence of local systemic infection.

Irrigation of a plugged catheter may embolize small catheter thrombi, some of which are infected. Contamination of the catheter may result from a break in aseptic technique, from contaminated fluid or set, from bacterial invasion of the puncture wound, or from clinically undetected bacteremia arising from an infection in a remote area of the body, such as a tracheostomy, the urinary tract, or a surgical wound. The clot around or in the catheter serves as an excellent trap for circulatory microorganisms and as a nutrient for bacterial proliferation.

Intravenous-associated Infections

Intravenous-associated sepsis is not always accompanied by phlebitis. Symptoms of infection consist of chills and fever, gastric symptoms, headache, hyperventilation, and shock. Should infection develop from an unknown source in a patient receiving intravenous therapy, the intravenous system should be suspected and the entire system, including the cannula, removed. The catheter and the infusion fluid should be cultured.

The following procedure should be used for culturing the catheter [17]:

1. Cleanse the skin about the cannula site with an effective antiseptic.
2. Maintaining asepsis, remove the catheter and with sterile scissors snip 1 cm of the catheter tip into blood culture or other appropriate culture medium.

The following procedure should be used for culturing the infusion fluid [17]:

1. Aseptically withdraw 20 ml of fluid from the intravenous line: 1 ml is used to prepare a pour plate; the remaining fluid is used to inoculate two blood culture bottles.
2. Add to the remaining intravenous fluid in the container an equal volume of brain-heart infusion broth enriched with 0.5 percent beef extract. Inoculate at 37° C; this is a more sensitive culture for detecting low-level contamination.

All containers of fluid previously administered to the patient should be suspected and, if possible, retained and cultured. All information and identification, including the lot number of the suspected solution, should be recorded on the culture requisition and the patient chart. The Food and Drug Administration should be notified if contamination during manufacturing is suspected and fluids bearing implicated lot number should be stored for investigation.

Particulate Matter

The literature concerning particulate matter in infusions and its clinical significance is increasing. Many articles indicate that intravenously administered particles can cause pathogenic states [40]. Particulate matter is defined as the mobile, undissolved substances unintentionally present in parenteral fluids [23]. Such foreign matter may consist of rubber, glass, cotton fibers, drug particles, molds, metal, or paper fibers.

Vascular Route of Infused Particles

The pulmonary vascular bed acts as a filter for infused particles. Particles introduced into the vein travel to the right atrium of the heart, down through the tricuspid valve, and into the right ventricle. From there they are pumped into the pulmonary artery and on through branches of arteries which decrease in size until the particles are trapped in the massive capillary bed in the lungs, where the capillaries measure 7 to 12 microns in diameter.

Five microns, the size of an erythrocyte suspended in fluid, has been suggested as the largest allowable size for a particle in the pulmonary capillary bed [18]. Particles larger than 5 microns are recognized as potentially dangerous since they are likely to become lodged. Particles as large as 300 microns can pass through an 18-gauge needle, and much larger particles may pass through an indwelling catheter with a larger lumen. See Table 4 for particle size comparisons. If occlusion of a small arteriole inhibits oxygenation or normal metabolic activities, cellular damage or tissue death may result. Where there is ample collateral circulation, the occlusion would have no appreciable biological effect. However, a particle that is not biologically inert may incite an inflammatory reaction, a neoplastic response, or an antigenic, sensitizing response [22].

Particles may gain access to the systemic circulation, where occlusion of a small arteriole in the brain, kidney or eye can be serious, in one of the following ways:

1. The pulmonary vascular bed does not filter out all particles. Prinzmetal and associates [33] demonstrated that glass beads up to 390 microns may pass through the pulmonary capillary bed and reach the systemic circulation.
2. Large arteriovenous shunts have been demonstrated to exist in the human lung [19, 24]. Particles bypass the pulmonary capillary bed and enter the systemic circulation, where a systemic occlusion could be serious.
3. Particles larger than 5 microns may reach the systemic circulation by interarterial injection or infusion.

Sources of Contamination
Recent studies [10] have shown that particulate contamination is present in all intravenous fluids and administration sets. Manufacturing and sterilizing processes are implicated. Great efforts are being made by manufacturers to produce high quality intravenous injections. Their efforts are being defeated by numerous manipulations before final infusion.

MEDICATION ADDITIVES. Drugs constitute a major source of contamination. Improper technique in the preparation of drugs results in the formation of insoluble particles. When personnel with no pharmaceutical knowledge add drugs to intravenous fluids, they contribute to incompatibilities which substantially increase the particle count. Rubber closures also have been implicated as a major source of contamination.

GLASS AMPULES. Glass ampules may be responsible for the injection of thousands of glass particles into the circulation. Turco and Davis [38],

Table 4. Particle Size Comparisons

Microns		Inches
175	=	.007
150	=	.006
125	=	.005
100	=	.004
75	=	.003
50	=	.002
25	=	.001

Note: One micron equals 40 millionths of an inch (approx.). A human hair is approximately 125 microns in thickness. Bacteria range in size from 0.3 to 0.5 micron. We cannot see a particle or hole smaller than 20 microns. A hole 25 microns in diameter in a HEPA filter is over 75 times larger than the contaminants and bacteria passing through.

Source: Contamination Control Laboratories [6].

in a study prompted by the frequency of high-dose administration of furosemide, showed that a dose of 400 mg, which at that time required the breaking of 20 ampules, could add to the injection 1085 glass particles larger than 5 microns. A dose of 600 mg, requiring 30 ampules, could result in 2387 particles larger than 5 microns.

ANTIBIOTIC INJECTABLES. Studies have been performed in relation to particulate matter in commercial antibiotic injectable products [27]. They showed particulate contamination levels of bulk-filled antibiotics to be two to ten times greater than those of stable antibiotic solutions and lyophilized antibiotics. Filtration is impossible since packaging by the sterile bulk-fill method involves extracting and processing the antibiotic in sterile bulk powder form and then aseptically placing the bulk antibiotic into dry presterilized vials. In the lyophilized and the stable liquid packaging processes the particulate matter can be terminally removed by filtration directly into presterilized vials. The majority of the antibiotics are packed by the bulk-fill method.

Particulate matter in intravenous injections may be responsible for much of the phlebitis that so often occurs with the infusion of these drugs. Russell [35] listed the major pathological conditions caused by particulate matter as (1) direct blockage of vessels, (2) platelet agglutination leading to formation of emboli, (3) local inflammation caused by impaction of particles, and (4) antigenic reactions with subsequent allergic consequence.

INTRAVENOUS FLUIDS. Walter [43] noted that critically ill patients who had received large amounts of intravenous fluid died of pulmonary insufficiency characterized by increased venous pressure and pulmonary hypertension. He observed that the lungs looked like leather and speculated that the cause of death might be the result of accumulated matter from the many liters of infused fluids.

111

MASSIVE INFUSIONS OF OLD BANKED BLOOD. Deaths caused by pulmonary emboli following massive transfusions have been reported [31]. Cellular debris in stored blood has been implicated; the standard blood filter of 170 microns has been found inadequate to remove the microaggregates that accumulate in stored bank blood. Commercially available blood filters*†‡ of small micropore size (under 40 microns) are now available and are recommended for use when more than 2 units of old banked blood is to be infused.

Reducing the Level of Contamination
Since particulate matter infused via intravenous fluids may produce pathological changes which could have an adverse effect on critically ill patients, every effort must be made to reduce the particulate count in intravenous injections. Until recently, nurses and doctors in general have been unaware of the potential dangers that exist and have unknowingly added to the contamination. Official agencies are developing standards for an acceptable limit for particles in intravenous fluids. Industry has provided the medical profession with filters to limit direct access of bacteria, fungus, and particulate matter to the bloodstream.

FILTER. A filter aspiration needle§ specially designed to remove particulate matter from intravenous medicaments is available. With this device attached to a syringe the medication is drawn from the vial, filtering out the particles. The filter needle must then be discarded to prevent the particles trapped on the filter from being injected when the medication is added to the intravenous fluid.

A double-ended filter needle‖ is available to facilitate the transfer and filtration of radiopharmaceuticals into a sterile evacuated vial.

FINAL FILTERS. Final filtration of intravenous fluids has been recommended. "Since the present USP standards for particulate matter in injectable solution and powder appear to be inadequate, injectable products known to contain a high level of particulate contamination should be terminally filtered or administered through infusion sets with in-line final filters" [27].

Wilmore and Dudrick [44] observed 250 0.45-micron membrane filters over a 6-month period. Seven positive bacterial cultures were ob-

* Ultipor Blood Transfusion Filter (Pall Corporation, Biomedical Products Division, Glen Cove, N.Y.).
† Microaggregate Blood Filter (Fenwal Laboratories, Morton Grove, Ill.; division of Travenol Laboratories, Inc.).
‡ Swank Transfusion Filter (Extracorporeal Medical Specialties, Inc., King of Prussia, Pa.).
§ Monoject Filter Aspiration Needle (Sherwood Medical Industries, St. Louis, Mo.).
‖ Paramedical Disposables, Inc., Needham Heights, Mass.

tained from the proximal surface of the membrane. No septic signs of bacteria, septicemia, or local signs of phlebitis were observed. Seventeen filters became obstructed: fourteen from microprecipitates resulting from drug incompatibilities, two from air lock, and one from the infusion of blood.

Turco and Davis [39] studied the effectiveness of commercially available filter devices. The study included the flow rate of intravenous infusion fluids with filter devices, flow-rate changes, and the effects of viscosity upon flow rates. "The 0.45 micron [filter] having a larger pore size yields flow rates approximately two to three times that of a 0.22 micron filter" [39]. Increasing the size of the diameter surface of the 0.22-micron filter could improve the flow rate.

Filters are manufactured in a variety of forms, sizes, and materials. Some, not all, when wet block the passage of air under normal pressure. Used in conjunction with infusion pumps, they play an important role in preventing air from being pumped into the bloodstream should the fluid container empty.

A knowledge of the characteristics of the filter, its use, and proper handling is important to the safety of the patient. Faulty handling can cause plugging of the filters, resulting in the patient's not receiving prescribed fluids and the necessity of performing a venipuncture to insert a new line, or in a ruptured filter which may go undetected and introduce filter fragments, bacteria, and air into the infusion line.

Two commonly used in-line filters are the depth filter and the membrane filter. The depth filter consists of fibers or fragmented material that have been pressed or bonded to form a tortuous maze. Fluid flows through a random path which absorbs and traps the particles. Because the pore size is not uniform, "depth filters cannot properly be given an absolute rating. Instead, they are assigned a nominal rating which, by definition, is the particle size above which 98 percent of the contaminants will be retained; for instance a depth filter rated at 5 microns will retain 98 percent of all particles larger than 5 microns, though 2 percent will pass through" [2]. Depth filters are efficient in removing particles; they do not block the passage of air.

Membrane filters are screen-type filters with uniformly sized pores which provide an absolute rating. A 0.45-micron filter will retain on the flat membrane all particles greater than 0.45 micron. These filters when wet block the passage of air under normal pressure. Membrane filters of 0.45 micron and 0.22 micron are bacteria particulate retention filters and are used to sterilize fluids. The 0.22-micron filter has the advantage of providing "absolute" sterilization, whereas the 0.45-micron filter can be used for sterile filtration when prior experience indicates that organisms smaller than 0.45 micron, e.g., *Pseudomonas* species, are not present in the solution to be filtered [39]. In-line filters do not filter out endotoxin, and conceivably, if contamination is present in hyperosmolar fluids containing penicillin derivatives, viable L forms could exist and pass [13].

HANDLING OF FILTERS. Although filters provide added protection for the patient, they are not a substitute for sterile technique. The manual addition or frequent changes of the filter increase the likelihood of contamination. An in-line membrane filter with a self-venting air filter (not yet developed) would reduce the risk of contamination by eliminating the need for (1) manual addition of the filter and (2) frequent changes due to obstruction of the filter by air block. Such a filter would require support against back pressure to prevent rupture of the filter and the introduction of air through the air vent.

PITFALLS IN THE USE OF MICROPORE MEMBRANE FILTERS. If not properly primed before use, in-line membrane filters will, upon becoming wet, block with air and prevent flow of the infusion. The following procedure is used for priming the filter:

1. Close clamp on the administration set containing the final filter.
2. Attach set to fluid container and suspend container.
3. Partially fill drip chamber.
4. Hold end of set with venipuncture needle pointed up or as recommended by the manufacturer; this inverts the filter.
5. Open clamp; the air will escape through the dry filter ahead of the fluid.
6. Tap the inverted filter to remove air bubbles.
7. Proceed with venipuncture.

Clamping off the set before the container is suspended, filling the drip chamber, and inverting the filter are important steps in preventing an air block in the line.

Some administration sets contain air vent filters which allow only sterile air to enter the container. Such sets are also available for the administration of salt-poor albumin. Misuse occasionally occurs, contributing to contamination. The drip chamber of the set *must be compressed* before it is introduced into the fluid bottle. This creates a vacuum which immediately causes the air vent to function, avoiding regurgitation of fluid and a wet filter which may cease to function. Occasionally a staff member inserts a needle into the air vent to provide a patent vent; however, this ruptures the filter and contributes to particulate contamination.

Administration sets are available with drip chambers located directly below the controlled volume chamber containing the micropore filter.

Once the intravenous system is filled, the drip chamber must not be compressed. If the drip chamber is inadvertently squeezed, the membrane may rupture, with the potential risk of introduction of filter particles and bacteria into the infusion. The ruptured membrane is not easily detected and false security results in the risk of air entering the line.

Final filters complicate a system by which viscous fluids, such as blood, and some drugs, such as amphotericin B, are infused. An injection site distal to the filter provides a means of infusion. A clamp located between the filter and the injection site plays an important role; if, through ignorance or carelessness, the injection is made without clamping off the tubing, the filter may become blocked by viscous fluid or back pressure from the injection may rupture the membrane and allow particulate matter and bacteria to enter the bloodstream.

In-line filters limit the access of bacteria, fungus, and particulate matter to the bloodstream, but their safety depends upon the knowledge of the individuals involved in their use.

References

1. Altemeier, W. A., Todd, J. C., and Inge, W. W. Gram-negative septicemia: A growing threat. *Annals of Surgery* 166:530–542, 1967.
2. Application Report AR-11. *Low Volume Sterilizing Filtration.* Bedford, Mass.: Millipore Corporation, 1969. P. 3.
3. Banks, D. C., Cawdreys, H. M., Yates, D. B., and Harries, M. G. *Lancet* 1:443, 1970.
4. Center for Disease Control. *Nosocomical Bacteremias Associated with Intravenous Fluid Therapy* (U.S.A. Morbidity and Mortality Weekly Report 20). (Special Suppl.) Vol. 20, No. 9, 1971.
5. Center for Disease Control. *Recommendations for the Prevention of I.V.-associated Infections* (for training purposes). Hospital Infections and Microbiological Control Sections, Bacterial Diseases Branch, Epidemiology Program, C.D.C., Atlanta, March 1973.
6. Contamination Control Laboratories. *Particle Size Comparisons* (information circular). Livonia, Mich., 1970.
7. Crossley, K., and Matsen, J. M. The scalp-vein needle: A prospective study of complications. *Journal of the American Medical Association* 220:985, 1972.
8. Curry, C. R., and Quie, P. G. Fungal septicemia in patients receiving parenteral hyperalimentation. *New England Journal of Medicine* 285: 1221, 1971.
9. Davis, N. M., and Turco, S. A study of particulate matter in I.V. infusion fluids—phase 2. *American Journal of Hospital Pharmacy* 28:620–623, 1971.
10. Davis, N. M., Turco, S., and Sivielly, E. A study of particulate matter in I.V. infusion fluids. *American Journal of Hospital Pharmacy* 27:822–826, 1970.

11. Deeb, E. N., and Natsios, G. A.   Contamination of intravenous fluids by bacteria and fungi during preparation and administration. *American Journal of Hospital Pharmacy* 28:764, 1971.
12. Dudrick, S. J.   Article in *Hospital Tribune* (University and Hospital Edition of *Medical Tribune and Medical News*) 8(3):1, 1974.
13. Duma, R. J., Warner, J. F., and Dalton, H. P.   Letter to the editor. *New England Journal of Medicine* 284:1038, 1971.
14. Felts, S. K., Shaffner, W., Melly, M. A., and Koenig, M. G.   Sepsis caused by contaminated intravenous fluids: Epidemiological clinical and laboratory investigation of an outbreak in one hospital. *Annals of Internal Medicine* 77:881, 1972.
15. Fonkalsrud, E. W., Murphy, J., and Smith, F. G., Jr.   Effect of pH in glucose infusions on development of thrombophlebitis. *Journal of Surgical Research* 8:539, 1968.
16. Fuchs, P. C.   Indwelling intravenous polyethylene catheters: Factors influencing the risk of microbial colonization and sepsis. *Journal of the American Medical Association* 216:1447–1450, 1971.
17. Goldmann, D. A., Maki, G. D., Rhame, F. S., and Kaiser, A. B.   Guidelines for infection control in intravenous therapy. *Annals of Internal Medicine* 79:849, 1973.
18. Groves, M. J.   Particles in intravenous fluids (letter). *Lancet* 2:344, 1965.
19. Hales, M. R.   Multiple small arteriovenous fistulae of the lungs. *American Journal of Pathology* 32:927, 1956.
20. Hansen, J. S., and Hepler, C. D.   Contamination of intravenous solutions by airborne microbes. *American Journal of Hospital Pharmacy* 30:326–331, 1973.
21. Hirshfield, J. W.   Bacterial contamination of wounds from the air, from the skin of the operator, and from the skin of the patient. *Surgery, Gynecology, and Obstetrics* 73:72–78, 1941.
22. Jonas, A. M.   Potentially Hazardous Effects of Introducing Particulate Matter into the Vascular System of Man and Animals. In *Safety of Large Volume Parenteral Solutions* (Proceedings of National Symposium of the U.S. Food and Drug Administration, Washington, D.C., 1966). Washington, D.C.: Government Printing Office, 1967.
23. Kruger, E. O., and Riggs, T. H.   Objectives: Pharmaceutical Manufacturers Association Parenteral Particulate Matter Committee. *Bulletin of the Parenteral Drug Association* 22:99–103, 1968.
24. Liebow, A. A., Hales, M. R., and Lindskog, G. B.   Enlargement of the bronchial arteries and their anastomoses with the pulmonary arteries in bronchiectasis. *American Journal of Pathology* 25:211–231, 1949.
25. Lillehei, R. C., Dietzman, R., Moras, S., and Block, J. H.   Treatment of septic shock. *Modern Treatment* 4(2):32–346, 1967. Cited in *Septic Shock: Pathogenesis and Treatment*. Kalamazoo, Mich.: Upjohn Co., December, 1973.
26. Maki, D. G., Goldman, D. A., and Rhama, F. S.   Infection control in intravenous therapy. *Annals of Internal Medicine* 79:869, 870, 872, 875, 876, 878, 880, 1973.
27. Masuda, J. V., and Beckerman, J. H.   Particulate matter in commercial antibiotic injectable products. *American Journal of Hospital Pharmacy* 30:72–76, 1973.
28. McDonough, J. J.   Preventing contamination in I.V. therapy. *Hospital Physician*, Nov. 1971, p. 70.

29. McGaw Laboratories. *McGaw Technical Information Bulletin #16.* Glendale, Calif., 1969.
30. Microbiological hazards of intravenous infusions. *Lancet* 1:43, 1974.
31. Moseley, R. V., and Doty, D. B. Death associated with multiple pulmonary emboli soon after battle. *Annals of Surgery* 171:336, 1970.
32. Motsay, G. J., Dietzman, R. H., Ersek, R. A., and Lillehei, R. C. Hemodynamic alterations and results of treatment in patients with Gram-negative septic shock. *Surgery* 67:577–583, 1970.
33. Prinzmetal, M., Ornitz, E. M., Jr., Simkin, B., and Bergman, H. C. Arteriovenous anastomoses in liver, spleen, and lungs. *American Journal of Physiology* 152:48–52, 1948.
34. Robertson, M. H. Fungi in fluids—A hazard of intravenous therapy. *Journal of Medical Microbiology* 3:99, 1970.
35. Russell, J. H. Pharmaceutical application of filtration, part 2. *Journal of Hospital Pharmacy* 28:125–126, 1970.
36. Tabers Cyclopedia Medical Dictionary. Revised and edited by Thomas, C. L. Philadelphia: Davis, 1973.
37. Thomas, E. T., Evers, W., and Racz, C. B. Post infusion phlebitis. *Anesthesia and Analgesia* 49:150–159, 1970.
38. Turco, S., and Davis, N. M. Glass particles in intravenous injections. *New England Journal of Medicine* 287:1264–1265, 1972.
39. Turco, S., and Davis, N. M. A comparison of commercial final filtration devices. *Lippincott's Hospital Pharmacy* 8:144, 1973.
40. Turco, S., and Davis, N. M. Clinical significance of particulate matter—A review of literature. *Lippincott's Hospital Pharmacy* 8:137, 1973.
41. Viaflex containers. *Medical Letter on Drugs and Therapeutics* 14:69–71, 1972.
42. Walter, C. W. *The Aseptic Treatment of Wounds.* New York: Macmillan, 1956.
43. Walter, C. W. *FDA Symposium on Safety of Large Volume Parenteral Solutions.* Washington, D.C.: U.S. Government Printing Office, 1967.
44. Wilmore, D. W., and Dudrick, S. J. An in-line filter for intravenous solutions. *Archives of Surgery* 99:462, 1969.

10. Fundamental Aspects of Fluid and Electrolyte Metabolism

Over the past fifteen years our knowledge of fluid and electrolyte balance has increased to the extent that we now recognize an imbalance as a threat to life. With this increased knowledge has come an increase in the nurse's responsibility in parenteral therapy. Not only is accurate recording of the patient's intake and output important, but so, too, is the ability to recognize symptoms of imbalance; prompt recognition of an imbalance may indicate adjustment in therapy which may be crucial to the safety of the patient.

Today electrolyte therapy is used extensively. About 70 percent of all fluids administered contain some electrolytes. A survey done at the Massachusetts General Hospital in 1967 by S. Shamsi, Staff Pharmacist, revealed that 48 percent of 1911 solutions administered intravenously were electrolyte solutions. Of the remaining 52 percent of nonelectrolyte solutions, potassium chloride was added to about 20 percent.

Electrolyte therapy is often a lifesaving procedure; its safe and successful administration is essential. Knowledge of the fundamentals of fluid and electrolyte metabolism contributes to safe electrolyte therapy. This knowledge alerts the nurse to (1) the necessity for accurate fluid and electrolyte administration, (2) the potential dangers of electrolyte therapy, and (3) a change in the patient's condition which could alter the therapy prescribed.

Abnormalities of body fluid and electrolyte metabolism present certain therapeutic problems. When the mechanisms normally regulating fluid volume, electrolyte composition, and osmolality are impaired, therapy becomes complicated. An understanding of these metabolic abnormalities enables the nurse to understand the problems involved. Such problems exist in patients with renal insufficiency, adrenal insufficiency, adrenal hyperactivity, and other kinds of impaired organ function. For example, correction of a severe potassium deficit resulting from vomiting and diarrhea presents a problem in the dehydrated patient. Potassium replacement is imperative. However, potassium administered to patients with renal insufficiency results in potassium toxicity; the kidneys are unable to excrete electrolytes. The adverse effects of excess potassium on the heart muscle are arrhythmia and heart block. The nurse must recognize the importance of (1) hydrating the patient before potassium can be administered safely and (2) watching for diminished diuresis which could necessitate a change in therapy. Once antidiuresis occurs the potassium infusion must be interrupted and the physician notified.

Therapeutic problems also exist in patients with impaired liver function. Gastric replacement is necessary when there has been an excessive loss of gastric fluid. Most deficits caused by gastric suction, unless severe, are treated with 0.85 percent sodium chloride in 5 percent dextrose in water. However, severe loss may call for gastric replacement solutions containing ammonium chloride, which can be potentially dangerous when administered to patients with impaired liver function. Ammonium chloride administered to a patient with severe liver damage may result in ammonia intoxication because of the liver's inability to convert ammonia to hydrogen ion and urea.

These examples illustrate the role that knowledge of fluid and electrolyte metabolism plays in contributing to safe and successful therapy in the critically ill patient.

Fluid Content of the Body

The total body water content of an individual varies with age, weight, and sex. The amount of water is dependent upon the amount of body fat. Body fat is essentially water-free; the greater the fat content, the less is the water content. In a normal male with an average amount of fat, the water weight is about 60 percent of the body weight. In a female, because of the normally larger degree of body fat, the proportion of water weight to body weight is less, about 54 percent of body weight.

Compartments

The total body fluid is functionally divided into two main compartments: the intracellular and the extracellular compartments. The intracellular compartment consists of the fluid inside the cells and comprises about two-thirds of the body fluid, or 40 percent of the body weight. The extracellular compartment consists of fluid outside the body cells—the plasma representing 5 percent of the body weight and the interstitial fluid (fluid in tissues) representing 15 percent of the body weight. See Table 5 for a schematic representation of compartments.

In newborn infants the proportion is approximately three-fifths intracellular and two-fifths extracellular. This ratio changes and reaches the adult level by the time the infant is about 30 months old.

Table 5. Total Body Water Composition

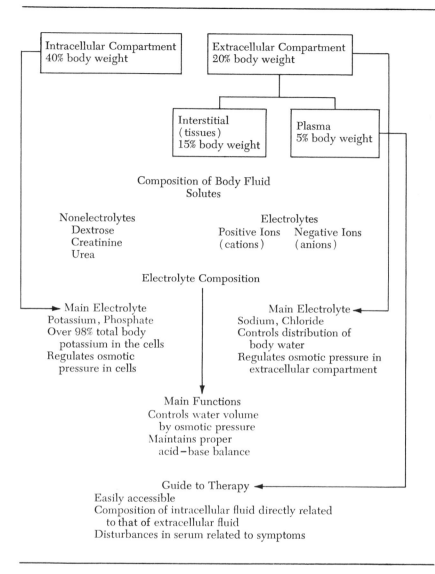

Intracellular Compartment
40% body weight

Extracellular Compartment
20% body weight

Interstitial
(tissues)
15% body weight

Plasma
5% body weight

Composition of Body Fluid
Solutes

Nonelectrolytes
Dextrose
Creatinine
Urea

Electrolytes
Positive Ions   Negative Ions
(cations)   (anions)

Electrolyte Composition

Main Electrolyte
Potassium, Phosphate
Over 98% total body
  potassium in the cells
Regulates osmotic
  pressure in cells

Main Electrolyte
Sodium, Chloride
Controls distribution of
  body water
Regulates osmotic pressure in
  extracellular compartment

Main Functions
Controls water volume
  by osmotic pressure
Maintains proper
  acid–base balance

Guide to Therapy
Easily accessible
Composition of intracellular fluid directly related
  to that of extracellular fluid
Disturbances in serum related to symptoms

There is one additional compartment, the transcellular compartment. The transcellular fluid is the product of cellular metabolism and consists of secretions such as gastrointestinal secretions and urine. Analysis of the secretions may assist the physician in tracing lost electrolytes and prescribing proper fluid and electrolyte replacement. Excessive fluid and electrolyte loss must be replaced to maintain fluid and electrolyte balance in the two main compartments. The amount of body water loss is easily computed by weighing the patient and noting loss of weight: 1 liter of body water is equivalent to 1 kg, or 2.2 pounds, of body weight. Up to 5 percent weight loss in a child or adult may signify moderate fluid volume deficit—over 5 percent may indicate severe fluid volume deficit [7]. Weight changes are also valuable as indicators of body water gains—acute weight gain may indicate water excess.

Composition of Body Fluid

The body fluid contains two types of solutes (dissolved substances): the electrolytes and the nonelectrolytes (see Table 5). The *nonelectrolytes* are molecules which do not break into particles in solution but remain intact. They consist of (1) dextrose, (2) urea, and (3) creatinine.

Electrolytes are molecules which break into electrically charged particles called ions. The ion carrying a positive charge is called a cation, the ion with a negative charge, an anion. Potassium chloride is an electrolyte which, dissolved in water, yields potassium cations and chloride anions. Chemical balance is always maintained; the total number of positive charges equals the total number of negative charges. The quantity of charges and their concentration is expressed as milliequivalents (mEq) per liter of fluid. As the number of negative charges must equal the number of positive charges for chemical balance, the milliequivalents of cations must equal the milliequivalents of anions [2] (see Table 6).

Electrolyte Composition

Each fluid compartment has its own electrolyte composition (see Table 5). The extracellular compartment (plasma and interstitial fluid) contains a high concentration of sodium, chloride, and bicarbonate and a low concentration of potassium. The composition of the intracellular fluid is quite different; the concentrations of potassium, magnesium, and phosphate are high, whereas the sodium and chloride concentrations are relatively low.

Electrolyte composition of the intracellular fluid is in part related to electrolyte composition of the plasma and interstitial fluids. Disturbances in the extracellular fluid are reflected in the patient's symptoms.

Table 6. Plasma Electrolytes Illustrate That Total mEq of Cations Must Equal Total mEq of Anions

Cations	mEq/L	Anions	mEq/L
Na^+	142	HCO_3^-	24
K^+	5	Cl^-	105
Ca^{++}	5	HPO_4^{--}	2
Mg^{++}	2	SO_4^{--}	1
		Organic acid$^-$	6
		Proteinate$^-$	16
Total	154	Total	154

Source: Baxter Laboratories [2].

These facts, combined with the accessibility of plasma, make the analysis of plasma a valuable guide to therapy. Occasionally, however, the electrolyte determination of plasma may be misleading. For example, concentration of potassium in plasma may be high while there is a body deficit. This surplus is due to the shift of potassium from intracellular to extracellular fluid in the process of large potassium losses through the kidneys. Determination of plasma sodium may also present a false picture. In the case of an edematous cardiac patient, the plasma concentration may be low in spite of excess body sodium. This is due to the fact that total body sodium is equal to the sum of the products of volume times concentration in the various compartments.

Electrolytes serve two main purposes: (1) to act in controlling body water volume by osmotic pressure and (2) to maintain the proper acid–alkaline balance of the body.

OSMOLALITY. Osmolality is the total solute concentration and reflects the relative water and total solute concentration since it is expressed per liter of serum. The osmotic pressure is determined by the number of solutes in solution. If the extracellular fluid contains a relatively large number of dissolved particles and the intracellular fluid contains a small amount of dissolved particles, the osmotic pressure would cause water to pass from the less concentrated fluid to the more concentrated. Therefore fluid from the intracellular compartment would pass into the extracellular compartment until the concentration became equal.

The unit of osmotic pressure is the osmole and the values are expressed in milliosmoles (mOsm). Normal blood plasma has an osmolality of 290 mOsm. The determination of serum osmolality is sometimes used to detect dehydration or overhydration. Because sodium chloride is the principal solute in the extracellular fluid, the osmolality reading usually parallels the sodium reading or is very close to two times the serum sodium plus 10. Therefore measurement of sodium concentration also indicates the water needs of the body. At times the osmolality reading may falsely indicate dehydration. Because the osmolality is the total solute concentration, nonelectrolytes are included in the reading. An elevated level of blood urea can therefore increase the osmolality without exerting osmotic pressure. A determination of the blood urea nitrogen may supply a correction to the osmolality reading in cases of increased serum urea.

Acid–Alkaline Balance

The alkalinity or acidity of a solution depends upon the degree of hydrogen ion concentration. An increase in the hydrogen ions results in a more acid solution; a decrease, in a more alkaline solution. Acidity is expressed by the symbol pH, which refers to the amount of hydrogen ion concentration. A solution having a pH of 7 is regarded as neutral.

The extracellular fluid has a pH ranging from 7.35 to 7.45 and is thus slightly alkaline. When the pH of the blood is higher than 7.45, an alkaline condition exists; when lower than 7.35, an acid condition exists.

The biological fluids, both extracellular and intracellular, contain a buffer system which maintains the proper acid–alkaline balance. This buffer system consists of fluid with salts of a weak acid or weak base. A base or hydroxide neutralizes the effect of an acid. These weak acids and bases maintain pH values by soaking up surplus ions or releasing them; acids yield hydrogen ions, bases accept hydrogen ions.

The carbonic acid–sodium bicarbonate system is the most important buffer system in the extracellular compartment. The normal ratio is 1 part of carbonic acid to 20 parts of base bicarbonate, which represents 1.33 mEq of carbonic acid to 27 mEq of base bicarbonate [7].

Acid–Base Imbalance

Acid–base imbalances are normally the result of an excess or a deficit in either base bicarbonate or carbonic acid. Deviations of pH from 7.35 to 7.45 are combated by the buffer system and by the respiratory and renal regulatory mechanisms. There are two types of disturbance that can affect the acid–base balance: respiratory and metabolic. Refer to Table 7 for a diagrammatic presentation of the material that follows.

RESPIRATORY DISTURBANCES. Respiratory disturbances affect the carbonic side of the balance by increasing or decreasing carbonic acid; when carbon dioxide unites with extracellular fluid, carbonic acid is produced.

Respiratory alkalosis is caused when excess carbon dioxide is exhaled during rapid or deep breathing. Carbonic acid is depleted, owing to the carbon dioxide loss. Respiratory alkalosis may occur as the result of emotional disturbances, such as anxiety and hysteria, and also from lack of oxygen or fever [6].

Symptoms are convulsions, tetany, and unconsciousness. Laboratory determination is a urinary pH above 7 and a plasma bicarbonate below 25 mEq per liter [7]. The body attempts to restore the ratio to normal by depressing the bicarbonate so as to compensate for the deficit in the carbonic acid.

Respiratory acidosis occurs when exhalation of carbon dioxide is depressed; the excess retention of carbon dioxide increases the carbonic acid. It may occur in conditions that interfere with normal breathing: emphysema, asthma, and pneumonia [6].

Symptoms are weakness, disorientation, depressed breathing, and coma. Urinary pH is below 6, and plasma bicarbonate is above 29 mEq per liter. The increase of the bicarbonate is due to the body's attempt to restore the carbonic acid–bicarbonate ratio [7].

METABOLIC DISTURBANCES. Metabolic disturbances affect the bicarbonate side of the balance. Kidney function controls the bicarbonate concentration by regulating the amount of cations (hydrogen, ammonium, and potassium) in exchange for sodium ions to combine with the reabsorbed bicarbonate in the distal tubular lumen. As hydrogen ions are excreted, bicarbonate is generated, maintaining the proper acid–base balance of the blood. Ammonia excretion is increased in response to a high acidity; bicarbonate replaces the ammonia.

Metabolic alkalosis is a condition associated with excess bicarbonate. This condition occurs when there is loss of chloride. Chloride and bicarbonate are both anions, which must equal the total number of cations. When the chloride anions are lost, the deficit must be made up by an equal number of anions to maintain electrolyte equilibrium; bicarbonate increases in compensation and alkalosis occurs.

Metabolic alkalosis is also associated with decreased levels of intracellular potassium. Potassium escapes from the cell into the extracellular fluid and is lost through the transcellular fluid. When body potassium is lost, the shift of the sodium and hydrogen ions from the extracellular fluid causes alkalosis, while the increase of hydrogen ions in the intracellular fluid causes acidosis of the cells.

Muscular hyperactivity, tetany, and depressed respiration are symptoms of metabolic alkalosis. The muscular hyperactivity and the tetany are symptoms of the deficit in ionized calcium which exists in alkalosis. Laboratory determinations are urinary pH above 7, plasma pH above 7.45, and bicarbonate above 29 mEq per liter in adults and 25 mEq per liter in children [7].

Treatment consists of the administration of solutions containing chloride to replace bicarbonate ions. Excess of bicarbonate ions is accompanied by potassium deficiency, so potassium must also be replaced.

Metabolic acidosis is a condition associated with a deficit in the bi-

Table 7. Acid–Base Imbalances

Result of

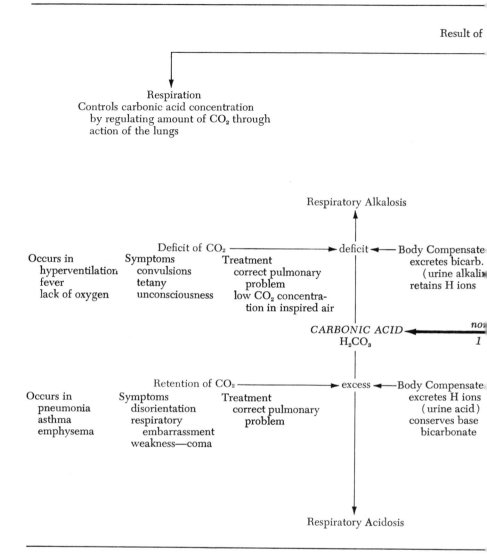

Respiration
Controls carbonic acid concentration
by regulating amount of CO_2 through
action of the lungs

Respiratory Alkalosis

Deficit of CO_2 ⟶ deficit ⟵ Body Compensate
excretes bicarb.
(urine alkali)
retains H ions

Occurs in	Symptoms	Treatment
hyperventilation	convulsions	correct pulmonary
fever	tetany	problem
lack of oxygen	unconsciousness	low CO_2 concentra-
		tion in inspired air

CARBONIC ACID ⟵ nor
H_2CO_3 1

Retention of CO_2 ⟶ excess ⟵ Body Compensate
excretes H ions
(urine acid)
conserves base
bicarbonate

Occurs in	Symptoms	Treatment
pneumonia	disorientation	correct pulmonary
asthma	respiratory	problem
emphysema	embarrassment	
	weakness—coma	

Respiratory Acidosis

urbances

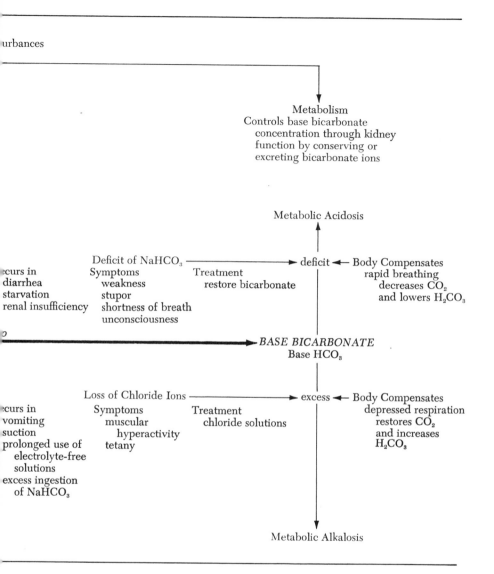

Metabolism
Controls base bicarbonate
concentration through kidney
function by conserving or
excreting bicarbonate ions

Metabolic Acidosis

Deficit of NaHCO₃ ⟶ deficit ⟵ Body Compensates
rapid breathing
decreases CO_2
and lowers H_2CO_3

	Symptoms	Treatment
ccurs in	weakness	restore bicarbonate
diarrhea	stupor	
starvation	shortness of breath	
renal insufficiency	unconsciousness	

BASE BICARBONATE
Base HCO₃

Loss of Chloride Ions ⟶ excess ⟵ Body Compensates
depressed respiration
restores CO_2
and increases
H_2CO_3

	Symptoms	Treatment
ccurs in	muscular	chloride solutions
vomiting	hyperactivity	
suction	tetany	
prolonged use of		
electrolyte-free		
solutions		
excess ingestion		
of NaHCO₃		

Metabolic Alkalosis

carbonate concentration. This occurs when (1) excessive amounts of ketone acids accumulate, as in uncontrolled diabetes or starvation, (2) inorganic acids like phosphate and sulphate accumulate, as in renal disease, and (3) excessive losses of bicarbonate occur from gastrointestinal drainage or diarrhea. Acidosis may occur also from intravenous administration of excessive amounts of sodium chloride or ammonium chloride, causing chloride ions to flood the extracellular fluid.

Stupor, shortness of breath, weakness, and unconsciousness are the symptoms of metabolic acidosis. Laboratory determination of urinary pH is below 6, plasma pH below 7.35, and plasma bicarbonate below 25 mEq per liter in adults and 20 mEq per liter in children [7].

Therapy consists of increasing the bicarbonate level. Solutions of sodium lactate are often employed, but since lactate ion must be oxidized to carbon dioxide before it can affect the acid–base balance, it is advisable to use sodium bicarbonate solutions which are effective even when the patient is suffering from oxygen lack.

Body Regulating Mechanisms

The body contains regulating mechanisms which maintain the constancy of body fluid volume, electrolyte composition, and osmolality. These mechanisms consist of the cardiovascular, renal, endocrine (adrenal, pituitary, and parathyroid), and respiratory systems. The kidneys, skin, and lungs are the main regulating agents [5].

The *kidney* plays a major role in fluid and electrolyte balance. To function adequately, the kidney depends upon its own soundness as well as on the coordination of all the regulating organs. The distal renal tubules in the kidney are important in regulating the body fluid. They selectively retain or reject electrolytes and other substances to maintain normal osmolality and blood volume; sodium is retained and potassium is excreted [2].

The kidneys also play an important part in acid–base regulation. The distal tubule has the ability to form ammonia and exchange hydrogen ion (in form of ammonia) for bicarbonate to maintain the carbonic acid–bicarbonate ratio.

The *lungs* and the *skin* play an important role in fluid balance–the skin in loss of fluid through insensible perspiration and the lungs in loss of fluid by expiration. It has been noted [3] that normal intake of 2500 ml from all sources will deliver a loss of about 1000 ml in breath and perspiration, 1400 ml in urine, and 100 ml in feces.

The *cardiovascular system* maintains fluid balance by regulating the amount and composition of urine. Renal disease, cardiac failure, shock, postoperative stress, and alarm impair this regulating mechanism [5].

The *adrenal glands* influence the retention or excretion of sodium, potassium, and water. These glands secrete aldosterone, a hormone that increases the reabsorption of sodium from the renal tubules in exchange for potassium, thus maintaining normal sodium concentration [5]. Any stress, such as surgery, increases the secretion of aldosterone, thus increasing the reabsorption of sodium bicarbonate. Adrenal hyperactivity also increases the secretions of the hormone and causes excess sodium retention. Excess loss of sodium occurs with adrenal insufficiency.

The *pituitary gland* is another important organ in the control of fluid and electrolyte balance. The posterior lobe of the pituitary releases antidiuretic hormone (ADH). This hormone inhibits diuresis by increasing water reabsorption in the distal tubule. "The release of ADH is influenced by the 'osmostat,' an auxiliary control located in the plexus of the internal carotid artery" [7]. Increased concentration of sodium in the extracellular fluid alerts the osmostat to signal the pituitary to release ADH. This hormone increases the reabsorption of water to dilute the sodium to the normal level of concentration. Increased body fluid osmolality, decreased body fluid volume, stress, and shock are conditions which increase ADH secretions. Increased body fluid volume, decreased osmolality, and alcohol inhibit ADH secretions.

The *pulmonary system* regulates acid–base balance by controlling the concentration of carbonic acid through exhalation or retention of carbon dioxide.

Electrolytes of Biological Fluids

Potassium

Potassium is one of the most important electrolytes in the body. An excess or deficiency of potassium can cause serious impairment of body function and even result in death.

It is the main electrolyte in the intracellular compartment, which houses over 98 percent of the body's total potassium. The healthy cell requires a high potassium concentration for cellular activity. When the cell dies, there is an exchange of potassium into the extracellular fluid with a transfer of sodium into the cell. This process also occurs to some degree when cellular metabolism is impaired, as in catabolism (breaking down) of cells from a crushing injury.

Plasma concentration of potassium is 4.0 to 5.5 mEq per liter. In the cell, the normal concentration is 115 to 150 mEq per liter of fluid. Variations from either of these levels can produce critical effects. High serum concentrations have an adverse effect on the heart muscle. At 7 mEq per liter an elevation of T waves in the electrocardiogram may be detected. With an extracellular level of 8 to 10 mEq per liter, arrhythmia and heart block may occur [1]. *Hyperkalemia* is the term which expresses serum potassium concentration above normal; *hypokalemia*, serum potassium below normal.

HYPOKALEMIA. Hypokalemia (serum potassium level below 4 mEq per liter) may result when any one of the following conditions occurs: (1) total body potassium is below normal, (2) concentration of potassium in cells is below normal, or (3) concentration of potassium in serum is below normal [4].

These conditions are often caused by variations in the intake or output of potassium. A decreased intake of potassium from prolonged fluid therapy (lacking potassium replacement) may result in hypokalemia. It may also occur during a "starvation diet," as the kidneys do not normally conserve potassium. An increased loss of potassium usually results from polyuria, vomiting, gastric suction (prolonged), diarrhea, and steroid therapy [4].

On the other hand, these conditions of potassium deficiency may be unrelated to intake and output. They can be caused by a sudden shift of potassium from extracellular fluid to intracellular fluid, such as that occurring from (1) anabolism (building up of cells), (2) healing processes, or (3) the use of insulin and glucose in the treatment of diabetic acidosis [4]. The shifts resulting from anabolism and healing processes are not usually of severe consequence unless accompanied by intervening factors. In the treatment of diabetic acidosis, the potassium shift may occur suddenly with grave consequences. When cells are anabolized, potassium shifts into the cells. During the use of glucose in the treatment of diabetic acidosis, the glucose in the cells is quickly metabolized into glycogen for storage, causing a sudden shift of potassium from the extracellular fluid to the intracellular fluid [4]. This process results in hypokalemia.

The signs and symptoms of hypokalemia are malaise, skeletal and smooth muscle atony, apathy, muscular cramps, and postural hypotension. Treatment consists of administration of potassium orally or parenterally.

HYPERKALEMIA. Hyperkalemia may result from renal failure with potassium retention or from excessive or rapid administration of potassium in fluid therapy. It may also occur in conditions unrelated to retention or excessive intake. A sudden shift of potassium from intracellular to extracellular fluid results when catabolism of cells takes place, as in a crushing injury; potassium shifts from cells to plasma.

The signs and symptoms of hyperkalemia are similar to those of hypokalemia. In addition to those signs already listed, the patient may experience tingling or numbness in the extremities, and the heart rate may be slow. A serum potassium level above 5.5 mEq per liter confirms the diagnosis.

Treatment consists of stopping the potassium intake. Dialysis may be necessary for a long-term renal problem. If the cause is a shift of potassium from cells to plasma, glucose and insulin therapy may be used.

Sodium

Sodium is the main electrolyte in the extracellular fluid; its normal concentration is 135 to 145 mEq per liter of plasma. The main role of sodium is to control the distribution of water throughout the body and to maintain a normal fluid balance. Alterations in sodium concentration markedly influence the fluid volume: the loss of sodium is accompanied by loss of water and dehydration; the gain of sodium, by retention of fluid.

The body, by regulating the urinary output, normally maintains a constant fluid volume and isotonicity of the plasma. The urinary output is controlled by ADH, secreted by the pituitary gland. If a hypotonic concentration results from a low sodium concentration, the fluid is drawn from the plasma into the cells. Nature attempts to correct this process; the pituitary inhibits ADH and diuresis results, with a loss of extracellular fluid. This loss of fluid increases sodium concentration to a normal level.

If a hypertonic concentration results from increased concentration of extracellular sodium, fluid is drawn from the cells. Again nature reacts, and the pituitary is stimulated to secrete ADH. This causes a retention of fluid diluting sodium to normal concentration.

Therefore increased sodium concentration stimulates the production of ADH, with retention of water thus diluting sodium to the normal level; a decrease in sodium concentration inhibits the production of ADH, resulting in a loss of water which raises the concentration of sodium to the normal level.

In the kidneys sodium is reabsorbed in exchange for potassium. Therefore with an increase in sodium there is loss of potassium; with a loss of sodium there is an increase in potassium.

A *sodium deficit* may be present when plasma sodium falls below 135 mEq per liter. It is caused by (1) excessive sweating with large intake of water by mouth (salt is lost and fluid increased, thus reducing sodium concentration), (2) excessive infusion of nonelectrolyte fluids, (3) gastrointestinal suction plus water by mouth, and (4) adrenal insufficiency, which causes large loss of electrolytes.

The symptoms of a sodium deficit are apprehension, abdominal cramps, diarrhea, and convulsions.

Dehydration results from loss of sodium and leads to peripheral circulatory failure. When sodium and water are lost from the plasma, the body attempts to replace them by a transfer of sodium and water from the interstitial fluid. Eventually the water will be drawn from the cells and circulation will fail; plasma volume will not be sustained [1].

Sodium excess may be present when the plasma sodium rises above 147 mEq per liter. Its causes are (1) excessive infusions of saline, (2) diarrhea, (3) insufficient water intake, (4) diabetes mellitus, and (5) tracheobronchitis (excess loss of water from lungs because of rapid breathing).

The symptoms of sodium excess are dry sticky mucous membranes, oliguria, excitement, and convulsions.

Calcium

Calcium is an electrolyte constituent of the plasma which is present in a concentration of about 5 mEq per liter. Calcium serves several purposes. It plays an important role in formation and function of bones and teeth. As ionized calcium, it is involved in (1) normal clotting of the blood and (2) regulation of neuromuscular irritability.

The parathyroid glands, located within the thyroid gland, control calcium metabolism. The parathyroid hormone, acting on the kidneys and bones, regulates the concentration of ionized calcium in the extracellular fluid. Impairment of this regulatory mechanism alters the calcium concentration. Hyperparathyroidism causes an elevation in the serum calcium level and a decrease in the serum phosphate level.

Calcium deficit may occur in patients with diarrhea or with problems in gastrointestinal absorption, in extensive infections of the subcutaneous tissue, and in burns [7]. This deficiency can result in muscle tremors and cramps, in excessive irritability, and even in convulsions.

Calcium ionization is influenced by pH; it is decreased in alkalosis and increased in acidosis. With no loss of calcium a patient in alkalosis may develop symptoms of calcium deficit: muscle cramps, tetany, and convulsions. This is due to the decreased ionization of calcium caused by the elevated pH.

A patient in acidosis may have a calcium deficit with no symptoms because the acid pH has caused an increased ionization of available calcium. Symptoms of calcium deficit may appear if acidosis is converted to alkalosis.

Other Electrolytes

Magnesium's primary role is in enzyme activity, contributing to the metabolism of both carbohydrates and proteins. Its serum concentration is 1.7 to 2.3 mEq per liter. A deficit in magnesium is not common but may occur from impaired gastrointestinal absorption.

Chloride, the chief anion of the extracellular fluid, has a plasma concentration of 100 to 106 mEq per liter. A deficiency of chloride leads to a deficiency of potassium and vice versa. There is also a loss of chloride with a loss of sodium, but because this loss can be compensated for by an increase in bicarbonate, the proportion will differ [2].

Phosphate is the chief anion of the intracellular fluid; its normal level in plasma is 1.7 to 2.3 mEq per liter.

References

1. Abbott Laboratories. *Fluid and Electrolytes.* North Chicago, Ill., 1960. Pp. 6–26.
2. Baxter Laboratories. *Fundamentals of Body Water and Electrolytes.* Morton Grove, Ill., 1967. Pp. 5, 35.
3. Burgess, R. E. Fluids and electrolytes. *American Journal of Nursing* 65:90–95, 1965.
4. Crowell, C. E., and Staff of Educational Design, Inc., N.Y. Potassium imbalance. *American Journal of Nursing* 67:343, 1967.
5. McGaw Laboratories. *Guide to Parenteral Fluid Therapy.* Glendale, Calif., 1963. Pp. 7–13.
6. Mead Johnson & Company. *Fluid Therapy.* Parenteral Division, Evansville, Ind., 1957–1959. Pp. 107–113.
7. Metheny, N. M., and Snively, W. D., Jr. *Nurses' Handbook of Fluid Balance.* Philadelphia: Lippincott, 1967. Pp. 27, 30, 107, 212–213.

11. Rationale of Fluid and Electrolyte Therapy

Objectives of Parenteral Therapy

Parenteral therapy has three main objectives: (1) to maintain daily requirements, (2) to restore previous losses, and (3) to replace present losses.

Maintenance Therapy

Maintenance therapy consists of provision of all the nutrient needs of the patient: water, electrolytes, dextrose, vitamins, and protein. Of these needs, water has the priority. The body may survive for a prolonged period without vitamins, dextrose, and protein, but without water, dehydration and death occur.

Water is needed by the body to replace the insensible loss which occurs with evaporation from the skin and evaporated moisture from the expired air. An average adult loses from 500 to 1000 ml of water per 24 hours through insensible loss [6]. The skin loss varies with the temperature and humidity.

Water must also be provided for kidney function; the amount needed depends upon the amount of waste products to be excreted as well as the concentrating ability of the kidneys [6]. Protein and salt increase the need for water.

Until 1925 parenteral fluids consisted solely of isotonic saline solutions [6]. Because water is hypotonic and cannot be given intravenously, salt was added to attain isotonicity. If given intravenously, distilled water causes hemolysis; the distilled water is drawn into the blood cells owing to the greater solute concentration, causing them to swell and burst. After 1925 glucose began to be used extensively to make water isotonic and to provide calories [6].

An individual's fluid requirements are based on age, height, weight, and amount of body fat. Because fat is water-free, a large amount of body fat contains a relatively low amount of water; as body fat increases, water decreases in inverse proportion to body weight [7]. The normal fluid and electrolyte requirements based on body surface area have been found to be more constant than when expressed in terms of body weight. Many of the essential physiological processes such as heat loss, blood volume, organ size, and respiration have a direct relationship to the body surface area [8]. The fluid and electrolyte requirements are also proportionate to surface area, regardless of the age of the patient [8]. These requirements are based on square meter of body surface area and calculated for a 24-hour period. Nomograms are available for determining surface area (see Figure 29).

Balanced solutions are available for maintenance. An estimate is made of the average requirements of fluid and electrolytes in a healthy person and applied to the patient. The balanced solutions contain electrolytes in proportion to the daily needs of the patient, but not in excess of the body's tolerance, as long as adequate kidney function exists. When a patient's water needs are provided by these maintenance solutions, the daily needs of sodium and potassium are also met. For maintenance, 1500 ml per square meter of body surface is administered over a 24-hour period [8].

Glucose, a necessary nutrient in maintenance therapy, has important functions. As it is converted into glycogen by the liver, it improves hepatic function. By supplying necessary calories for energy, it spares body protein and minimizes the development of ketosis occasioned by the oxidation of fat stores for essential energy in the absence of added glucose.

The basic daily caloric requirement of a 70-kg adult at rest is about 1600 calories. However, the administration of 100 gm of glucose a day is considered sufficient to help prevent ketosis [8]; 100 gm is contained in 2 liters of 5 percent dextrose in water or 1 liter of 10 percent dextrose in water.

Protein is another nutrient important to maintenance therapy. Though a patient may be adequately maintained on glucose, water, vitamins, and electrolytes over a limited time, protein may be required to replace normal protein losses over an extended period of time. It is necessary for cellular repair, healing of wounds, and synthesis of vitamins and some enzymes. The usual daily requirement for a healthy adult is 1 gm of protein per kilogram of body weight [8]. Protein is available as amino acids; taken orally, it is broken down into amino acids before being absorbed into the blood.

Vitamins, though not nutrients in the true sense of the word, are necessary for the utilization of other nutrients. Vitamin C and the various B complex vitamins are the most frequently used in parenteral therapy. As these vitamins are water soluble, they are not retained by the body but lost through urinary excretion. Because of this loss, larger amounts are required parenterally to ensure adequate maintenance than may be required when administered orally. Vitamin B complex vitamins play an important role in the metabolism of carbohydrates and in maintaining gastrointestinal function. As vitamin C promotes wound healing, it is frequently used for the surgical patient.

Vitamins A and D are fat-soluble vitamins, better retained by the body and not generally required by the patient on maintenance therapy.

Restoration of Previous Losses

Restoration of previous losses is essential when past maintenance has not been met—when the output has exceeded the intake. Severe dehydration may occur from failure to replace these losses. Therapy consists of replacing losses from previous deficits in addition to providing fluid and electrolytes for daily maintenance. The status of the kidneys must be considered before electrolyte replacement and maintenance can be initiated; urinary suppression may result from decreased fluid volume or renal impairment. A hydrating solution such as 5 percent dextrose in 0.2 percent (34.2 mEq) sodium chloride is administered. Urinary flow will be restored if the retention is functional. The patient must be rehydrated rapidly to establish an adequate urinary output. Only after kidney function is proved adequate can large electrolyte losses be replaced. Potassium chloride must be used with considerable caution and is considered potentially dangerous if administered when renal function is impaired. A buildup of potassium, owing to the kidney's inability to excrete salts, can prove hazardous; arrhythmia and heart block can result from the effect of excess potassium on the heart muscle.

Replacement of Present Losses

Replacement of present losses of fluid and electrolytes is as necessary as daily maintenance and replacement of previous losses. The importance of accurate measurement of all intake and output cannot be underestimated as a means of calculating fluid loss. Fluid loss may also be estimated by determining loss of body weight; 1 liter of body water equals 1 kg, or 2.2 pounds, of body weight. An osmolality determination may indicate the water needs of the body. If necessary a corrective blood urea nitrogen determination may be done in conjunction with the osmolality.

The type of replacement is dependent upon the type of fluid being lost. A choice of appropriate replacement solutions is available. Excessive loss of gastric fluid must be replaced by solutions resembling the fluid lost, such as gastric replacement solutions. Excessive loss of intestinal fluid must be replaced by an intestinal replacement fluid.

Examples of conditions that may result from current losses are alkalosis and acidosis (see Table 7, Chapter 10). *Alkalosis* may occur from an excessive loss of gastric fluid, either by vomiting or suction. Gastric

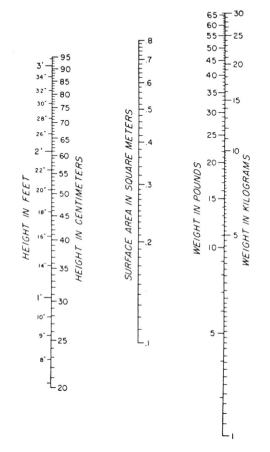

a

Fig. 29. Body surface area nomograms for (a) infants and young children, and (b) older children and adults. To determine the surface area of the patient draw a straight line between the point representing his height on the left vertical scale to the point representing his weight on the right vertical scale. The point at which this line intersects the middle vertical scale represents the patient's body surface area in square meters. (From Talbot, N. B., Sobel, E. H., McArthur, J. W. and Crawford, J. D. *Functional Endocrinology from Birth Through Adolescence.* Cambridge, Mass.: Harvard University Press, © 1952 by the President and Fellows of Harvard College.)

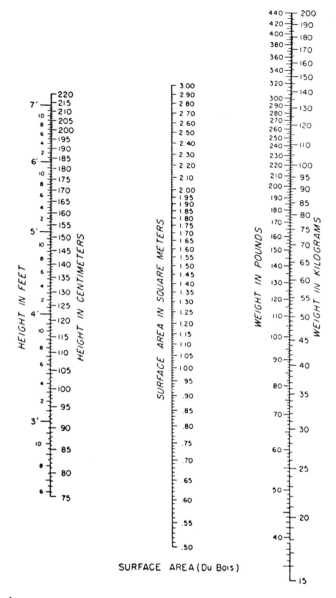

HEIGHT IN FEET

HEIGHT IN CENTIMETERS

SURFACE AREA IN SQUARE METERS

WEIGHT IN POUNDS

WEIGHT IN KILOGRAMS

SURFACE AREA (Du Bois)

b

juices, with a pH of 1 to 3, are the most acid of the body secretions [8]. Excess loss of chloride causes an increase in the bicarbonate ions; total anions must always equal total cations. The patient's respiration becomes slow and shallow; the body attempts to correct alkalosis by retaining carbon dioxide. Because of the body's inability to ionize calcium in the presence of a high pH, muscular hyperactivity and tetany occur. The patient may become irritable, uncooperative, and disoriented.

Prompt recognition of symptoms is important for early treatment or for altering current treatment. Most alkalotic states secondary to gastric suction are corrected by sodium chloride and potassium chloride solutions. Special gastric replacement solutions are available. They contain ammonium chloride, which replaces the chloride without increasing the sodium. The hydrogen ions, liberated by urea in the conversion of ammonium chloride, correct alkalosis. These solutions, invaluable in certain conditions, can be potentially dangerous if given to patients with impaired liver or kidney function. Ammonia, metabolized by the liver, is converted into urea and hydrogen ion. If the liver fails to convert the ammonia to urea, ammonia retention and toxicity will result. Symptoms of ammonia toxicity include pallor, sweating, tetany, and coma, and death may ensue.

Acidosis may occur when the excessive fluid loss is alkaline, as are intestinal secretions, bile, and pancreatic juices. Intestinal secretions contain large amounts of bicarbonate ions; with the loss of these ions, there is an increase in the chloride ions—and acidosis occurs. Symptoms include shortness of breath with rapid breathing (respiratory compensation to reduce carbon dioxide and correct acidosis). Weakness and coma occur. In order to replace lost alkaline secretions and correct acidosis, specific parenteral solutions containing base salts, such as sodium lactate or sodium bicarbonate, are employed.

Electrolyte and Fluid Disturbances

Fluid and electrolyte imbalances occurring in the ill patient are serious complications which can threaten life. The correction of these imbalances is of vital concern to the welfare of the patient. A discussion follows of a few of the most common clinical cases in which fluid disturbances contribute to serious complications, with emphasis on the physiological changes accompanying these imbalances and the parenteral therapy necessary to correct them.

Parenteral Therapy for the Surgical Patient

A knowledge of the endocrine response to stress assists the nurse in a better understanding of imbalances and problems associated with them. It also contributes to safe and successful parenteral therapy: the nurse knows what to expect, is alert to the possible dangers of imbalances, and recognizes early symptoms.

Endocrine Response to Stress

The endocrine homeostatic controls are affected by stress. At times stress from preoperative apprehension triggers an undesirable endocrine response, making it necessary to postpone an operation. Apprehension, pain, and duration and severity of trauma give rise to surgical stress and cause an increased endocrine response during the first 2 to 5 days following surgery. On the whole the stress reaction is normal and is nature's way of protecting the body from hypotension resulting from trauma and shock. Correction is often unnecessary and may, in fact, be harmful.

The two major endocrine homeostatic controls affected by stress are the pituitary gland and the adrenal gland (see Table 8). The posterior pituitary controls quantitative secretions of ADH (antidiuretic hormone); the anterior pituitary controls secretions of ACTH (adrenocorticotropic hormone). ACTH stimulates the adrenal gland to increase (1) mineralocorticoid secretions (aldosterone) and (2) glucocorticoid secretions (hydrocortisone) [8]. The adrenal medulla secretes vasopressors (epinephrine and norepinephrine) to help maintain the blood pressure.

A direct physiological effect is produced when stress increases the secretions of these various hormones. When the posterior pituitary increases ADH secretions, antidiuresis is effected, thus helping maintain blood volume. When the anterior pituitary increases ACTH secretions, the adrenal gland is stimulated to increase the secretions of aldosterone and hydrocortisone. These two adrenal hormones help maintain blood volume by (1) causing the retention of sodium ions and chloride anions, thereby causing water retention, and (2) promoting the excretion of potassium (loss of cellular potassium ions causes loss of cellular water into extracellular space, where it is retained by ADH to maintain blood volume) [8].

Hydrocortisone also promotes the catabolism of protein to provide necessary amino acids for healing and stimulates the conversion of protein and fat to glucose for metabolism during the stress period. This metabolic activity may elevate the blood sugar level, a finding which may mistakenly suggest diabetes mellitus. A drop in the eosinophil count indicates increased adrenal activity [8].

Fluid Therapy

Accurate records of intake and output measurements are important for assessing the proper fluid requirements and preventing serious fluid im-

Table 8. Endocrine Response to Stress

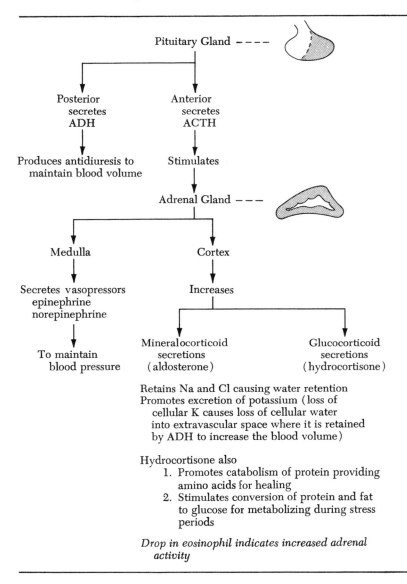

Retains Na and Cl causing water retention
Promotes excretion of potassium (loss of
    cellular K causes loss of cellular water
    into extravascular space where it is retained
    by ADH to increase the blood volume)

Hydrocortisone also
    1. Promotes catabolism of protein providing
       amino acids for healing
    2. Stimulates conversion of protein and fat
       to glucose for metabolizing during stress
       periods

*Drop in eosinophil indicates increased adrenal
activity*

balances during the early postoperative period. The daily requirement of 1500 to 2000 ml varies with the patient's needs. Caution must be taken not to overhydrate the patient—the intake should be adequate but should not exceed the fluid losses.

We have seen how the adrenocortical secretions, increased by trauma and stress of surgery, cause some water and sodium retention. This retention may be severe enough to give a false picture of oliguria. Excessive quantities of nonelectrolyte solutions, such as 5 percent dextrose in water, administered at a time when antidiuresis is occurring may cause a serious fluid imbalance, hyponatremia.

Hyponatremia is a condition in which the serum sodium concentration is less than normal. Water-yielding solutions, infused in excess of the body's tolerance, expand the extracellular compartment, lowering the electrolyte concentration. By the process of osmosis water invades the cells, with a resulting excess accumulation of intracellular fluid. Usually there is no edema, as edema is the result of an excess accumulation of fluid in the extracellular compartment [3].

Symptoms of water excess include confusion, hallucinations, delirium, weight gain, hyperventilation, muscular weakness, twitching, and convulsions. If these occur during the early postoperative stages, the nurse should suspect water excess. This is of particular concern in the young and the aged. Serious consequences, even death, can result.

Restricting the fluid intake may correct mild water excess, but for the more severe cases the administration of high concentrations of sodium chloride may be indicated. The electrolyte concentration of the plasma, increased by the concentrated saline, causes an increase in the osmotic pressure, drawing fluid from the cells for excretion by the kidneys.

Often parenteral therapy during the stress period consists of administering conservative amounts of 5 percent dextrose in water. As some sodium retention results from the endocrine response to stress, caution is taken to avoid administration of excessive quantities of saline at a time when there is an interference in the elimination of salt. During this early period, the physician frequently gives 5 percent dextrose in quarter- or half-strength saline to avoid sodium excess.

Hypernatremia is a condition in which the serum sodium concentration is higher than normal. This excess can cause (1) expanded extracellular fluid volume or edema and (2) possible disruption of cellular function (in potassium-depleted patients the sodium may replace the intracellular potassium).

Symptoms of sodium excess include flushed skin, elevation in temperature, dry sticky mucous membranes, thirst, and a decrease or absence of urinary output. Treatment consists of reducing the intake of salt and water and promoting diuresis to eliminate the excess of salt and water from the plasma.

Nutrients

CARBOHYDRATES. Carbohydrates provide an indispensable source of calories for the postoperative patient unable to receive oral sustenance. When carbohydrates are inadequate, the body will utilize its own fat to supply calories; the by-products are ketone bodies. These acid bodies neutralize bicarbonate and produce metabolic acidosis. The only by-products excreted in the utilization of carbohydrates are water and carbon dioxide.

Carbohydrates, by providing calories for essential energy, also reduce catabolism of protein. During the stress response the renal excretion of nitrogen (from the catabolism of protein) exceeds the intake. By reducing the protein breakdown, glucose helps prevent a negative nitrogen balance. The administration of as little as 100 gm of carbohydrate (2 liters of 5 percent dextrose or 1 liter of 10 percent dextrose) daily can reduce catabolism by as much as one-half [8].

Carbohydrates do not provide adequate calories for the patient receiving prolonged therapy. One liter of 5 percent dextrose in water provides 170 calories. Many liters, a volume too great for most patients to tolerate, would be required to provide a patient with 1600 calories. Greater concentrations of glucose, 20 percent and 50 percent, may be administered to provide calories for patients unable to tolerate large volumes of fluid (e.g., patients with renal insufficiency). The concentrated solutions must be administered slowly for utilization of the glucose to take place. Rapid administration results in diuresis; the concentrated glucose acts as a diuretic, drawing interstitial fluid into the plasma for excretion by the kidneys. Glucose may be administered to normal individuals at a maximum speed of about 0.5 gm per kilogram per hour without producing glycosuria [8].

ALCOHOL. Alcohol solutions may be administered to the postoperative patient for nutritional and physiological benefits. Nutritionally the alcohol supplements calories provided by the glucose, 1 gm of ethyl alcohol yielding 6 to 8 calories [8]. Because alcohol is quickly and completely metabolized, it provides calories for essential energy, sparing fat and protein. Metabolized in preference to glucose, alcohol allows the infused glucose to be stored as glycogen.

Physiologically, alcohol produces a sedative effect, reducing pain; 200 to 300 ml of a 5 percent solution per hour produces sedation without intoxication in the average adult [8]. Alcohol also inhibits the secretion of ADH, promoting water excretion.

It is well to bear in mind that the solutions containing alcohol, particularly hypertonic solutions, can cause phlebitis. These solutions, if allowed to infiltrate, may cause tissue necrosis. The needle should be carefully inserted within the vein and inspected frequently to detect any infiltration.

AMINO ACIDS. Amino acids are beneficial to the surgical patient after the catabolic state has passed. They are usually used in conjunction with alcohol and glucose; alcohol and glucose provide calories for metabolism, while the protein is made available for tissue repairs.

Before amino acids are administered, the patient should be questioned regarding allergies, and the infusion should be started slowly and cautiously. Sometimes rapid infusion causes nausea, flushed face, and a feeling of warmth. Reducing the speed should alleviate these symptoms.

Commercial solutions containing alcohol, dextrose, and amino acids are available in varying strengths and caloric values. No solutions should be used which are cloudy or contain precipitate [2]. These solutions, once opened, must be used immediately. Storing a partially used bottle in the refrigerator for later use may provide a culture medium for the growth of bacteria. Use of such contaminated solutions has been known to lead to death.

POTASSIUM. Once the stress period is past, adrenal activity decreases and diuresis begins. At this time, usually after the second to the fifth postoperative day, potassium is given daily to prevent a deficit; potassium is not conserved by the body but lost in the urine. Electrolyte maintenance fluids may be used or potassium may be added to parenteral solutions; usually 40 mEq per liter daily is sufficient to replace normal loss. Potassium should be well diluted and the rate should not exceed 20 to 30 mEq per hour. A slower rate of administration is preferred for older patients. Usually 40 mEq is infused over an 8-hour period. The solution containing potassium should be conspicuously labeled and must never be used when positive pressure is indicated —rapid infusion may result in cardiac arrest.

Potassium is irritating to the vein and may cause a great deal of pain, especially if infused into a vein where a previous venipuncture has been performed. Slowing the rate may decrease the pain.

VITAMINS. Vitamins B complex and C are usually added to parenteral solutions if, after 2 or 3 days, the patient is unable to take fluids orally. Vitamin C is important in promoting healing in the surgical patient and vitamin B complex is helpful in aiding in carbohydrate metabolism.

Parenteral Therapy for the Burned Patient
The body mechanisms that regulate fluid and electrolyte balance are altered when severe burns occur. The changes that take place during

the first 48 hours must be recognized and dealt with. Fluid and electrolyte therapy sufficient to replace losses and maintain a status quo increase the patient's chances of survival. Awareness of these physiological changes contributes to intelligent therapy and aids in the patient's recovery.

Fluid and Electrolyte Changes

INTRAVASCULAR TO INTERSTITIAL FLUID SHIFT. The shift from intravascular to interstitial fluid, followed by shock, begins immediately following the burn. This fluid shift represents the water, electrolyte, and protein that are lost through the damaged capillaries, resulting in edema and a marked reduction in plasma volume. The severity of the shift depends upon the degree and extent of the burn. In an adult with a 50 percent burn, the edema may exceed the total plasma volume of the patient. Parenteral fluids must be given immediately to replace the fluid loss and combat shock.

DEHYDRATION. In the early phases of fluid shift from plasma to tissues, water and electrolyte are lost in larger quantities than is the protein (protein, because of its larger molecular size, does not readily pass through the capillary walls). The osmotic pressure, increased by the higher protein concentration of the plasma, draws fluid from the undamaged tissues and generalized tissue dehydration occurs.

A much more significant fluid loss occurs as (1) exudate from the burned area, (2) water in the form of vapor at the burned area, and (3) blood lost through the damaged capillaries. These losses further contribute to dehydration and hypovolemia.

DECREASED URINARY OUTPUT. Decreased urinary output occurs when the lowered blood volume causes a diminished renal blood flow. Increased endocrine secretions further contribute to the decrease in urinary output: adrenal cortical secretions cause sodium and water absorption; ADH causes increased water reabsorption by the kidneys.

In deep burns free hemoglobin, released by destruction of red cells, may produce renal damage.

POTASSIUM EXCESS. When excessive amounts of potassium build up in the extracellular fluid, potassium excess occurs: cell destruction releases potassium and decreased renal flow obstructs normal excretion of potassium. Plasma potassium concentrations may rise to a dangerously high level. Because of the tendency to plasma potassium excess and the uncertainty of the extent of renal impairment in the burned patient, administration of potassium is contraindicated.

SODIUM DEFICIT. When plasma is lost in edema and exudate, sodium, the chief electrolyte of the extracellular fluid, is lost with the plasma, and sodium deficit occurs. Further loss may occur as sodium moves into the cells to replace lost potassium.

METABOLIC ACIDOSIS. Acidosis results from a loss of bicarbonate ions accompanying the loss of sodium ions as well as from altered aerobic metabolized tissue destruction.

Fluid Therapy

When moderate or severe burns occur, immediate fluid therapy is necessary to combat hypovolemic shock and prevent renal depression. An indwelling venous catheter is inserted to ensure parenteral therapy during this critical period. As the measurement of venous pressure is an important guide against overinfusion, a second catheter may be inserted for venous pressure determination.

In small burns that require parenteral therapy, solutions such as isotonic saline, Ringer's solution, or 5 percent dextrose in water or saline may be sufficient, but in severe burns a colloid is usually employed. Colloids, because of their tendency to hold fluids in the vascular compartment, are used to maintain blood volume and combat shock. Plasma, albumin, and dextran are the most common of the colloidal solutions used. Whole blood is added when indicated.

Fluid therapy consists in supplying (1) the normal daily fluid requirements and (2) additional amounts of fluid for replacement of burn losses. The amount of fluid necessary to replace burn losses is calculated in relation to the extent and severity of the burn. The "rule of nines" is the most common used to estimate the burned area. The surface area of the body is divided into areas of 9 percent or its multiples (see Table 9).

During the first 24 hours, a great deal more fluid is required to replace the marked reduction in plasma volume caused by the rapid shift of intravascular to interstitial fluid. This fluid replacement increases the total body water content, secondary to the burn edema, and results in a weight gain. This gain may be as much as 10 percent of the normal body weight [4].

Caution must be taken to avoid overzealous fluid therapy. Later, when fluid shifts back into the plasma, excess parenteral fluid could cause overburdened circulation and pulmonary edema. If smoke and heat damage to the lungs have impaired their capacity to function, the threat of pulmonary edema is further increased. Only enough fluid to maintain blood volume and urinary output is administered.

The shift from interstitial fluid to plasma begins on the second to third day after the burn and accounts for the large reduction in paren-

147

Table 9. "Rule of Nines" for Estimating Burned Body Area in Adults

Part of Body	Percentage of Body
Head and neck	9
Anterior trunk	18
Each arm	9
Posterior trunk	18
Genitalia	1
Each leg	18

teral fluids. An increase in the urinary output should alert the nurse to the edema mobilization taking place and the need to decrease fluid therapy.

Massachusetts General Hospital's Principles of Fluid Replacement
Various formulas based on fluid needs for the first 24 hours have been developed to serve as a guide to fluid therapy. Such estimates are helpful in reducing the danger of overhydration or underhydration that exists during the critical period.

In the years following the fire in 1942 at the Coconut Grove (a Boston nightclub), the Massachusetts General Hospital made great strides in introducing theory and principles beneficial to burn therapy. Immediately after a burn, edema begins to develop in the involved area. The description of the nature of this fluid and protein loss into the interstitial compartment was accomplished to a great extent by Oliver Cope.

The Massachusetts General Hospital and the Shriners Burns Institute employ their own formula and principles of fluid replacement based upon the belief that "the normal fluid environment of the tissues is the optimal one and there is no good evidence that healing or survival is improved by any variations" [4]. Consequently the fluid program is based upon an attempt to replace fluid loss with similar fluid.

In severe burns a large amount of water is lost through the damaged skin and this must be replaced. The fluid lost in edema contains about 4.5 gm of protein per 100 ml, which is less protein than the 6 to 7 gm normally present in plasma [4]. The concentration of electrolytes generally remains about the same. The blood bank plasma that is available usually has a protein content slightly higher (between 4.5 and 5 gm per 100 ml) than the burn edema fluid and, in some cases, a sodium content somewhat lower [4]. Therefore plasma is used either alone or with small amounts of saline to make an isotonic solution with a protein content of about 4.5 gm per 100 ml.

Because of the potential risk of serum hepatitis to the patient infused with pooled plasma, the amount of available plasma is limited; only single-donor plasma is used. Other colloids such as albumin and dextran may be substituted. Frequently normal human albumin prepared in a 5 percent solution is used. However, if other protein fractions, such as gamma globulin, are indicated they must be given as a supplement.

Whole blood is used cautiously during the first 48 hours in the belief that only proved blood losses should be replaced. A decreased red blood cell volume usually is not apparent until 48 hours after the burn when the red cells damaged by the heat become increasingly more fragile and hemolyze. Slow administration of blood during the critical period may delay the urgent need for the more vitally needed fluid.

Fluid Requirements Based on Massachusetts General Hospital's Replacement Principles
The following schedule of fluid replacement is followed at Massachusetts General Hospital in accord with the principles [4] just elucidated:

FIRST 24 HOURS
Normal fluid requirements
2000 ml of nonelectrolyte solution (5 percent dextrose in water)
Replacement of burn loss
Plasma with approximately 5 gm protein per 100 ml, amount determined by degree of burn (125 ml plasma per percentage of body area burned)
Saline amount determined by degree of burn (15 ml saline per percentage of body area burned)
One-half of the first 24-hour total amount infused in first 8 hours and the rest in 16 remaining hours

SECOND 24 HOURS
Normal fluid requirements
2000 ml of 5 percent dextrose in water
Replacement of burn loss
One-half of the previous 24-hour requirement

Because it is believed that each patient should be treated on an individual basis, the formula gives only a rough approximation of amount of fluid that should be infused and is used only while the critical period exists. Physicians still vary in their opinions on replacement fluid. Some prefer to treat the patient clinically, relying on lactated Ringer's injection. At Massachusetts General Hospital the Brooke formula is being used frequently, with lactated Ringer's injection replacing the nonelectrolyte fluid.

Brooke Army Hospital Formula
The Brooke Army Hospital formula [5] is one of the most widely used.

Normal fluid requirements

2000 ml of nonelectrolyte solution (5 percent dextrose in water)

Replacement of burn loss

Colloid and electrolyte solution in ratio of 1 to 3 with amount of replacement fluid equaling 2 ml × kg body weight × percentage of body area burned

One-half of this total amount infused in first 8 hours and the rest in 16 remaining hours

SECOND 24 HOURS

Normal fluid requirements

2000 ml of 5 percent dextrose in water

Replacement of burn loss

One-half the amount of colloid and electrolyte solution of the first 24 hours

The Evans formula is probably considered one of the best known. It is much the same as the Brooke formula with the exception that equal proportions of colloid and electrolyte solutions are used. This ratio was originally based on the belief that the fluid lost in edema contained 50 percent plasma.

Parenteral Therapy after Critical Phase

After 48 hours, when the edema remobilization period is reached, colloids are stopped and parenteral fluids are curtailed or discontinued to prevent expanded fluid volume with pulmonary edema. The amount of fluid then administered parenterally depends upon the patient's ability to take fluid orally.

During the convalescent phase care is taken to provide necessary electrolytes to prevent or correct a deficit of sodium, potassium, and calcium.

Fluid Therapy for the Burned Child

Fluid replacement for the burned child is essentially the same as for the adult with the exception of the calculation of the percentage of surface area involved. See Table 10 for estimations of these percentages.

The tentative plan of fluid therapy for the burned child is 90 ml of plasma and 10 ml of saline for each percentage of burned area times the body surface area in square meters [4]. Ringer's Lactate is being used more frequently with colloid being withheld for the first 48 hours depending on the patient's condition. Greater accuracy in fluid administration is necessary than for the adult, as the child is more sensitive to minor errors, developing pulmonary edema and shock more quickly.

Table 10. Estimating Burned Area in Children

Part of Body	Percentage of Body	
	0–4 yr	4–10 yr
Head	16	12
Neck	2	2
Trunk (whole)	32	32
Each arm	8	9
Each leg	16	18

Source: Abbott Laboratories [1], based on work of Charles L. Fox, Jr., M.D., Columbia University College of Physicians and Surgeons, New York.

Diabetic Acidosis

Diabetic acidosis is an endocrine disorder causing complex fluid and electrolyte disturbances. It occurs when a lack of insulin prevents the metabolism of glucose, and essential calories are provided instead by the catabolism of fat and protein. Acidosis results from the accumulation of acid by-products. Knowledge of the physiological changes in diabetic acidosis aids the nurse in early detection of imbalances and in an understanding of the treatment involved.

Physiological Changes

Lack of insulin prevents cellular metabolism of glucose and its conversion into glycogen. Glucose accumulates in the bloodstream (*hyperglycemia*). When the blood sugar rises above 180 mg per 100 ml, glucose spills over into the urine (*glycosuria*). The kidneys require 10 to 20 ml of water to excrete 1 gm of glucose; water excretion increases (*polyuria*).

The body's fat and protein are utilized to provide necessary calories for energy. Ketone bodies, metabolic by-products, reduce plasma bicarbonate, and acidosis occurs.

Fluid and Electrolyte Disturbances

DEHYDRATION. Dehydration results from excessive fluid and electrolyte losses. Cellular fluid deficit occurs when water is drawn from the cells by the hyperosmolality of the blood. Extracellular deficit occurs when (1) glycosuria increases the urinary output, (2) ketone bodies increase the load on the kidneys and the water to excrete them, (3) vomiting causes loss of fluid and electrolytes, (4) oral intake is reduced because of the patient's condition, and (5) hyperventilation is induced by the acidotic state.

DECREASED KIDNEY FUNCTION. Dehydration lowers the blood volume, decreasing renal blood flow, and the kidneys produce less of the ammonia needed to maintain acid–base balance. Severe dehydration may lower the blood volume enough to cause circulatory shock and oliguria.

KETOSIS. Ketosis is the excessive production of ketone bodies in the blood stream. Electrolytes and ketone bodies, retained in high serum concentration, increase the acidosis; the increase in the number of hydrogen ions, from the retention of ketone bodies, may drop the blood pH to as low as 6.9. The bicarbonate anions decrease to compensate for the increase in ketone anions and may drop the bicarbonate level as low as 5 mEq per liter [8].

ELECTROLYTE CHANGES. Cellular potassium deficit occurs when cells, unable to metabolize glucose, break down and release potassium into the serum. Normal or high serum potassium concentration may exist in spite of a body deficit (98 percent of the body's potassium is contained in the cells). Increase in the concentration of serum potassium is the result of the large amounts of potassium released from the cells plus the increased retention of potassium due to impaired kidney function. In severe diabetic acidosis, serious sodium and chloride deficits may occur when these electrolytes are lost through diuresis, vomiting, and gastric dilatation.

Signs and Symptoms of Diabetic Acidosis
The nurse should be familiar with the signs and symptoms that characterize diabetic acidosis. By recognizing impending diabetic acidosis, early treatment may be initiated and complications prevented.

1. *Hyperglycemia* occurs when a lack of insulin prevents glucose metabolism; glucose accumulates in the bloodstream.
2. *Glycosuria* occurs when the accumulation of glucose exceeds the renal tolerance and spills over into the urine.
3. *Polyuria.* Osmotic diuresis occurs when the heavy load of nonmetabolized glucose and the metabolic end products increase the osmolality of the blood, and the increased renal solute load requires more fluid for excretion.
4. *Thirst* is prompted by cellular dehydration due to the osmotic effect produced by hyperglycemia.
5. *Weakness* and *tiredness* come from the inability of the body to utilize glucose and from a potassium deficit.
6. *Flushed face* results from the acid condition.
7. *Rapid deep breathing* is the body's defense against acidosis; expiration of large amounts of carbon dioxide reduces carbonic acid and increases the pH of the blood.
8. *Acetone breath* results from an increased accumulation of acetone bodies.

9. *Nausea* and *vomiting* are caused by distention due to atony of gastric muscles.
10. *Weight loss* accompanies an excess loss of fluid (1 liter of body water equals 2.2 pounds, or 1 kg, body weight) and a lack of glucose metabolism.
11. *Low blood pressure* results from a severe fluid deficit.
12. *Oliguria* follows the decreased renal blood flow that results from a severe deficit in fluid volume.

Parenteral Therapy

Insulin is given to metabolize the excess glucose and combat diabetic acidosis. Since absorption is quickest by the bloodstream, insulin is administered intravenously. When given subcutaneously or intramuscularly, the slower rate of absorption of insulin may be further decreased by peripheral vascular collapse in the presence of shock.

Parenteral fluids are administered to increase the blood volume and restore kidney function. Hypotonic solutions with sodium chloride (usually containing sodium lactate or bicarbonate) are employed. These provide the basic needs for water, sodium, and alkali of the acidotic patient, thus hydrating him and reducing the acidosis. Solutions of glucose may be needed to prevent hypoglycemia and are sometimes used at the onset of treatment. Some physicians feel that the glucose increases the hyperglycemia, causing increased diuresis with further loss of water and electrolytes [8]. For this reason they prefer to wait 4 to 6 hours until the available glucose has been metabolized before administering glucose solutions.

Frequently isotonic solutions of sodium chloride are used to replace sodium and chloride losses and expand the blood volume.

Potassium administration is contraindicated in the early treatment of diabetic acidosis. During the later stages (10 to 24 hours after treatment) the plasma potassium level falls; improved renal function increases potassium excretion and, in anabolic states, as the glucose is converted into glycogen, a sudden shift of potassium from extracellular fluid to intracellular fluid further lowers the plasma potassium level. If the patient is hydrated, potassium should be administered when the plasma potassium concentration falls.

A severe potassium deficit may occur if symptoms are not recognized and early treatment begun. Symptoms include weak grip, irregular pulse, weak picking at the bedclothes, shallow respiration, and abdominal distension.

References
1. Abbott Laboratories. *Fluid and Electrolytes.* North Chicago, Ill., 1960. Pp. 45–46.
2. Adriani, J. Venipuncture. *American Journal of Nursing* 62:66, 1962.

3. Burgess, R. E.   Fluid and electrolytes. *American Journal of Nursing* 65:90, 1965.
4. Burke, J. F., and Constable, J. D.   Systemic changes and replacement therapy in burns. *Journal of Trauma* 5:242–253, 1965.
5. Collentine, G. E., Jr.   How to calculate fluids for burned patients. *American Journal of Nursing* 62:77, 1962.
6. Elman, R.   Fluid balance from the nurse's point of view. *American Journal of Nursing* 49:222, 1949.
7. McGaw Laboratories.   *Guide to Parenteral Fluid Therapy.* Glendale, Calif., 1963. P. 63.
8. Metheny, N. M., and Snively, W. D., Jr.   *Nurses' Handbook of Fluid Balance.* Philadelphia: Lippincott, 1967. Pp. 103, 122, 147–154, 157–169, 177, 218.
9. Talbot, N. B., Sobel, E. H., McArthur, J. W., and Crawford, J. D. *Functional Endocrinology from Birth Through Adolescence.* Cambridge, Mass.: Harvard University Press, 1952.

12. Parenteral Fluids and Related Fluid and Electrolyte Abnormalities

Parenteral Fluids

A knowledge of parenteral fluids is essential if the patient is to be protected from the rapid and critical changes in fluid and electrolyte balance caused by infusions.

Until the 1930s, intravenous fluids consisted of dextrose and saline; little was known regarding electrolyte therapy. Today, with over 200 types of commercially prepared fluids available and with the great increase in their use, fluid and electrolyte disturbances are more common. Intravenous fluids are being taken for granted. It is assumed that the nurse who works daily with infusions is familiar with them; yet bottles of fluid are being hung daily by nurses who know little of the chemical composition and the physical effects of the infusions they administer. With the increase in fluids and in the knowledge concerning them, more rational intravenous therapy must be practiced.

The nurse has a legal and professional responsibility to know the normal amount and the desired and untoward effects of any intravenous infusion she administers. The type of fluid, the amount, and the rate of flow are arrived at only after the physician has carefully assessed the patient's clinical condition. Welt [17] stated, "One of the most important lessons to be learned with regard to the problem of fluid and electrolyte imbalances is that the physician must examine the details of management as carefully as would be the case in the prescription of a drug or any other therapy in clinical medicine." The nurse must follow the orders as carefully as she would in administering a medication, thereby ensuring that the patient receives only the quantity of fluid ordered at the rate of flow prescribed.

Definition of Intravenous Infusion

An infusion is usually regarded as an amount of fluid in excess of 100 ml designated for parenteral infusion, since the volume must be administered over a long period of time.

Intravenous fluids are mistakenly referred to as *intravenous solu-*

tions. The term *solution* is defined in the U.S.P. (United States Pharmacopeia) [15] as "liquid preparations that contain one or more soluble chemical substances usually dissolved in water. They are distinguished from injection, for example, because they are not intended for administration by infusion or injection." They may vary widely in methods of preparation. The U.S.P. refers to parenteral fluids as injections, and methods of preparation must follow standards for injection.

Official Requirements of Intravenous Fluids

Intravenous injections must meet the tests, standards, and all specifications of the U.S.P. applicable to injections. This includes quantitative and qualitative assays of infusions, including tests for pyrogens and sterility.

PARTICULATE MATTER. To date there has been no reliable and objective system for detecting particulate matter in parenteral fluids. The final responsibility falls on the pharmacist and the nurse who administers the fluid. Each container must be carefully examined to detect cracks and the fluid examined for cloudiness or presence of particles. Tests to detect the presence of particulate matter and standards for an acceptable limit of particles are now being established by the U.S.P.

pH. The pH indicates hydrogen ion concentration or free acid activity in solution [11]. All intravenous fluids must meet the pH requirements set forth by the U.S.P. Most of these requirements call for a solution that is slightly acid, usually ranging in pH from 3.5 to 6.2.

Dextrose requires a slightly acid pH to yield a stable solution. Heat sterilization, used for all commercial solutions, contributes to the acidity. The pH is often adjusted by the manufacturer to even lower levels during processing to yield a more stable solution. A few intravenous fluids have a more physiological pH.

It is important to know the pH of the commonly used intravenous fluids since it may affect the stability of an added drug and cause the drug to deteriorate. The acidity of dextrose solutions has been criticized for its corrosive effect on veins (see Chapter 8).

Tonicity

Parenteral fluids are classified according to the tonicity of the fluid in relation to the normal blood plasma. The osmolality of blood plasma is 290 mOsm per liter. Fluid that approximates 290 mOsm per liter is considered isotonic. Intravenous fluids with an osmolality significantly higher than 290 mOsm (+50 mOsm) are considered hypertonic, while those with an osmolality significantly lower than 290 mOsm (−50 mOsm) are hypotonic [6]. Parenteral fluids range largely from approximately one-half isotonic (0.45 percent sodium chloride) to five to ten times isotonic (25 to 50 percent dextrose).

The tonicity of the fluid when infused into the circulation has a direct physical effect on the patient. It affects fluid and electrolyte metabolism and may result in disastrous clinical disturbances. Hypertonic fluids increase the osmotic pressure of the blood plasma, drawing fluid from the cells; excessive infusions of such fluid can cause cellular dehydration. Hypotonic fluids lower the osmotic pressure, causing fluid to invade the cells; when such fluid is infused beyond the patient's tolerance for water, water intoxication results. Isotonic fluids cause increased extracellular fluid volume, which can result in circulatory overload. By knowing the osmolality of the infusion and the physical effect it produces, the nurse is alerted to the potential fluid and electrolyte imbalances.

The choice of veins used for an infusion is affected by the tonicity of the fluid; hyperosmolar fluids must be infused through veins with a large blood volume in order to dilute the fluid and prevent trauma to the vessel.

The tonicity of the fluid affects the rate at which it can be infused; hypertonic dextrose infused rapidly may result in diuresis and dehydration.

Because of the direct and effective role osmolality plays in intravenous therapy, it is helpful for the nurse involved in the administration of intravenous fluids to be able to determine their osmolality. The osmotic pressure is proportional to the total number of particles in the fluid. The milliosmole is the unit that measures the particles or the osmotic pressure. By converting milliequivalents to milliosmoles, an approximate osmolality may be determined. A quick method for approximating the tonicity of intravenous injections follows [16].

FLUIDS CONTAINING UNIVALENT ELECTROLYTES. Each milliequivalent is approximately equal to a milliosmole since univalent electrolytes, when ionized, carry one charge per particle. Normal saline injection (0.9 percent sodium chloride) contains 154 mEq of sodium and 154 mEq of chloride per liter, making a total of 308 mEq per liter, or approximately 308 mOsm per liter.

FLUIDS CONTAINING DIVALENT ELECTROLYTES. Since each particle carries two charges when ionized, the milliequivalents per liter or the number of electrical charges per liter when divided by the charge per ion (two) will give the approximate number of particles or milliosmoles per liter. As an example, when 20 mEq of magnesium sulfate is introduced into a liter of fluid, each particle ionized will carry two charges. By dividing 20 mEq or 20 charges by 2, an approximate 10 particles or

10 mOsm per liter is reached for each component, or 20 mOsm per liter total.

The osmolality of electrolytes in solution may be accurately computed, but involves the use of the atomic weight and the concentration of the given electrolytes in milligrams per liter. The methods for accurately computing the osmolality of an electrolyte in solution and a whole electrolyte in solution follow [5]:

OSMOLALITY OF A GIVEN ELECTROLYTE IN SOLUTION:

$$\text{Formula} = \frac{\text{milligrams of electrolyte/liter}}{(\text{atomic weight}) \ (\text{valence})} = \text{milliosmoles/liter}$$

Example = 39 mg K/liter

$$\frac{39}{39 \times 1} = 1 \text{ mOsm/liter}$$

Example = 40 mg Ca/liter

$$\frac{40}{40 \times 2} = \text{½ mOsm/liter}$$

OSMOLALITY OF A WHOLE ELECTROLYTE IN SOLUTION. The milliosmolar value of the whole electrolyte in solution is equal to the sum of the milliosmolar values of the separate ions. For example, determine the number of milliosmoles in 1 liter of a 0.9 percent sodium chloride (NaCl) solution.

Formula (atomic) weight of NaCl = 58.5 gm (58,500 mg)

1 millimole NaCl = $\frac{1}{1000}$ formula weight = 58.5 mg

Assuming complete dissociation,

1 millimole NaCl = 2 mOsm of total particles *or* each 58.5 mg of the whole electrolyte (NaCl) = 2 mOsm of total particles

To calculate the osmotic activity (expressed as milliosmoles) for 9000 mg (0.9 percent NaCl) use the following proportion:

$$\frac{58.5 \text{ mg (weight of 1 mOsm of whole electrolytes)}}{9000 \text{ mg (weight of whole electrolyte/liter)}} = \frac{2 \text{ mOsm (number of particles from whole electrolyte)}}{X \text{ (mOsm)}}$$

X = 307.7 mOsm

Specific Intravenous Fluids

Dextrose in Water Fluids

Glucose is usually referred to as *dextrose* when it occurs as part of a parenteral solution because it is U.S.P. designation for glucose of requisite purity [14]. Dextrose is available in concentrations of 2½, 5, 10, 20, and 50 percent in water. In order to determine the osmolality or the caloric value of a dextrose solution, it is necessary to know the total number of grams or milligrams per liter. Because 1 ml of water weighs 1 gm, and 1 ml is 1 percent of 100 ml, milliliters, grams, and percentages can be used interchangeably when calculating solution strength [3]. Thus, 5 percent dextrose in water = 5 gm dextrose in 100 ml = 50 gm dextrose in 1 liter.

CALORIES. "It should be noted that hexoses (glucose or dextrose and fructose) do not yield 4 calories per gram as do dietary carbohydrates (e.g., starches) but only 3.75 calories per gram. Thus one liter of a 10% solution yields 375 calories. In addition, U.S.P. standards require the use of monohydrated glucose in glucose solutions, per se, so that only 91 percent is actually glucose, i.e., one liter of 10% glucose solution will yield $0.91 \times 375 = 340$ calories" [18, 19].

TONICITY OF 5 PERCENT DEXTROSE IN WATER. Five percent dextrose in water is considered an isotonic solution because its tonicity approximates that of normal blood plasma, 290 mOsm per liter. Since dextrose is a nonelectrolyte and the total number of particles in solution does not depend upon ionization, the osmolality of dextrose solutions is determined differently than that of electrolyte solutions. One millimole (one formula weight in milligrams) of dextrose represents 1 mOsm (unit of osmotic pressure). One millimole of monohydrated glucose is 198 mg, and 1 liter of 5 percent dextrose in water contains 50,000 mg. Thus,

$$\frac{50,000 \text{ mg}}{198 \text{ mg}} = 252 \text{ mOsm/liter}$$

pH. The U.S.P. requirement for pH of dextrose solutions is 3.5 to 6.0. This broad pH range may at times contribute to an incompatibility in one bottle of dextrose and not in another when an additive is involved (see Chapter 14).

METABOLIC EFFECT OF DEXTROSE [10]

1. Provides calories for essential energy.
2. Since glucose is converted into glycogen by synthesis in the liver, it improves hepatic function.

3. Spares body protein (prevents unnecessary breakdown of protein tissue).
4. Prevents ketosis or excretion of organic acid which frequently occurs when fat is burned by the body without an adequate supply of glucose.
5. When deposited intracellularly in the liver as glycogen, dextrose causes a shift of potassium from the extracellular to the intracellular fluid compartment. This effect is used in the treatment of hyperkalemia by infusing dextrose and insulin.

INDICATIONS FOR USE

1. *Dehydration.* Dextrose 2½ percent in Water and Dextrose 5 percent in Water provide immediate hydration to the dehydrated patient and are often used for hydrating the medical and surgical patient. Five percent dextrose in water is considered isotonic only in the bottle; once infused into the vascular system, the dextrose is rapidly metabolized, leaving the water; "also the glucose itself yields water by its own oxidation, being 0.6 ml. of water per gram of glucose oxidized" [4]. The water decreases the osmotic pressure of the blood plasma and invades the cells, providing immediately available water to dehydrated tissues.

2. *Hypernatremia.* If the patient is not in circulatory difficulty with extracellular expansion, 5 percent dextrose may be administered to decrease the concentration of sodium.

3. *Vehicle for administration of drugs.* Many of the drugs for intravenous use are added to infusions of 5 percent dextrose in water.

4. *Nutrition.* Concentrations of 20 and 50 percent dextrose in conjunction with electrolytes provide long-term nutrition. Insulin is frequently added to prevent overtaxing of the islet tissue of the pancreas.

5. *Hyperkalemia.* Infusions of dextrose in high concentration with insulin cause anabolism (build-up of body cells), which results in a shift of potassium from the extracellular to the intracellular compartment, thereby lowering the serum potassium concentration.

UNDESIRABLE EFFECTS

1. *Hypokalemia.* Since the kidneys do not store potassium, prolonged fluid therapy with electrolyte-free fluids may result in hypokalemia. When cells are anabolized by the metabolism of glucose, a shift of potassium from extracellular to intracellular fluid may occur, resulting in hypokalemia.

2. *Dehydration.* Osmotic diuresis occurs when dextrose is infused at a rate faster than the patient's ability to metabolize it. A heavy load of nonmetabolized glucose increases the osmolality of the blood and acts

as a diuretic; the increased solute load requires more fluid for excretion, 10 to 20 ml of water being required to excrete each gram of dextrose [14].

3. *Hyperinsulinism.* This condition may occur from a rapid infusion of hypertonic carbohydrate solutes. In response to a rise in blood sugar, extra insulin pours from the beta islet cells of the pancreas in its attempt to metabolize the infused carbohydrate. Termination of the infusion may leave excess insulin in the body, causing such symptoms as nervousness, sweating, and weakness due to the severe hypoglycemia that may be induced. Frequently, after infusion of hypertonic dextrose, a small amount of isotonic dextrose is administered to cover the excess insulin [14].

4. *Water intoxication.* This imbalance results from an increase in the volume of the extracellular fluid from water alone. Prolonged infusions of isotonic or hypotonic dextrose in water may cause water intoxication. This condition is compounded by stress, which leads to inappropriate release of antidiuretic hormone and fluid retention. The average adult can metabolize water at a rate of about 35 to 40 ml per kilogram per day and the kidney can safely metabolize only about 2500 to 3000 ml per day in an average patient receiving intravenous therapy [9]. Under stress, the patient's ability to metabolize water is decreased.

ADMINISTRATION. Isotonic dextrose may be administered through a peripheral vein. Hyperosmolar fluids such as 50 percent dextrose in water should be infused into the superior vena cava through a central venous catheter or a subclavian line. Hypertonic dextrose administered through a peripheral vein with small blood volume may traumatize the vein and cause thrombophlebitis; infiltration can result in necrosis of the tissues.

Sodium-free dextrose injections should not be administered by hyperdermoclysis. Dextrose solutions, by attracting body electrolytes in the pooled area of infusions, may cause peripheral circulatory collapse and anuria in sodium-depleted patients.

Electrolyte-free dextrose injections should not be used in conjunction with blood infusions. Dextrose mixed with blood causes hemolysis of the red cells.

The amount of water required for hydration depends upon the condition and the needs of the patient. The average adult patient requires 1500 to 2500 ml of water per day. In patients with fever or loss of excess water from undue perspiration, the water requirement may amount to 2000 to 3000 ml above the requirement for urinary loss, which averages between 600 to 1500 ml. Patients in a hypermetabolic state or with high fever and excessive sweating may require as much as 5000 ml daily [4].

The rate of administration depends upon the condition of the patient and the purpose of therapy. When the infusion is used to supply calories, the rate must be slow enough to allow complete metabolism of the glucose (0.5 gm per kilogram per hour in normal adults). When the infusion is used to produce diuresis, the rate must be fast enough to prevent complete metabolism of the dextrose, thereby increasing the osmolality of the extracellular fluid.

Isotonic Sodium Chloride Infusions

Sodium Chloride Injection (0.9 percent), U.S.P. (normal saline) contains 308 mOsm per liter (Na, 154 mEq per liter; Cl, 154 mEq per liter), has a pH between 4.5 and 7.0, and is usually supplied in volumes of 1000, 500, 250, and 100 ml. The term *normal* or *physiological* is misleading since the chloride in normal saline is 154 mEq per liter, compared to the normal plasma chloride value of 103 mEq per liter, while the sodium is 154 mEq per liter, or about 9 percent higher than the normal plasma value of 140 mEq per liter. Since the other electrolytes present in plasma are lacking in normal saline, the isotonicity of the solution depends upon the sodium and chloride ions, resulting in a higher concentration of these ions.

INDICATIONS FOR USE

1. Extracellular fluid replacement when chloride loss has been relatively greater than or equal to sodium loss.
2. Treatment of metabolic alkalosis in the presence of fluid loss; the increase in chloride ions provided by the infusion causes a compensatory decrease in the number of bicarbonate ions.
3. Sodium depletion. Mild sodium depletion (200 to 400 mEq) may be treated with 3 or more liters of isotonic saline solution with 100 gm of glucose [4]. To avoid infusion of excess chloride ions and prevent acidosis, Bland [4] suggested the use of 700 ml of isotonic saline solution with 300 ml of sixth-molar sodium lactate solution. This fluid increases the sodium to 167 mEq per liter and decreases the chloride to 108.5 mEq per liter.
4. Initiation and termination of blood transfusions. When isotonic saline is used to precede a blood transfusion, the hemolysis of red cells, which occurs with dextrose in water, is avoided.

DANGERS. Normal sodium chloride provides more sodium and chloride than the patient needs. Marked electrolyte imbalances have resulted from the almost exclusive use of normal saline. Untoward effects include the following:

1. *Hypernatremia.* An adult's dietary requirement for sodium is about 90 to 250 mEq per day, with a minimum requirement of 15 mEq and a maximum tolerance of 400 mEq [7]. When 3 liters of normal saline or 5 percent dextrose in normal saline is administered, the patient receives 462 mEq of sodium (154 mEq per liter × 3), a level that exceeds his normal tolerance. Such an infusion at a time when sodium retention is occurring, as during stress, can result in hypernatremia.

There is an increased danger in the elderly, in patients with severe dehydration, and in patients with chronic glomerulonephritis; these patients require more water to excrete the salt than do patients with normal renal function. Isotonic saline does not provide water but requires most of its volume for the excretion of salt.

2. *Acidosis.* One liter of normal saline contains one-third more chloride than is present in the extracellular fluid; when infused in large quantities, the excess chloride ions cause a loss of bicarbonate ions and result in an acidifying effect.

3. *Hypokalemia.* Infusion of saline increases potassium excretion and at the same time expands the volume of extracellular fluid, further decreasing the concentration of the extracellular potassium ion [4].

4. *Circulatory overload.* Continuous infusions of isotonic fluids expand the extracellular compartment and lead to circulatory overload.

REQUIREMENTS. In an average adult, the daily requirements of sodium chloride are met by infusing a liter of 0.9 percent sodium chloride, but the dosage is dependent upon the size of the patient, his needs, and his clinical condition.

Isotonic Saline with Dextrose

FIVE PERCENT DEXTROSE IN NORMAL SALINE. Five percent dextrose in normal saline contains 252 mOsm of dextrose (Cl, 154 mEq per liter; Na, 154 mEq per liter), has a pH of 3.5 to 6.0 and is available in volumes of 1000, 500, 250, and 150 ml.

When normal saline is infused, the addition of 100 gm of dextrose prevents formation of ketone bodies and the increased demand for water the ketone bodies impose for renal excretion. The dextrose prevents catabolism and, consequently, loss of potassium and intracellular water.

INDICATIONS FOR USE

1. Temporary treatment of circulatory insufficiency and shock due to hypovolemia in the immediate absence of a plasma expander.

2. Early treatment along with plasma or albumin for replacement of loss due to burn.
3. Early treatment of acute adrenocortical insufficiency.

DANGERS. The hazards are the same as those for normal saline (see preceding section).

Ten Percent Dextrose in Normal Saline
Ten percent dextrose in normal isotonic saline contains 504 mOsm per liter of dextrose (Na, 154 mEq per liter; Cl, 154 mEq per liter), has a pH of 3.5 to 6.0 and is usually supplied in volumes of 1000 and 500 ml.

INDICATIONS FOR USE. This fluid is used as a nutrient and an electrolyte (Na and Cl) replenisher.

DANGERS. Hypernatremia, acidosis, and circulatory overload may result when normal saline is administered in excess of the patient's tolerance.

ADMINISTRATION. Ten percent dextrose in normal saline, because of its hypertonicity, must be administered intravenously, preferably through a vein of large diameter to dilute the fluid and reduce the risk of trauma to the vessel. Close observation and precautions are necessary to prevent infiltration and damage to the tissues.

Hypertonic Sodium Chloride Infusions
These infusions include 3 percent sodium chloride (Na, 513 mEq per liter; Cl, 513 mEq per liter) and 5 percent sodium chloride (Na, 850 mEq per liter; Cl, 850 mEq per liter).

INDICATIONS FOR USE

1. *Severe dilutional hyponatremia* (water intoxication). Hypertonic sodium chloride, upon infusion, increases the osmotic pressure of the extracellular fluid, drawing water from the cells for excretion by the kidneys.
2. *Severe sodium depletion.* Infusions of hypertonic saline replenish sodium stores. An estimate of the sodium deficit can be made by taking the difference between the normal sodium concentration and the patient's current sodium concentration and multiplying it by 60 percent of the body weight in kilograms; sodium depletion is based on total body water and not on extracellular fluid [4].

ADMINISTRATION. Hypertonic saline infusions must be administered carefully and slowly to prevent pulmonary edema. Frequent reevaluation of the clinical and electrolyte picture during administration is advised. A dose of 200 to 300 ml of 3 to 5 percent saline solution may be given, with reevaluation before further saline is infused [4].

The rate of infusion of 5 percent saline should not exceed 100 ml per hour [12], and the patient should be observed constantly. The fluid must be infused by vein, with great care to prevent infiltration and trauma to the tissues.

Hypotonic Sodium Chloride in Water

One-half hypotonic saline (0.45 percent saline containing 77 mEq per liter of Na and 77 mEq per liter of Cl) is used as an electrolyte replenisher. When there is a question regarding the amount of saline required, hypotonic saline is preferred over isotonic saline. In general, 0.45 percent sodium chloride is preferable to normal saline [13].

Hydrating Fluids

Since solutions consisting of dextrose with hypotonic saline provide more water than is required for excretion of salt, they are useful as hydrating fluids. These solutions include: 2.5 percent dextrose in 0.45 percent saline (126 mOsm per liter of dextrose, with 77 mEq per liter of Na and 77 mEq per liter of Cl), 5 percent dextrose in 0.45 percent saline (252 mOsm per liter of dextrose, with 77 mEq per liter of Na and 77 mEq per liter of Cl), and 5 percent dextrose in 0.2 percent saline (252 mOsm per liter of dextrose, with 34.2 mEq per liter of Na and 34.2 mEq per liter of Cl).

INDICATIONS FOR USE

1. Commonly called *initial hydrating solutions,* hypotonic saline dextrose infusions are used to assess the status of the kidneys before electrolyte replacement and maintenance are initiated.
2. Hydration of medical and surgical patients.
3. Promotion of diuresis in dehydrated patients.

ADMINISTRATION. To assess the status of the kidneys, the fluid is administered at the rate of 8 ml per square meter of body surface per minute (see the nomograms in Figure 29, pp. 138–39) for 45 minutes. The restoration of urinary flow shows that the kidneys have begun to function; the hydrating fluid may be replaced by more specifically needed electrolytes. If after 45 minutes the urinary flow is not restored, the rate of infusion is reduced to 2 ml per square meter of body surface per minute for another hour. If this does not produce diuresis, renal impairment is assumed [14].

Initial hydrating fluids must be used cautiously in edematous pa-

Table 11. Individual Electrolyte Composition of Hypotonic Multiple Electrolyte Fluids (Milliequivalents per Liter)

Fluid	Manufacturer	Na	K	Ca	Mg++	Cl	Lactate	Acetate
Isolyte R	Baxter	40	16	5	3	40	12	12
Normosol-M	Abbott	40	13	0	3	40	0	16
Polysal M	Cutter	40	16	5	3	40	12	12
Plasma-Lyte M	Travenol	40	16	5	3	40	12	12

tients with cardiac, renal, or hepatic disease. Once good renal function is obtained, appropriate electrolytes should be administered to prevent hypokalemia.

Hypotonic Multiple Electrolyte Fluids
Hypotonic multiple electrolyte fluids (Table 11) are patterned after the type devised by Butler. Butler, with his co-workers at the Massachusetts General Hospital, was the first to emphasize the fact that basic water and electrolyte requirements are proportionate to the body surface area. Butler-type fluids are one-third to one-half as concentrated as plasma. They provide fluid to meet the patient's fluid volume requirement and in so doing provide cellular and extracellular electrolytes in quantities balanced between the minimal needs and the maximal tolerance of the patient. These fluids, because of their hypotonicity, provide water for urinary and metabolic needs and take advantage of the body's homeostatic mechanisms to retain the electrolytes and reject those not needed, thus maintaining water and electrolyte balance [14].

Hypotonic fluids should contain 5 percent dextrose for its protein-sparing and anti-ketogenic effect [8]. The dextrose will increase the tonicity of the fluid "in the bottle," but since it is metabolized in the body, leaving the water and salt, the electrolyte tonicity is obtained by disregarding the osmotic effect of dextrose [1]. Whether the patient has received too much or too little water depends upon the tonicity of the electrolyte and not the dextrose.

A balanced solution of hypotonic electrolytes is ideal for routine maintenance [1]. There are several modifications of the Butler-type fluids. Those containing 75 mEq of total cation are used for adult patients.

ADMINISTRATION. "A useful formula for maintenance water requirements, based on studies by Crawford, Butler and Talbot is: Maintenance Water = 1600 ml./square meter of body surface area/day" [8]. In the case of obese or edematous patients this should be calculated on ideal weight rather than actual weight. The water requirement must be patterned after the condition of the patient. When infection, trauma

Table 12. Individual Electrolyte Composition of Isotonic Multiple Electrolyte Fluids (Milliequivalents per Liter)

Fluid	Manufacturer	Na	K	Cl	HCO₃	Ca	Mg	NH₄	pH
Plasma-Lyte Polysal	Baxter Cutter	140	10	103	55	5	3	0	0
Electrolyte No. 3	Baxter Cutter	63	17	150	0	0	0	70	3.3–3.7
Lactated Ringer's injection (Hartmann's)		130	4	109	28	3	0	0	6.75

involving the brain, or stress lead to inappropriate release of antidiuretic hormone, maintenance requirements are less. Excessive fluid losses through urine, stool, expired air, and so forth require increased water. The rate of infusion is usually 3 ml per square meter of body surface per minute.

DANGERS

1. *Hyperkalemia.* When renal function is impaired, intravenous potassium should be used cautiously. The nurse should be alert to signs of hyperkalemia. If such signs develop, the physician should be notified and the fluid replaced by more appropriate electrolytes.

2. *Water intoxication.* The patient's tolerance limits for water can be exceeded. Care should be exercised in maintaining the prescribed flow rate and in ensuring that the patient receives the prescribed volume of fluid. Water intoxication is more likely to occur when inappropriate release of antidiuretic hormone, in response to stress, causes water retention. These patients should be carefully watched to detect any early signs of an imbalance, so that a change in therapy can be initiated before the condition becomes precarious. Weighing the patient is the best way to monitor the status of water balance. Daily weights are extremely important in following the state of hydration in very ill patients.

Isotonic Multiple Electrolyte Fluids

Many types of commercial replacement fluids are available; three such fluids are listed in Table 12. When severe vomiting, diarrhea, or diuresis result in a heavy loss of water and electrolytes, replacement therapy is necessary. Balanced fluids of isotonic electrolytes (Plasma-Lyte* and Polysal†) having an ionic composition similar to plasma are used.

Rapid initial replacement is seldom necessary. However, if impaired

* Baxter Laboratories, Morton Grove, Ill.; division of Travenol Laboratories, Inc.
† Cutter Laboratories, Berkeley, Calif.

circulation and renal function of a severely dehydrated patient become evident and it is necessary to restore the patient's blood pressure quickly, 30 ml per kilogram of an isotonic fluid may be provided in the first hour or two [8]. Fluid overload must be prevented. Central venous pressure monitoring is especially helpful in the elderly patient and in patients with renal or cardiovascular disorders.

Extracellular replacement can generally be assumed to be complete after 48 hours of replacement therapy unless proved otherwise by clinical or laboratory evidence. To continue replacement fluids after deficits have been corrected may result in sodium excess leading to pulmonary edema or heart failure [8]. Patients receiving replacement therapy should be observed closely to detect any signs of circulatory overload.

Gastric replacement fluids, such as Electrolyte No. 3 by Baxter and Cutter, provide the usual electrolytes lost by vomiting or gastric suction. They contain ammonium ions which are metabolized in the liver to hydrogen ion and urea, replacing the hydrogen ion lost in gastric juices. They are useful in metabolic alkalosis due to excessive ingestion of sodium bicarbonate. The usual adult dose is 500 to 2000 ml and the infusion should not be faster than 500 ml per hour (check with physician).

Gastric replacement fluids are contraindicated in the presence of hepatic insufficiency or renal failure. They require the same precautions as any fluid containing potassium, and should be avoided in patients with renal damage or Addison's disease. Also, the low pH causes incompatibilities with many additives.

Lactated Ringer's injection is a popular fluid and is considered safe in certain conditions. Since the electrolyte concentration very closely resembles that of the extracellular fluid, it may be used to replace fluid loss from burns and fluid lost as bile and diarrhea. Lactated Ringer's injection has been useful in mild acidosis, the lactate ion being metabolized in the liver to bicarbonate.

DANGERS. Three liters contains about 390 mEq of sodium, which can quickly elevate the sodium level in a patient who is not deficient [7]. Lactated Ringer's injection is contraindicated in severe metabolic acidosis or alkalosis and in liver disease or anoxic states which influence lactate metabolism.

ADMINISTRATION. Usually 1 to 3 liters per day corrects fluid deficits and replaces recurrent losses. The rate of infusion is 5 to 10 ml per kilogram of body weight per hour. If there are no cardiac or other contraindications to rapid infusion, 30 ml per kilogram per hour may be given (check with physician) [12].

Alkalizing Fluids

When anesthesia or disorders such as dehydration, shock, liver disease, starvation, and diabetes cause retention of chlorides, ketone bodies, or organic salts, or when excessive bicarbonate is lost, metabolic acidosis occurs. Treatment consists of infusion with an appropriate alkalizing fluid. These fluids include one-sixth molar isotonic sodium lactate (1.9 percent, with 167 mEq Na per liter, 167 mEq lactate ions per liter, and a pH of 6.0 to 7.3), one-sixth molar Sodium Bicarbonate Injection, U.S.P. (1.5 percent, with 178 mEq Na per liter, 178 mEq bicarbonate per liter, and a pH of 7.0 to 8.0), and hypertonic sodium bicarbonate injection (7.5 or 5 percent).

ONE-SIXTH MOLAR SODIUM LACTATE. The lactate ion must be oxidized in the body to carbon dioxide before it can effect acid–base balance; the complete conversion of sodium lactate to bicarbonate requires about 1 to 2 hours [2]. Since oxidation is necessary to increase the bicarbonate concentration, sodium lactate is not used for patients suffering from oxygen lack, as in congenital heart disease with persistent cyanosis.

One-sixth molar sodium lactate is used when acidosis results from a sodium deficiency in such disorders as vomiting, starvation, uncontrolled diabetes mellitus, acute infections, and renal failure [2].

In order to supply concentrated sodium and avoid the large doses of chloride present in hypertonic saline, a mixture may be made by using 650 ml of isotonic saline solution and 350 ml of one-sixth molar sodium lactate [4].

The usual dose is 1 liter of a one-sixth molar solution, but the dosage depends upon the patient's condition and the serum sodium level. One-sixth molar infusion may be administered by venoclysis or hyperdermoclysis and usually at a rate not greater than 300 ml per hour [2]. The patient should be observed closely for any evidence of alkalosis.

SODIUM BICARBONATE. Sodium Bicarbonate Injection, U.S.P. (1.5 percent, with 178 mEq per liter Na, 178 mEq per liter bicarbonate) is an isotonic solution that provides bicarbonate ions in conditions in which excess depletion has occurred. It is used for severe hyperpnea early in the treatment of severe acidosis until the signs of dyspnea and hyperpnea are relieved. The bicarbonate ion is released in the form of carbon dioxide through the lungs, leaving an excess of sodium cation behind to exert its electrolyte effect [2].

The usual dose is 500 ml in a 1.5 percent solution. The dosage is dependent upon the patient's weight, condition, and carbon dioxide content. If the isotonic infusion is not available it may be made by adding two 50-ml ampules containing 3.75 gm each of sodium bicarbonate to 400 ml of hypotonic saline. The fluid should be infused slowly intravenously. Rapid injection may induce cellular acidity and death. The patient should be watched for signs of hypocalcemic tetany, and calcium supplement should be administered if required; calcium does not ionize well in an alkaline medium.

Acidifying Infusions

Normal saline (0.9 percent sodium chloride injection, U.S.P.) is not usually listed among the acidifying infusions. However, since metabolic alkalosis is a condition associated with excess bicarbonate and loss of chloride, isotonic saline provides conservative treatment. When the chloride ions are infused, the bicarbonate decreases in compensation and the alkalosis is relieved.

Ammonium chloride, the usual acidifying agent, is available as isotonic 0.9 percent ammonium chloride injection (167 mEq NH_4 per liter and 167 mEq Cl per liter) and hypertonic 2.14 percent ammonium chloride injection (400 mEq NH_4 per liter and 400 mEq Cl per liter). The pH range is 4.0 to 6.0. Both concentrations are supplied in 1-liter bottles.

INDICATIONS FOR USE. Ammonium chloride is used as an acidifying infusion in severe metabolic alkalosis due to loss of gastric secretions, pyloric stenosis, or other causes. The ammonium ion is converted by the liver to hydrogen ion and to ammonia, which is excreted as urea.

ADMINISTRATION. The 2.14 percent ammonium chloride is usually used in the treatment of the adult patient; 0.9 percent ammonium chloride is used for children [14].

The dosage depends upon the condition of the patient and upon an accurate chemical picture, including plasma carbon dioxide–combining power. Ammonium chloride must be infused at a very slow rate to enable the liver to metabolize the ammonium ion. Rapid injection can result in toxic effects causing irregular breathing, bradycardia, and twitching [2].

PRECAUTIONS. Since the acidifying effect of ammonium chloride depends upon the liver for conversion, it must not be administered to patients with severe hepatic disease or renal failure. It is contraindicated in any condition with a high ammonium level.

Evaluation of Water and Electrolyte Balance

A rational approach is necessary if the patient is to receive safe and successful intravenous therapy. In the past, emphasis was placed on the technical responsibility of the nurse in maintaining the infusion and in keeping the needle patent. With the increase in the use of intravenous therapy, clinical disturbances in fluid and electrolyte metabolism are more common. Changes can occur quickly and in the absence of the physician. Today the nurse's responsibility consists of monitoring the fluid and electrolyte status of the patient as well as the progress of the infusion. Greater emphasis must be placed on the causes and effects of fluid and electrolyte abnormalities so that these imbalances may be anticipated and recognized before they become disastrous. The nurse should be familiar with the parameters used in evaluating fluid and electrolyte imbalances and in supplying fluid and electrolyte requirements.

Clinical Parameters

CENTRAL VENOUS PRESSURE. Monitoring of the central venous pressure provides a simple, accurate, and valuable guide in detecting changes in blood volume and in assessing fluid requirements. It is particularly valuable in assessing the ability of the heart to tolerate the infusion. The importance of a properly functioning central venous pressure line must be stressed; many erroneous conclusions are drawn from false values recorded when the line is not properly responsive to right atrial pressures.

A normal venous pressure indicates an adequate circulatory blood volume.

An elevated venous pressure may mean an increase in circulatory volume and right heart pressure, with the possibility of circulatory overload. It may also indicate other problems such as a pulmonary embolus, myocardial infarction, or lack of digitalis. Determination of the hematocrit value will supplement clinical information [9].

A low venous pressure, too low to measure, indicates that the patient has probably lost fluid or blood. One must not overlook the fact that fluid loss can result from the improper administration of intravenous fluids. If rapid infusion of dextrose exceeds the patient's tolerance, massive diuresis with dehydration and diminished circulatory volume may occur. The decreased venous blood return into the right atrium is reflected by a decrease in the central venous pressure.

PULSE. The quality and the rate of the pulse provide clinical information valuable in assessing fluid and electrolyte changes in the patient. A high pulse pressure, bounding and not easily obliterated by pressure, indicates a high cardiac output caused by circulatory overload. A regular pulse, easily obliterated by pressure, indicates low cardiac output resulting from a lowered blood volume. A bounding, easily obliterated pressure signifies a drop in blood pressure with a wide pulse pressure, indicative of impending circulatory collapse. As the patient's condition deteriorates the pulse will become rapid, weak, thready, and easily obliterated, signifying circulatory collapse [4].

PERIPHERAL VEINS. Examination of the peripheral veins provides a means of evaluating the plasma volume. The peripheral veins will usually empty in 3 to 5 seconds when the hand is elevated and will fill in the same length of time when the hand is lowered to a dependent position. Peripheral vein filling may take as long as 10 to 12 seconds in patients with sodium depletion and extracellular dehydration [4]. Slow emptying of the peripheral veins indicates overhydration and an excessive blood volume, while slow filling indicates a low blood volume and often precedes hypotension. Peripheral veins which become engorged and clearly visible indicate an increase in the plasma volume secondary to an interstitial to vascular fluid shift or an increase in extracellular fluid volume [14].

WEIGHT. A sudden gain or loss in weight is a significant sign of a change in the fluid volume. A change in the volume of body fluid can be computed by weighing the patient daily at the same time of day, on the same scales, with the same amount of clothing. A loss or gain of 1 kilogram of body weight reflects a loss or gain of 1 liter of body fluid. A weight loss of up to 5 percent in a child or an adult indicates a moderate fluid volume deficit, and a weight loss of over 5 percent indicates a serious fluid volume deficit [14].

Weisburg [20] stated: "The weight in pounds can be converted to kilograms by a simple mental calculation. Divide pounds by 2; 10 percent of this quotient is subtracted from the quotient to obtain the weight in kilograms. For example, a 180 pound patient weighs 81 kg.; 180 divided by 2 equals 90, and 10 percent of 90 is 9, which is subtracted from the 90 to give 81 kg."

THIRST. Thirst is an important and valuable symptom denoting a deficit in body fluid or, more specifically, cellular dehydration. This type of dehydration occurs when the extracellular fluid becomes hypertonic, either as a result of water deprivation or the infusion of hypertonic saline. The increase in osmotic pressure causes fluid to be drawn from the cells, resulting in cellular dehydration, the stimulus to thirst. "Thirst is the prime symptom and occurs early. Thirst is present with a loss of only 2 per cent of body weight or 1.4 Kg., equivalent to a deficit of only 1.4 liters of water" [4].

Normally thirst governs the need for water, but in certain conditions the lack of thirst may accompany dehydration. This is especially true in the aged, in whom thirst is not urgent. These patients may lose their thirst and as a result become severely dehydrated before the condition is recognized.

In the severely burned patient, the great thirst experienced may lead to ingestion of excess water and to a serious sodium deficit.

INTAKE AND OUTPUT. Water intake and output should be carefully measured and recorded. Hourly urine output measurements may be particularly important. A urine output of 200 ml per hour indicates that too much water is being infused too rapidly. Dudrick [9] stated, "By regulating the urine output between 30 and 50 ml./hr. the patient receives at least enough fluid for his kidneys to work efficiently."

A decreased urinary output accompanies a decreased blood volume; changes in the arterial pressure and pressure in the glomeruli result in the oliguria or anuria of profound shock. The increase in urinary output accompanying an increase in blood volume is primarily due to changes in arterial pressure and pressure in the glomeruli [14].

SKIN. Observing changes in skin turgor (elasticity) and texture is helpful in assessing the state of water balance. To test skin turgor, pick up the skin of the forearm and then release it; in the normal individual, the pinched skin will return to its original position. Skin that remains in a raised position for several seconds indicates a deficit in fluid volume.

A dry, leathery tongue may indicate a fluid volume deficit or mouth breathing. To differentiate between the two, the mucous membrane may be checked for moisture by running the finger between the gums and the cheek; dryness indicates a fluid volume deficit.

EDEMA. Edema reflects an increase in the extracellular fluid volume outside the circulating intravascular compartment. It depends upon an imbalance or a disturbance in (1) the exchange of water and electrolytes between the patient and his environment or (2) the exchange of water and electrolytes between the compartments of the body. The fluid and electrolyte exchange between the body compartments may be affected by an alteration in (1) the circulatory system, (2) the lymphatic system, or (3) the concentration of albumin in the serum; water and electrolytes escape from the circulation faster than they enter, and edema ensues. Edema may be (1) generalized, as in congestive failure, (2) localized, as with ascites, or (3) peripheral [4].

By detecting edema early, a clinical imbalance may be corrected before the patient's condition deteriorates. Early peripheral edema may be detected by finger printing, a procedure in which the finger is rolled over the bony prominence of the sternum or tibia. As edema increases, pitting edema will occur and may be detected by pressure of the fingers on the subcutaneous tissue.

In generalized edema, such as that seen in cardiac failure, there is an increase in total extracellular water volume as well as interstitial edema. Symptoms such as venous engorgement, restlessness, dyspnea, cyanosis, and pulmonary rales indicate generalized edema.

Laboratory Values

Laboratory values, when used to supplement clinical observations, aid in forming diagnostic and therapeutic guidelines.

Electrolyte studies (serum sodium, potassium, chloride, bicarbonate, and pH) performed daily are important in assessing the fluid and electrolyte status of the patient receiving intravenous fluids. In patients with massive electrolyte losses such studies may be required two or three times a day.

Blood cell count and hematocrit determinations are helpful in detecting hemoconcentration or hemodilution; hemoconcentration reflects a diminished plasma volume due to dehydration, and hemodilution, an increased volume from overtreatment with water.

Measurement of *serum protein with the albumin–globulin* ratio helps in detecting a change in fluid volume; large quantities of parenteral fluid rapidly administered dilute and decrease the serum protein concentration. This determination is helpful when used to supplement clinical observation—otherwise it may be misleading and interpreted as showing actual depletion. A decrease in serum protein reduces the osmotic pressure of the extracellular compartment, causing some edema and loss of plasma volume (see Chapter 14).

Blood urea nitrogen should be measured frequently to evaluate kidney function, an important parameter in treating fluid and electrolyte imbalances.

Clinical Disturbances of Water and Electrolyte Metabolism

Most of the common clinical disturbances in water and electrolyte balance result from changes in the volume of total body water or in one or more of the fluid compartments of the body. Bland [4] classified clinical disturbances in water and electrolyte metabolism into six types: isotonic, hypertonic, and hypotonic expansion and contraction. These are discussed in the following pages and are summarized in Tables 13 and 14.

Isotonic Expansion

Isotonic expansion (circulatory overload) occurs when fluids of the same tonicity as plasma are infused into the vascular circulation. Because solutions isotonic to plasma do not affect the osmolality, there is no flow of water from the extracellular compartment to the intracellular compartment. The extracellular compartment expands in proportion to the fluid infused and is the only compartment affected. The increase in the volume of fluid dilutes the concentration of hemoglobin and lowers the hematocrit and total protein levels, but the serum sodium level remains the same.

Isotonic expansion is a critical complication of intravenous therapy. Patients who receive isotonic fluids around the clock are prime targets and should be observed closely for early signs of circulatory overload. Normal saline or solutions containing balanced isotonic multiple electrolytes are used for preexisting or continuing fluid and electrolyte losses and are not the ideal fluids for maintenance therapy. The electrolyte isotonicity of these solutions causes expansion of the extracellular compartment and does not provide the extra water that balanced hypotonic solutions provide for the kidney to retain or secrete as needed [7].

The early postoperative or post-trauma patient is prone to this critical complication. The increased endocrine response to stress during the first 2 to 5 days following surgery results in retention of sodium chloride and water [14]. When a patient under stress is receiving isotonic infusions, the nurse must anticipate and watch for signs of circulatory overload.

Elderly patients receiving isotonic fluids must be carefully monitored as they have a lower tolerance to fluids and electrolytes. Because they are also likely to have some degree of cardiac and renal impairment, the ability of the kidneys to eliminate fluid is apt to be diminished. The status of these patients can change quickly.

In the patient who has had a craniotomy, large-volume isotonic infusions can increase the intracranial pressure and prove detrimental.

Patients who are potential candidates for isotonic expansion must be watched carefully and turned frequently to prevent fluid from settling in the lungs. Pulmonary edema can result from the cardiac and pulmonary side-effects of intravenous therapy. Dudrick [9] stated, "The apices of the lungs which are high will tend to be fairly dry, but the bases of their lungs, posteriorly and inferiorly, can be fairly wet." As a result, hypostatic pneumonia secondary to gravity may develop.

MANIFESTATIONS. The nurse who monitors intravenous infusions must be familiar with the early clinical manifestations that accompany isotonic expansion in order to recognize and prevent its development; mild pulmonary edema progressing to severe pulmonary edema is a late stage that must be prevented. Early clinical manifestations consist of: (1) weight gain, (2) increase in fluid intake over output, (3) a high

Table 13. Comparison of Three Types of Dehydration

	Isotonic	Hypertonic	Hypotonic
Cause	Loss of blood or isotonic fluid	Excess loss of water or insufficient intake	Loss of salt
Effect on fluid compartments	ECF volume ↓	ICF and ECF volume ↓	ICF volume ↑ ECF volume ↓
Clinical signs			
Weight	↓	↓	↓
Rate of H_2O excretion	↓	↓	↑
Rate of Na excretion	↓	↓	↓
Thirst	. . .	Early sign, due to cellular dehydration	. . .
Pulse rate	Regular, easily obliterated by pressure	Regular and normal in early stages	Increased, weak and thready, easily obliterated by pressure
Hand vein filling time (normal = 3–5 sec)	May increase	May be normal	Normal to ↑
Behavior	. . .	Irritability, restlessness, possibly confusion	Possibly vomiting and cramps
Signs in late stages	Developing shock with pulse weak and thready	Skin turgor diminished; dry, furrowed tongue; death, possibly due to rise of osmotic pressure	Skin turgor may be diminished; thready pulse; possibly confusion and apathy; death from peripheral circulatory failure
Laboratory values			
Hematocrit	↑	↑	↑
Hemoglobin	↑	↑	↑
Total protein and albumin–globulin ratio	↑	↑	↑
Sodium concentration	. . .	↑	↓

Table 14. Comparison of Three Types of Fluid Expansion

	Isotonic	Hypertonic	Hypotonic
Cause	Infusion of excess quantities of isotonic fluids	Infusion of excess quantities of hypertonic saline	Increased intake or infusion of water in excess of patient's tolerance
Effects on fluid compartments	ECF volume ↑	ECF volume ↑ ICF volume ↓	ECF and ICF volume ↑
Clinical signs			
Weight	↑	↑ depending on amount infused	↑
Rate of H_2O excretion	↑	↓	↑
Rate of Na excretion	↑	↑	↑
Thirst	. . .	Present	. . .
Pulse rate	Bounding, not easily obliterated by pressure	Full, bounding (significant)	May be regular and not easily obliterated by pressure
Hand vein emptying time (normal = 3–5 sec)	↑	↑	↑
Edema	May be present	Early, tibial edema; later, pitting edema; diminished skin turgor	Tibial edema with finger printing
Signs of intracranial pressure	. . .	. . .	Irritability, headache, confusion
Signs in late stages	Hoarseness, pulmonary edema, cyanosis, coughing, dyspnea	Water rales, pulmonary edema	Pulmonary edema
Other signs	. . .	Hoarseness (a frequent early sign)	Cramping of exercised muscles
Laboratory values			
Hematocrit	↓	↓	↓
Hemoglobin	↓	↓	↓
Total protein and albumin–globulin ratio	↓	↓	↓
Sodium concentration	. . .	↑	↓

pulse pressure, bounding and not easily obliterated, showing signs of high cardiac output, (4) increase in central venous pressure, (5) peripheral hand vein emptying time longer than the normal 3 to 5 seconds when the hand is elevated from a dependent position, (6) peripheral edema, depending on the extent of fluid expansion, and (7) hoarseness. If intravenous therapy is allowed to continue, isotonic expansion becomes more apparent and dangerous, with easily recognized signs: cyanosis, dyspnea, coughing, and neck vein engorgement.

Laboratory characteristics include a drop in the hematocrit value and reduced concentration of hemoglobin and total protein.

TREATMENT. Treatment for circulatory overload when detected early is relatively simple and consists of withholding all fluids until excess water and electrolytes have been eliminated by the body. After the condition is rectified, hypotonic maintenance fluids will provide the patient with fluid and a minimum daily requirement of electrolytes. The hypotonicity of the fluid allows the kidneys to maintain the needed amount and selectively retain or excrete the excess.

Isotonic Contraction

Isotonic contraction occurs when there is loss of fluid and electrolytes isotonic to the extracellular fluid, such as whole blood or large volumes of fluid from diarrhea or vomiting. The extracellular compartment contracts. Since the fluid lost is isotonic, the osmolality of the extracellular compartment remains unchanged and there is no movement of water between the compartments; only the extracellular volume is affected.

MANIFESTATIONS. Because of the loss of fluid, the hematocrit level and the concentration of hemoglobin and total protein are increased. There is no change in the serum sodium concentration.

Clinical manifestations are: (1) weight loss, (2) negative fluid balance (a decrease in urinary output but a greater output than total fluid intake), (3) pulse that is regular in rate and easily obliterated by pressure; as the patient's condition deteriorates the pulse becomes weak and thready, and (4) possible increase in peripheral hand filling time above the normal 3 to 5 seconds when the hand is moved from an elevated to a dependent position.

TREATMENT. Treatment consists of replacing the fluid loss with isotonic solutions containing balanced electrolytes (see Table 12).

Hypertonic Expansion

Hypertonic expansion occurs when the volume of body water is increased by the intravenous infusion of hypertonic saline. Three or 5 percent sodium chloride is used to replace a massive sodium loss or to remove excess accumulation of body fluids, but if it is rapidly infused hypertonic expansion can result. The saline increases the osmotic pressure of the extracellular compartment, causing water to be drawn from the intracellular compartment until both compartments are isosmotic. There is an increase in the volume of the extracellular compartment and a decrease in the volume of the cellular compartment. The osmolality of the extracellular fluid is higher than before the infusion but lower than the high level after the infusion because of the increased extracellular fluid volume [4].

Caution must be used in the intravenous administration of hypertonic saline. Circulatory overload with hypernatremia can occur. The nurse must understand the reason for the infusion, the condition of the patient, the proper rate of administration, and the signs and symptoms of hypertonic expansion.

MANIFESTATIONS. Clinical manifestations include a gain in body weight dependent upon the volume infused. A small volume (500 ml) will not contribute to a significant weight gain [16]. An increased sodium load results in a decreased rate of water excretion; however, the abrupt increase in plasma volume may cause an increase in the rate of water excretion as the body attempts to excrete the excess salt and water. The degree of thirst will be dependent upon the hypertonicity of the plasma and consequently the amount of cellular dehydration. Peripheral hand vein emptying time may be increased beyond the normal 5 seconds when the hand is elevated, but is dependent upon the degree of expansion of the extracellular compartment. A bounding pulse is significant in detecting hypertonic expansion. The serum sodium concentration is increased. The hematocrit level and the concentration of hemoglobin and total serum protein are decreased as a result of the expanded fluid volume in the extracellular compartment.

TREATMENT. Treatment consists of stopping the infusion to allow the kidneys to eliminate the overload of salt and water. If there are no cardiovascular side-effects, five percent dextrose in water may be infused slowly to reduce the tonicity of the extracellular fluid and replace body water.

Hypertonic Contraction
Hypertonic contraction (hypertonic or cellular dehydration) occurs when there is a loss of water without a corresponding loss of salt. This condition occurs in patients who are unable to take sufficient fluid for a prolonged period of time or in patients with excess insensible water loss through the lungs and skin.

In the elderly, hypertonic dehydration is a common clinical disturbance; there is frequently a decrease in the thirst stimuli in response to hypertonicity of body fluids, and adequate intake of fluid is not met. In the unconscious or incontinent, frequency and excess urination may go undetected or may be recognized as a sign of good renal function. "The aged patient frequently manifests loss of tubular ability to concentrate urine, as well as diminished responsiveness to antidiuretic hormone" [4]. Because of this, large amounts of dilute urine may be lost, resulting in hypertonic dehydration.

To prevent fluid imbalance the nurse must recognize that individuals differ widely in the water they require; patients whose kidneys do not concentrate well require more water than those whose kidneys concentrate well. The daily fluid requirement must be met.

In hypertonic contraction, the loss of water from the extracellular compartment results in an increase in the osmolality, causing water to flow from the cells to the extracellular compartment. Cellular dehydration occurs as water leaves the cellular compartment to replace the plasma volume. Both compartments, the intracellular and the extracellular, are affected by the water loss; there is a decrease in volume and an increase in osmolality in both compartments. In contrast, in isotonic contraction only the extracellular compartment is affected and the contraction is more serious.

Because signs of hypertonic contraction are not obvious in the early stages, the nurse must anticipate such an imbalance and be alert to any changes.

MANIFESTATIONS. Clinically, thirst is an early and reliable sign of hypertonic contraction but may be absent in the elderly, complicating early recognition of this imbalance. Weight loss occurs. Negative fluid balance (output greater than intake) is present. Hourly output measurements show a decrease in the rate of excretion of water. The pulse has a normal quality and is regular in the early stages of hypertonic contraction. The hand vein filling time may be within the normal limits; cellular fluid has partly replenished the plasma. Irritability, restlessness, and possibly confusion may be present. Skin turgor diminishes and is a sign of dehydration in the later stages. A dry mouth with a furrowed tongue shows dehydration.

Laboratory studies show an increase in serum sodium concentration, hematocrit level, hemoglobin concentration, and total serum protein concentration.

TREATMENT. Treatment consists of hydrating the patient by administering 2400 ml of a hypotonic solution per square meter of body surface per day for moderate preexisting deficit, and 3000 ml per square meter of body surface per day for severe preexisting deficit [14]. A therapeutic test for functional renal depression may be necessary before infusing water and electrolytes for maintenance.

Hypotonic Expansion

Hypotonic expansion (water intoxication, dilutional hyponatremia) occurs when the increase in the volume of body fluids is due to water alone. Water expands the extracellular compartment, causing a decrease in the concentration. Water then diffuses into the cells until both compartments are isosmotic. Both the extracellular and the intracellular compartments are affected; the volume is increased and the concentration is decreased. The serum sodium concentration and the hematocrit, hemoglobin, and total serum protein levels are reduced.

Hypotonic expansion occurs in patients who are receiving large quantities of electrolyte-free water to replace excessive fluid and electrolytes lost from gastric suction, vomiting, diarrhea, or diuresis, or insensibly through the skin.

Patients receiving continuous infusion of 5 percent dextrose in water are particularly prone to water intoxication. This solution contains 252 mOsm of dextrose per liter, making it an isotonic solution in the bottle. Once introduced into the circulation, the dextrose is quickly metabolized, leaving the water free to dilute and expand the extracellular compartment. With the decreased osmolality of the extracellular fluid, water diffuses into the cells and hypotonic expansion occurs.

The patient's tolerance to water can be exceeded by infusion of excess amounts of hypotonic fluids. The kidneys of the normal adult can metabolize water in amounts of 35 to 45 ml per kilogram per day, but the kidneys of the average patient can metabolize only 2500 to 3000 ml per day; above these volumes abnormal accumulation of water occurs [9].

Hypotonic expansion is more likely to occur during the early postoperative period when retention of water is being affected by the response to stress. It is particularly likely in the elderly patient in whom the response to stress is compounded by impairment in renal function. Small amounts of adjusted hypotonic saline (sodium 90 mEq, chloride 60 mEq, and lactate 30 mEq per liter) have a real place in the early postoperative management of the aged [4].

MANIFESTATIONS. When acute onset of behavioral changes, such as confusion, apathy, and disorientation, occurs in the elderly patient postoperatively, overhydration should be suspected. Central nervous system disturbances such as weakness, muscle twitching, and convulsions are seen, as are headaches, nausea, and vomiting. There is an increase in fluid intake over fluid output. Weight gain is always present.

Blood pressure usually is normal but may be elevated. Peripheral hand veins are usually full and hand emptying time is increased beyond the normal 5 seconds when the hand is elevated from a dependent position. The pulse may be regular and not easily obliterated when pressure is applied.

TREATMENT. Treatment consists of withholding all fluids until the excess water is excreted. In severe hyponatremia it may be necessary to administer small quantities of hypertonic saline to increase the osmotic pressure and the flow of water from the cells to the extracellular compartment for excretion by the kidneys. Hypertonic saline must be used cautiously and not administered to patients with congestive heart failure.

Hypotonic Contraction

Hypotonic contraction (hypotonic dehydration) occurs when fluids containing relatively more salt than water are lost from the body. This loss results in a decrease in the effective osmolality of the extracellular compartment. Water is drawn into the cells until osmotic equilibrium is established. Owing to the invasion of water the intracellular compartment is expanded and the extracellular compartment is contracted.

This imbalance may result from the loss of salt from any one of several sources: urine of patients receiving diuretics, fistula drainage, severe burns, vomitus, and sweat. A loss of up to 500 mEq of sodium has been shown to effect little change in the plasma sodium concentration in normal persons since the kidneys maintain the effective osmolality of the extracellular fluid by excreting an amount of water equivalent to the loss of sodium. The elderly are affected by the loss of much smaller quantities of sodium [4].

MANIFESTATIONS. Clinical manifestations include (1) weight loss, (2) negative fluid balance, (3) pulse rate increased, weak or thready, and easily obliterated, (4) increased hand filling time, and (5) decreased skin turgor.

Laboratory studies show a decrease in serum sodium concentration and an increase in hematocrit, hemoglobin, and total serum protein levels.

TREATMENT. Treatment of hypotonic contraction consists of replacing the fluids and electrolytes that have been lost. Because other electrolytes are usually lost along with the sodium loss, a balanced electrolyte solution may be administered.

References

1. Abbott Laboratories. *Fluid and Electrolytes.* North Chicago, Ill., 1970. Pp. 27, 28.
2. American Society of Hospital Pharmacists. *American Hospital Formulary Service.* Washington, D.C., 1969. Pp. 40:04, 40:08.
3. Asperheim, M. K. *Pharmacology for Practical Nurses* (3d ed.). Philadelphia: Saunders, 1971. P. 47.
4. Bland, J. H. *Clinical Metabolism of Body Water and Electrolytes.* Philadelphia: Saunders, 1963. Pp. 165, 170, 180, 184, 193, 205, 206, 217, 218, 220, 327, 329, 330.
5. Bradley, W. T., Gustafson, C. B., and Stoklosa, M. J. *Pharmaceutical Calculations* (5th ed.). Philadelphia: Lea & Febiger, 1968. Pp. 248, 249.
6. Burgess, R. E. Fluid and electrolytes. *American Journal of Nursing* 65:90, 1965.
7. Burns, W. Indications for I.V. therapy (Proceedings of Clinical Seminar, San Francisco, 1968). In *Health Care World Wide.* North Chicago, Ill.: Abbott Laboratories, 1972. Pp. 7, 8, 12.
8. Drug and Therapeutic Information, Inc. Parenteral water and electrolyte solutions. *Medical Letter* 12(19):77, 1970.
9. Dudrick, S. J. Rational I.V. therapy. *American Journal of Hospital Pharmacy* 28:83–85, 1971.
10. Elman, R. Fluid balance from the nurse's point of view. *American Journal of Nursing* 49:223, 1949.
11. Lebowitz, M. H., MaSuda, J. V., and Beckerman, J. H. The pH and acidity of intravenous infusion solutions. *Journal of the American Medical Association* 215:1937, 1971.
12. McGaw Laboratories. *Guide to Parenteral Fluid Therapy.* Glendale, Calif., 1963. Pp. 37, 45.
13. McGaw Laboratories. *McGaw Solutions Usage Chart.* Glendale, Calif., 1968.
14. Metheny, N. M., and Snively, W. D., Jr. *Nurses' Handbook of Fluid Balance.* Philadelphia: Lippincott, 1967. Pp. 2, 48, 58, 106, 107, 121, 129, 147, 217.
15. *United States Pharmacopeia* (18th ed.). Easton, Pa.: Mack Publishing, 1970. P. 810.
16. Voda, A. M. Body water dynamics. *American Journal of Nursing* 70: 2597, 2598, 2600, 2601.
17. Welt, L. G. Agent Affecting Volume and Composition of Body Fluids. In L. Goodman and A. Gilman (Eds.), *The Pharmacological Basis of Therapeutics* (3d ed.). New York: Macmillan, 1965. P. 793.
18. Weisberg, H. F. *Water, Electrolyte, and Acid-Base Balance* (2d ed.). Baltimore: Williams & Wilkins, 1962. P. 296.
19. Weisberg, H. F. Pit falls in fluid and electrolyte therapy. *Journal of St. Barnabas Medical Center* 2:106, 1964.
20. Weisberg, H. F. Parenteral Fluid Therapy in Adults. In H. F. Conn (Ed.), *Current Therapy.* Philadelphia: Saunders, 1969. P. 414.

13. Total Parenteral Nutrition—Nursing Practice

Rita Colley*

Total parenteral nutrition is the administration of sufficient nutrients by vein to support life and maintain growth and development. An exciting concept of care, the topic appears frequently in the medical literature. In the early 1960s, the Harrison Department of Surgical Research at the University of Pennsylvania Hospital demonstrated that animals could maintain positive nitrogen balance, that is to say, gain weight and grow normally, while being fed totally by vein.

Stanley Dudrick is recognized as being chiefly responsible for the remarkable advances in surgical nutrition that this technique has fostered. While still a surgical resident at the University of Pennsylvania, Dudrick developed an intravenous feeding method which achieved normal weight gain and growth in beagle puppies. These successful experiments in intravenous feeding, which totally bypassed the gastrointestinal tract, quickly led to human application. Shortly after the puppy experiments, Dudrick successfully treated a severely ill infant. He also treated starving adults, who would have been unable to survive by gastrointestinal feeding. From these early beginnings, total parenteral nutrition has reached the status of universal acceptance as a feasible method of maintaining positive nutritional balance in the absence of gastrointestinal tract feeding [6].

Patients are starving in hospitals throughout the world. When the gastrointestinal tract is functioning inadequately, and only routine intravenous fluids are administered, a caloric deficit quickly develops. When sufficient energy calories are not supplied in the daily diet, glyconeogenesis occurs. This means that body proteins are converted to carbohydrate (for energy) and a protein (nitrogen) deficit occurs. In order to spare protein from this conversion, to leave it free for the ongoing, daily process of protein synthesis, varying amounts of energy calories are needed. Fever, stress, certain catabolic drugs, trauma, and hypermetabolic disease processes may elevate a patient's basal caloric requirement to more than 10,000 calories a day.

* Registered Nurse, Massachusetts General Hospital School of Nursing; Nurse Clinician, Hyperalimentation Unit, Massachusetts General Hospital.

Since isotonic fluids provide few calories, e.g., a liter of 5 percent dextrose contains only 170 calories, it becomes obvious that fluid volumes necessary to meet even the usual hospitalized patient's requirements exceed renal, cardiac, and pulmonary tolerances. Therefore, until Dudrick's work, persons with prolonged periods of nutritional deprivation caused by a nonfunctioning gastrointestinal tract were destined to starve. They were catabolic (in negative nitrogen balance).

Solutions

Types

Total parenteral nutrition is now available to American patients in a wide variety of solution types. Investigational solutions will be discussed later. Most patients receive commercially available solutions containing hydrolyzed protein or synthetic amino acids. The protein hydrolysates are derived from either casein (a major milk protein) or fibrin (which has beef blood as its source). Hydrolyzed protein is a mixture of essential and nonessential amino acids bonded together as polypeptides. The polypeptides are broken down and probably excreted as nitrogen waste during protein metabolism. Synthetic amino acids may be thought of as a purer form of protein. They are a mixture of essential and nonessential amino acids without the polypeptide bonding. When the body metabolizes synthetic amino acids, there is less nitrogen waste, because the need for polypeptide breakdown and excretion has been eliminated. These protein sources are known by many different trade names. Some examples of the hydrolysate solutions available are Hyprotigen, Amigen, and Aminosol. Synthetic amino acid solutions are currently available as Freamine, although other preparations will soon be released in the United States.

Preparations of total parenteral nutrition solutions are highly concentrated. Large amounts of energy calories, usually in the form of dextrose, are combined with the nitrogen source. This aspect of solution content is very important. To spare the supplied protein for protein synthesis, a calorie–nitrogen ratio of 125 to 150 calories per gram of nitrogen is recommended. Solutions also contain a basic electrolyte and vitamin profile which is necessary for balanced nutrition. This requirement varies individually, depending upon each person's nutritional needs. Most patients in the Massachusetts General Hospital receive water-soluble vitamins daily and fat-soluble vitamins weekly.

Preparation

Because hyperalimentation solutions cannot be sterilized terminally (they "caramelize" if autoclaved), they should be prepared in the pharmacy with stringently controlled aseptic practice. Ideally the solutions should be mixed under a laminar flow hood by trained technicians, who are supervised by a clinical pharmacologist. The use of headgear, mask, and sterile gloves is desirable.

All additives should be placed in the dextrose–protein mixture at the time of initial mixing. The pharmacist should inspect the bottles adequately for turbidity, particulate matter, and cracks. The intravenous tubing should be inserted into the bottle under the laminar flow hood. These procedures should be done as close to the time of infusion as possible and not longer than 24 hours beforehand. Prepared solutions may be refrigerated until use. Of course, if this is done, it will become necessary to warm the solutions to room temperature before they are administered.

Many institutions cannot practice the ideal method of solution preparation just described. Some adaptations of technique are acceptable and others are not. It is acceptable to prepare the solutions in a clean environment, using a completely closed system. Commercially available solution kits are supplied with a closed transfer system of intravenous tubing to facilitate sterile preparation. When using McGaw parenteral fluids, additives should be placed through the latex diaphragm so that the vacuum is not broken. Prepared solutions must be sealed with a sterile occlusive cap. Mixture of these solutions should be done immediately prior to infusion.

The obvious need to be familiar with the necessary equipment prompts a reminder—directions for equipment use should be made available, posted, and understood by all who mix hyperalimentation solutions. Workshops that allow nurses and pharmacy technicians leisurely practice sessions with this equipment also are helpful.

It is not acceptable to have total parenteral nutrition solutions prepared by an inexperienced, untrained person. An unclean environment is also forbidden. Remember that an active nurses' station, a utility room or area proximal to the bedpan flusher, or even a clean, designated intravenous admixture area receiving a high-velocity breeze are unclean areas. It is easy to forget the principles of asepsis when one is busy. Solution contamination and admixture incompatibilities are easily possible when proper education in techniques and rules of preparation are not utilized.

At the Massachusetts General Hospital basic solution formulations are prepared with alternative solution mixtures. The alternative solutions contain additional salt, insulin, or decreased potassium, in any combination. Additional modifications are made by the placement of additives, in the clinical area, immediately before infusion [9]. Only the highly skilled intravenous nursing team is allowed to do this. Tailor-made solutions for each patient would be ideal, but this is not possible owing to the large volume of patients in the hospital.

Administration

Total parenteral nutrition solutions are highly concentrated and usually contain 20 to 27 percent dextrose. These hypertonic, hyperosmolar solutions must be delivered into a blood vessel of wide diameter so that they may be rapidly diluted before reaching the peripheral circulation. The only veins acceptable for the catheter tip are the superior vena cava, the innominate vein, and the intrathoracic subclavian vein. The ideal location for the catheter tip is the middle of the superior vena cava.

Early attempts to administer total parenteral nutrition solutions often employed the brachial approach to a central vein. The 24-inch long catheters used frequently irritated the vein wall, causing painful thrombophlebitis. Arm veins are narrow and the walls of these veins often do not tolerate long-term catheterization. The approach of choice, then, to the superior vena cava is percutaneously, via the subclavian or internal jugular vein. These vessels are close to the superior vena cava and require only an 8- to 12-inch catheter. The external jugular vein is usually too narrow for easy catheterization.

Catheter Insertion

Patient Considerations

Before the subclavian vein catheterization procedure is begun, the nurse should explain to the patient what is about to occur. Proper teaching beforehand seems to increase patient tolerance and markedly decrease the actual level of pain experienced during the procedure. Patients seem to appreciate knowing beforehand:

1. That they will be placed in Trendelenburg position. ["We will place you in a head-down position. This is so that the doctor can find your vein easily, because it fills up more when you are in this position."]

2. That the doctor will be wearing a mask, gown, and gloves and that all personnel at the head of the bed will also wear a mask. ["We want to prevent infection so we are very careful not to give you any of our germs. We all have some bacteria naturally occurring in our mouths, you know, and wearing masks is a clean way to go about this procedure. It's quite routine."]

3. That they will be draped surgically. ["For the same reason that we all wear masks and the surgeon wears a gown and gloves, sterile towels (about the size of dishcloths) will be placed around the area where the catheter is to be inserted. Your face will be turned away and loosely covered, but you will be able to breathe normally and see."]

4. That the physician will place a short towel roll beneath the cervical vertebrae to hyperextend the neck and elevate the clavicles. ["This raises your shoulder blades and puts them out of the way for the doctor. When he places the needle beneath your collarbone (clavicle) to puncture the vein, he needs your shoulders up. It's easier for you to be supported than to try keeping your neck arched and shoulders up for the whole time by yourself."]

5. That they will be washed with acetone, iodine, and alcohol with surgical technique. ["The doctor will wash you with some strange-smelling solutions. He applies these solutions by using large gauze pads held with a pair of tongs. The solutions are acetone, iodine, and alcohol, but if you didn't know this, you could imagine that the acetone is ether! It's not; it's just one of the three solutions we use to really clean the area."]

6. That the anesthetic will be administered a few minutes ahead of time and will probably hurt. ["The doctor will give you an injection of Xylocaine. That's a lot like the Novocain your dentist uses. It will help to numb your shoulder. A lot of patients have said that this is the most unpleasant part of the whole procedure—that the Xylocaine stings, sort of like a bee sting, until it starts to work."]

7. That the search for the subclavian vein produces a bizarre sensation, causing a lot of pressure, if not pain. ["Now, when the doctor searches for your vein with the needle, you will have been given Xylocaine, but you'll probably feel a strange sensation, sort of a pressure, inside your chest. Everybody feels this, there's nothing wrong. It's just a new experience to have anything from outside of you inside of your chest."]

When this teaching is done in a calm, matter-of-fact way, it usually results in an atraumatic experience for the patient. When it is not done, consider that the patient is experiencing something totally foreign which he cannot anticipate. Also realize that it would be quite possible to fantasize that one were having emergency surgery performed without warning, "right in my own bed!" The acetone smells like ether, and the surgeon is dressed as he is in the operating room. He uses drapes and instruments. He is assisted by a nurse who watches his every move intently. The procedure is easily misinterpreted. Elicit feedback from the patient as you teach, so that you may be able to determine if he understands what is about to happen and if he has great fear.

The patient also appreciates knowing that only a very thin tubing ["about one-third as thin as regular intravenous tubing"—and demonstrate this] remains inside him, and that the needle is removed immediately. He wonders about catheter removal and is relieved to know that this is a quick, simple, and painless procedure. ["It's not anything like having the catheter inserted; we just snip one suture, outside you, and slide the little tubing out."]

If the patient seems to be especially apprehensive, even after the preinsertion teaching has been done, suggest the use of an analgesic or psychotropic medication to the physician.

If possible, hold the patient's hand during the procedure. If the nurse is familiar with the equipment and has set up everything ahead of time, she is free to support the patient while the physician places the catheter.

It is a nursing responsibility to take an active role in sterile technique. This means that if a glove is contaminated, offer the physician another pair of gloves, rather than hope he will notice that he has contaminated the first pair. The procedure is either sterile or unsterile. Nurses should feel responsibility for maintaining asepsis in order to protect their patients.

The intracatheter is placed in a standard fashion. When the needle is open to the air, as the catheter is threaded, the patient is asked to perform the Valsalva maneuver (forced expiration with a closed glottis). This maneuver is a precaution against air embolism and is easily accomplished by instructing the patient to "bear down with your mouth closed." If the patient is unable to do this, the nurse may produce the Valsalva maneuver by compressing the patient's abdomen or by carefully maintaining inspiration with an Ambu bag for 3 to 5 seconds.

After the catheter is placed, the needle is withdrawn and its point is covered with a plastic needle guard to prevent accidental puncture of the external catheter tubing. One suture is placed at the catheter insertion site. This prevents in-and-out motion of the catheter, which could introduce skin organisms into the puncture wound, and also prevents accidental catheter dislodgment. This procedure should be performed only by an experienced physician. Since there are potential complications associated with this procedure and since it is uncomfortable at best, repeated unsuccessful attempts to catheterize a specific vessel are unjustified.

Immediate Postcatheterization Management

After the catheter has been sutured, the routine dressing is applied (this will be described later in detail). A chest roentgenogram is taken immediately. An isotonic solution should be infused at a slow keep-open (10 to 20 ml per hour) rate until the chest x-ray film confirms central venous location [7]. It is nursing responsibility at the Massachusetts General Hospital to receive and document the initial chest x-ray wet reading. If the catheter tip is located in the superior vena cava, innominate, or intrathoracic subclavian vein, a hypertonic infusion such as 20 percent dextrose is usually begun until the first bottle of hyperalimentation solution is available.

It is unacceptable to have the catheter tip located in the atrium or ventricle or in an extrathoracic vessel or the inferior vena cava. Atrial rupture, valvular damage, myocardial irritability, and cardiac tamponade are possible and have been reported when catheter tips are located in the heart. Extrathoracic veins are too narrow to dilute hypertonic solutions and will become sclerosed if used for hyperalimentation. Although the inferior vena cava has a wide diameter, its use is contraindicated because it has been associated with catheter-induced thrombosis and occlusion [5].

Technical Complications

Although complications are infrequent, placement of a subclavian catheter can be followed by devastating events. Because of this possibility, the nurse should carefully observe the patient for signs of respiratory distress, pain, a slowly increasing hematoma, or *any unexplainable symptom*. Some of the possible complications following a subclavian puncture are listed below [5, 6, 10].

PNEUMOTHORAX. The pleura is near the subclavian vein and may be punctured. Diagnosis is made by clinical signs and symptoms (sharp chest pain and decreased breath sounds) and by x-ray films. Treatment is symptomatic. Sometimes a chest tube is indicated, although smaller pneumothoraces often resolve spontaneously.

HEMOTHORAX. The subclavian vein or adjacent vessels may be traumatized during the needle puncture. Slow, constant bleeding into the thorax from these leaking vessels is possible. Symptoms and treatment are as for pneumothorax.

HYDROTHORAX. The catheter may transect the vein and rest freely in the thorax. If this is the case, intravenous solutions will be infused directly into the chest. Symptoms and treatment are as for pneumothorax.

INADVERTENT ARTERIAL PUNCTURE. It is possible to enter an artery during attempted venipuncture. This is not a problem when clinically observed and treated immediately. Measurement of arterial blood gases is commonly performed in hospitals today. After a puncture, arteries must receive direct pressure for at least 5 full minutes in order to stop bleeding. If the patient has a bleeding disorder or platelet abnormality, direct pressure must be applied for an even longer period of time. Therefore, one must be on the alert for a rapidly expanding hematoma, signs and symptoms of tracheal compression, or respiratory distress, or a combination of these. If these symptoms occur, direct pressure is placed on the site and the physician is called immediately.

BRACHIAL PLEXUS INJURY. Tingling sensation of the fingers, pain shooting down the arm, or paralysis may indicate brachial plexus injury. This is a rare complication of subclavian puncture. The treatment is symptomatic and may not always resolve the injury. Physical therapy is indicated for paralysis.

THORACIC DUCT INJURY (CHYLOTHORAX). The thoracic duct is enlarged in cirrhotic patients owing to alterations in lymph flow. Therefore it is more easily entered, accidentally, during catheter placement. A left-sided subclavian puncture should be avoided in cirrhotic patients.

SHEARED CATHETER WITH DISTAL EMBOLIZATION. Although this is the physician's responsibility, it is mentioned here because it may be prevented by active nursing intervention. When the needle is internal and the catheter is being threaded, *the catheter should not be pulled back for redirection.* The entire unit is removed and a new catheter set is utilized for insertion. If the catheter pulls back against the needle, it may shear off and travel in the circulatory system. In such cases, cardiac catheterization, with snaring of the catheter embolus under fluoroscopic control, may be necessary [4].

Dressing Change Procedures

The procedure we follow at the Massachusetts General Hospital in changing dressings is one of many that are considered safe and acceptable [14]. It is based on the procedure Dudrick found effective [10]. Other ways of changing dressings also maintain the principles of infection control. The dressing change procedure is also illustrated for increased clarity.

A kit prepared by the Central Service Department is brought to the bedside and opened immediately before use. The use of prepackaged kits is efficient; it eliminates collecting and preparing material in an unclean area and automatically provides the correct equipment in a standard fashion. If procedural instructions are enclosed in the kits, the additional advantage of a teaching tool is also afforded.

Bottles of acetone, tincture of iodine and alcohol, and a spray container of tincture of benzoin are also brought to the bedside. The bedside table is cleansed with an antiseptic solution. The nurse puts on a mask and washes her hands before beginning. If it will not compromise his respiratory function, the patient also wears a mask. This decreases exposure of the catheter insertion site to the normal flora of the respiratory tract, not to mention the pathogens that may be present in an infected respiratory tract.

The nurse first prepares the catheter insertion site with acetone, a defatting agent. It should be applied repeatedly until the prepping sponges are free of debris. The next prepping solution is iodine. It is used because of its antifungal as well as antibacterial properties. It is applied for 2 minutes, timed by a watch, and allowed to air dry before removal. This facilitates absorption. Next, alcohol completes the defatting process and also removes the iodine. Alcohol should be applied until all the iodine is removed. If left on the skin, iodine may cause a skin irritation or burn. The alcohol should be allowed to air dry naturally (without fanning or blotting).

The method of prepping should emphasize the "clean-to-dirty" technique (see Figure 30). Instruments and gloves are used to prepare the area in concentric circles, beginning at the catheter insertion site and moving out to the periphery (see Figure 31). One should never return to the center with a sponge that has touched the periphery. If the brand of intracatheter which has a fixed needle and needle guard is being used, careful attention is given to cleaning the catheter of all foreign bodies attached to it.

Topical antibacterial and antifungal ointment is applied to the catheter insertion site and part way down the catheter, usually about 2 cm (see Figure 32). The insertion site is covered with two small gauze sponges; the needle (or part of the intracatheter) is left partially uncovered. The exposed skin is sprayed with tincture of benzoin (see Figure 33); this is allowed to dry partially, until it becomes tacky. Benzoin toughens the skin and prevents breakdown of tissue. Some catheters are left in for a long time; even with dressing changes every 48 hours, there will be little trouble with skin irritation if benzoin has been applied.

An elasticized adhesive bandage is cut in such a way that the part that will be placed over the sterile gauze bandage is not touched (see Figure 34). It is placed over the sponges in an air-occlusive fashion and the edges are sealed with adhesive tape. The bandage and tape are from unused rolls; the outer edges are discarded and they are not cut ahead of time (e.g., attached to the bedside table or intravenous pole). This is the cleanest way to handle unsterile, aseptic equipment.

A slit piece of tape is placed up under the catheter hub (see Figure 35). It helps ensure air occlusion and allows the nurse easy access to the hub when she changes the intravenous tubing each evening. All tubing junctions are firmly sealed with adhesive tape to prevent accidental tubing and catheter separation (see Figure 36). The intravenous filter is anchored to the dressing; this prevents traction on the catheter insertion site (see Figures 37 and 38).

The hyperalimentation dressing is changed every 48 hours, or more frequently if necessary. The dressing is changed immediately if it becomes contaminated or wet. If the seal is broken, the dressing should

193

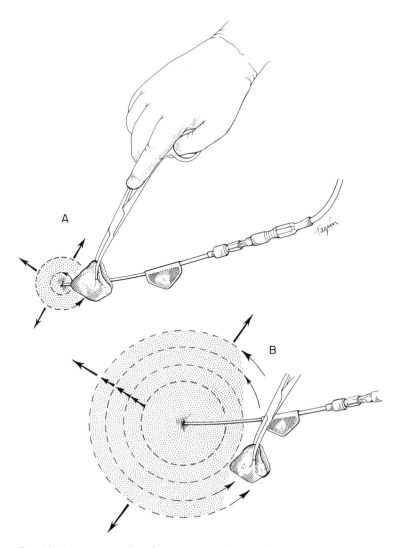

Fig. 30. Preparation of catheter site for change of dressing. Antiseptic solution is applied in concentric circles, starting at the site of catheter insertion and moving out toward the periphery ("clean-to-dirty" technique).

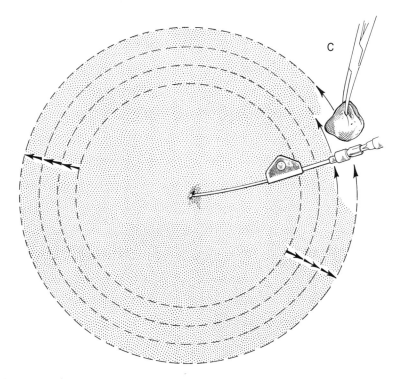

Fig. 31. The prepared area of the catheter site extends to the middle of the catheter hub.

not be reinforced; it should be changed. If the patient has a draining wound or is in a high-humidity area (such as that caused by an oxygen face tent), or if the bandage is likely to become wet for any reason, the dressing is waterproofed. Sterile plastic drapes, similar to those used in the operating room, are used to waterproof these dressings. The drape is simply placed over the completed dressing. When this special drape is used, paper tape, rather than adhesive, must join the catheter hub and intravenous tubing junction. When adhesive tape is stuck onto a plastic drape, it tears a hole which breaks the seal at tubing change time.

When the procedure is completed, the nurse writes a note in the patient's chart. Any relevant condition is mentioned and the appropriate plan of care is recorded. If erythema, edema, skin ulceration, or drainage exists, action must be taken immediately. Occasionally skin irritation subsides when application of a sterile, nonallergic adhesive bandage is substituted for the usual elasticized adhesive. If skin ulceration or drainage exists, the physician should order appropriate cultures and remove the catheter immediately.

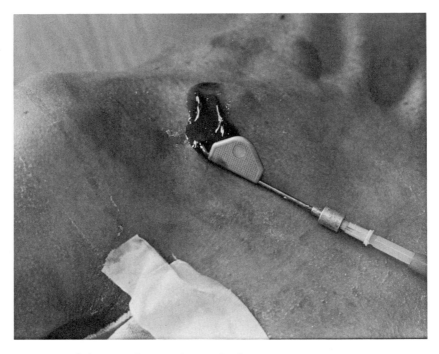

Fig. 32. A subclavian catheter with topical iodophor ointment.

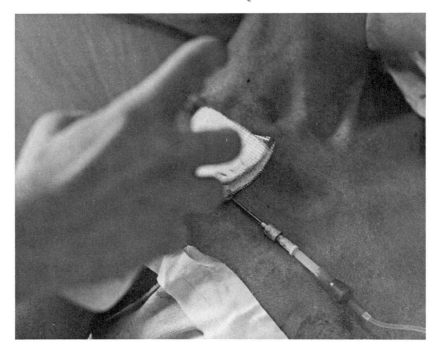

Fig. 33. The catheter insertion site is covered with two small gauze sponges. The needle (or part of the intracatheter) is left partially uncovered. The surrounding skin is being sprayed with tincture of benzoin.

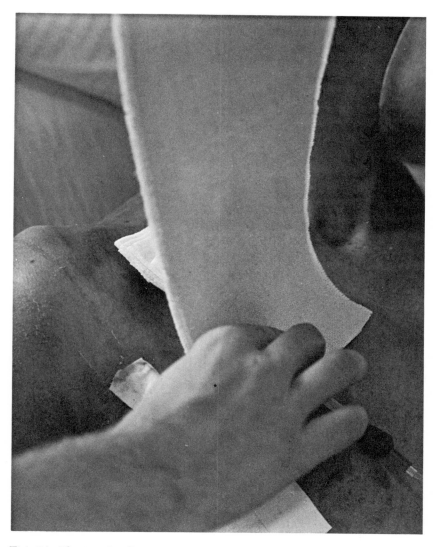

Fig. 34. Elasticized adhesive bandage is placed over the sponges in an air-occlusive fashion.

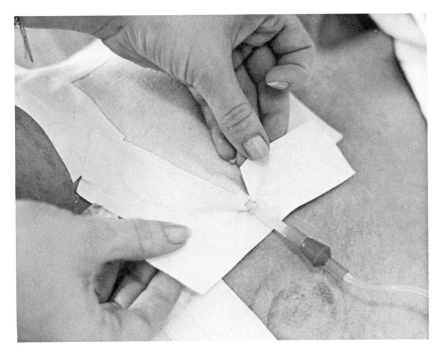

Fig. 35. Adhesive tape placed on the edges of the elasticized bandage and a slit piece of tape placed up under the catheter hub helps ensure air occlusion.

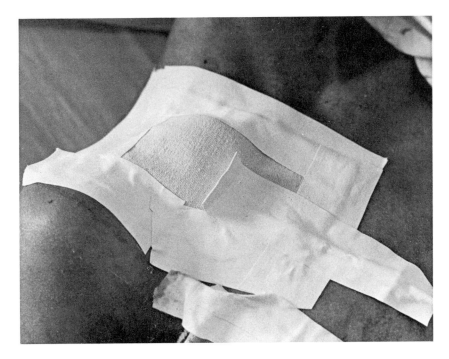

Fig. 36. All tubing junctions are firmly sealed with adhesive tape to prevent accidental separation of tubing and catheter.

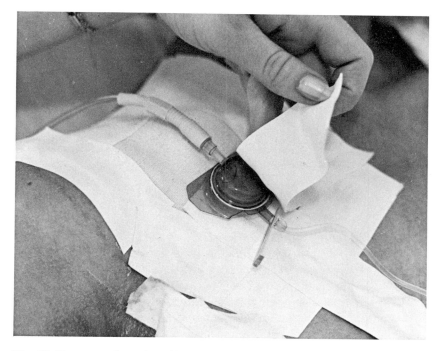

Fig. 37. Tape securely anchors filter. (Micropore filter, Travenol Laboratories, Inc., Morton Grove, Ill.)

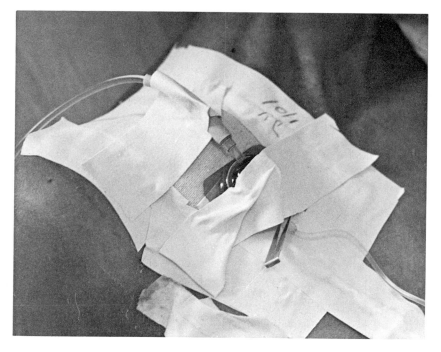

Fig. 38. Complete dressing of a subclavian catheter. Note the inscription of date the dressing has been changed.

Certification

All nurses at the Massachusetts General Hospital may apply these dressings, but only after they have been "certified." After each nurse has witnessed a dressing change, read the hyperalimentation literature, and attended an orientation session, she then performs a dressing change under the supervision of one of the hyperalimentation nurses or her chosen delegate. The nurse achieves certification when she has performed the procedure satisfactorily. Some physicians feel strongly that all dressing changes should be done by one or two hyperalimentation nurses. This does seem desirable whenever possible. When it is impossible, a method of certification may be helpful in ensuring rigidly controlled, standardized care.

Intravenous Tubing and Filter Change

The intravenous tubing is changed at least every 24 hours, preferably on a standardized time basis. We have standardized the time of tubing, filter, and bottle change at 6 P.M. each evening. At this time, the current day's supply expires and new solutions have arrived in the clinical area. By changing the tubing and filter along with the new bottles, an additional break in the line is eliminated.

If a filter is used, its porosity should be 0.45 micron or less. This size will trap most bacteria, fungi, and particulate matter. The method of filling the filter varies with different brands. Directions should be carefully read so that all goes smoothly at the time of tubing change.

It cannot be overemphasized that contamination is easily possible when intravenous tubing is changed. Extreme precautions should be taken in order to prevent this. A method of tubing change we have found helpful is to gently grasp the intracatheter hub (using a clamp for leverage), carefully rotate out the used intravenous tubing, and quickly replace this with the new tubing. If the tubing has touched anything other than the inside of the catheter hub, it is contaminated. If the nurse has difficulty in changing the intravenous tubing, a small sterile sponge placed beneath the catheter hub helps to prevent accidental contamination of the intravenous tubing. This is a small but very important aspect of asepsis in the care of these patients.

During intravenous tubing change, the patient should be flat in bed. When the catheter is open to the air, he should perform the Valsalva maneuver. Both of these conditions enhance positive pressure of the central vessels, decreasing the chance of accidental air embolism.

Other Aspects of Infection Control

Nutritional intravenous lines are placed specifically for hyperalimentation. At the Massachusetts General Hospital nurses infuse total parenteral nutrition solutions only through a new catheter placed specifically for these solutions. The nutritional intravenous system is used for nothing but hyperalimentation. It is not used for central venous pressure monitoring, withdrawal of blood for testing purposes, "piggyback" infusions of medication, or intravenous bolus injection of drugs [7].

Nurses play an important role here because they are often the first to witness a violation in the use of the catheter. Violations render the catheter unacceptable for hyperalimentation. At the Massachusetts General Hospital a method of surveillance has been initiated which encourages staff nurses to call the Hyperalimentation Unit and report any such violations. The physicians in the Hyperalimentation Unit then rule that the catheter is unacceptable for administration of nutrient solutions. This method of watchfulness seems to encourage inviolate catheters and has worked fairly well. If one attempts such a method of surveillance, it is important to tell the persons involved that this is not a name-calling issue, that it is of primary importance for patient safety, and that sources of information are anonymous.

Teaching programs in the Massachusetts General Hospital constantly remind the staff that hyperalimentation patients are very susceptible to infection, especially *Candida* septicemia. This reminder keeps the general level of awareness high. Every few months there is a Hyperalimentation Workshop, which is an 8-hour day devoted to these principles of care. Many nurses from outside hospitals also attend these staff education programs. Infection control is one of the primary topics of the lectures by physicians, pharmacists, and nurses. The Infection Control Team at the Massachusetts General Hospital participates in the workshops and in the daily surveillance which is necessary for these patients. The importance of prevention is given particular emphasis; the physicians and nurse epidemiologists are involved clinically and academically for the benefit of the patient.

A study of 200 patients at Massachusetts General Hospital [18] demonstrated that when routine standards of catheter care were practiced by general-duty nurses and staff physicians the catheter infection rate was 3 percent. On the other hand, in patients whose catheter care did not follow the standard protocol, the catheter infection rate was 20 percent, or seven times greater. This finding is statistically significant. It demonstrates that nursing care greatly influences the safety of this technique.

Unexplained fever necessitates immediate attention. Initially a temperature elevation should be dealt with by discontinuing the solution, tubing, and filter. A physical history, examination, and fever work-up should also be instituted. If the source of temperature elevation becomes obvious and is other than the hyperalimentation system, therapy may be resumed. If the cause of temperature elevation is unknown and the patient becomes afebrile, hyperalimentation may be cautiously resumed.

If a fever of unknown origin persists or recurs, the catheter must be removed and cultured. Total parenteral nutrition should never be administered to a patient with a fever of unknown origin. Unrecognized catheter-induced septicemia is a dangerous possibility [7, 13, 18]. Because fungal septicemia is a special danger of total parenteral nutrition therapy, all specimens sent for culture should be marked with clear instructions requesting fungal studies.

Metabolic Considerations

Body response to glucose varies. In most adults the rate of glucose utilization reaches its maximum at 0.8 to 1.0 gm of glucose per kilogram of body weight. This means that most patients can tolerate constant intravenous infusion of the large glucose load found in hyperalimentation solutions. As the highly concentrated glucose infusion is initiated, a pancreatic response to the elevated serum glucose level occurs. Increased serum insulin levels are found in patients receiving total parenteral nutrition therapy if causes of glucose intolerance are not a clinical entity in the patient's diagnosis [17]. Initial infusions of the hyperosmolar nutrient should begin slowly, usually at a rate of 60 to 80 ml per hour in the adult of average weight. A gradual increase in flow rate allows time for the pancreas to establish and maintain the elevated serum insulin levels which correlate with the amount of glucose being infused.

This response to large amounts of intravenous glucose is compromised by sepsis, stress, shock, hepatic and renal failure, starvation, diabetes, pancreatic disease, and administration of certain catabolic drugs (especially steroids). When these conditions exist, administration of exogenous insulin often is necessary. Conversely, when the patient's illness induces a hypermetabolic state, and daily caloric utilization is accelerated, glucose tolerance often exceeds 0.8 to 1.0 gm per kilogram per hour [17].

Urinary Glucose Measurement

Urine should be tested for sugar and acetone content every 6 hours, around the clock [7]. During the initial period of hyperalimentation, as glucose tolerance becomes established, it is not unusual for sugar to "spill" into the urine.

Glycosuria should not be allowed to persist without clinical evaluation and treatment. Until elevated serum insulin levels are established, a urine spill of 2^+ (or less) usually is not alarming. Urinary sugar content greater than 2^+ requires a serum glucose test to determine the exact concentration of sugar present. Because 4^+ urinary sugar is an open-ended value, the serum glucose level should be measured immediately whenever this condition exists.

Treatment is directed to the cause of the glucose intolerance. Many patients require a reduction in initial infusion rates and then proceed to establish a level of glucose tolerance which never requires exogenous insulin during hyperalimentation therapy. Others require periodic administration of insulin, provided as needed, during the initial few days of therapy.

Glycosuria with a normal serum glucose level may exist secondary to hypokalemia. Potassium is utilized during glucose metabolism. As tissue mass breaks down, which is often the case in chronically depleted hyperalimentation patients, potassium leaves the intracellular compartment. Intracellular potassium depletion leads to decreased renal excretion of this cation as the body attempts to conserve it. If hypokalemia coexists with decreased urinary potassium levels (and renal function is normal), more potassium is needed in the intravenous diet [13].

The nurse should bear in mind that certain drugs render a false-positive result when urinary sugar test tablets (e.g., Clinitest*) are used. Cephalosporins, acetylsalicylic acid, or other reducing agents also may give a false-positive result. When a patient is receiving these drugs, it is advisable to use a glucose-specific indicator, e.g., Tes-Tape.†

Urinary sugar measurements are continued every 6 hours throughout the therapy. A patient who has established adequate glucose levels may at any time become glucose intolerant because of the previously mentioned conditions. Without this testing, hyperglycemia could exist undetected. Serum glucose levels should be determined daily until the maintenance flow rate has been achieved, and twice a week thereafter.

Insulin Administration

When exogenous insulin is required, the dosage may be based on the urinary sugar level. This, of course, presupposes that the physician has determined the patient's renal threshold and knows the serum correlate for the particular level of glycosuria. Some forms of renal disease (e.g., acute tubular necrosis) render urinary glucose measurements meaningless as indicators of serum glucose levels. A person with acute tubular necrosis could have a blood glucose level over 1000 mg per 100 ml and yield a negative urinary sugar test.

Regular insulin may also be added directly to the hyperalimentation solution. Contrary to published reports, it does not stick to the glass of the hyperalimentation intravenous bottle, because the insulin is bound

* Ames Company, Elkhart, Ind.
† Lilly and Company, Eli, Indianapolis, Ind.

to the protein [8]. Many physicians prefer this method of insulin administration because it provides a more constant serum insulin level than does periodic subcutaneous administration.

Flow Rates

Total parenteral nutrition solutions must be infused at a *constant rate*, around the clock. The flow rate must be checked at least every 30 minutes and *reset to the rate ordered*, as necessary. Too rapid infusion of these highly concentrated dextrose solutions can cause a hyperglycemic reaction. The flow rate should not be adjusted to make up for past losses or excesses, but always should be reset to the rate ordered. It is helpful to mark the bottle in hourly time allotments of prescribed fluid volume. When this is done, the nurse can easily see whether the patient is off schedule in administration of fluids.

When fluids are administered by gravity drip, a double clamping system fixed to the intravenous tubing provides increased patient protection. After the regular intravenous clamp is set, a second clamp is applied to function as a safeguard in case the first one fails.

It is both safer and more accurate to infuse these solutions via a mechanical device. There are many varieties of infusion apparatus commercially available. Use of a machine that delivers a prescribed volume of fluid, as opposed to one which delivers a prescribed number of drops, eliminates the frequent necessity for readjustment (of the machine) which occurs as drop size changes. Although infusion machines sometimes cause a patient to feel less mobile, they are a great help in preventing accidental fluid overload and in consistently delivering the exact amount of solution prescribed.

Accurate Charting

Accurate daily weights, measured at the same time of day, with the same clothing, are important. The intake and output sheets should also be scrupulously maintained. Without these data, it is extremely difficult for the physician to calculate and prescribe the proper nutritional needs of his patient.

Hypoglycemia

Blood sugar levels less than 50 mg per 100 ml chemically define hypoglycemia. Many patients are asymptomatic at this level and are identified only during routine blood chemistry studies. If a patient complains of weakness, headache, chills, hunger, or apprehension or all of these, he may be manifesting initial signs of hypoglycemia. Other symptoms are diaphoresis, decreased levels of consciousness, and changes in vital signs. Hypoglycemia can progress to a seizure disorder if untreated.

Treatment depends on the cause. Hypoglycemia often occurs in the total parenteral nutrition patient whose glucose infusion has been abruptly decreased or terminated. After solution flow interruption, serum insulin levels remain elevated longer than serum glucose levels, and this leads to an insulin rebound phenomenon. Frequently a catheter becomes kinked beneath the bandage, decreasing the flow rate. If a patient unknowingly kinks the intravenous tubing during a position change, the flow rate will decrease and may even stop. This can add the complication of a clotted catheter (which necessitates catheter change) to the hypoglycemic reaction.

When a patient is transported to another area of the hospital (e.g., for testing), it is important to ensure continuity of solution flow rate. If a nurse cannot accompany the patient and he is unable to time and reset his own hyperalimentation fluid, the nursing personnel in the area of destination should be alerted so that they may check and adjust the rate. Remember that this is not "just another IV"; if no one is able to assume responsibility for the patient's flow rate, it is unfair to send the patient out of his clinical area. Another possibility would be use of a battery-operated flow regulator, if one is available.

Hyperglycemia and Hyperosmolarity

When the body's ability to metabolize the glucose content of total parenteral nutrition solutions is inadequate, hyperglycemia occurs. Initial glucose intolerance has been discussed. However, hyperglycemia may progress to serious proportions in these patients. Osmotic diuresis causing dehydration of the central nervous system and coma is possible if severely elevated serum glucose levels are allowed to persist untreated. This happens because the renal threshold for sugar is exceeded and the elevated serum glucose levels act as an osmotic diuretic. Metabolic imbalance is also caused by this serum hyperosmolarity; during the diuresis, the metabolic derangement is exacerbated as molecules of sodium, potassium, and chloride are excreted.

Psychological Aspects

Until the 1960s, when Dudrick began hyperalimenting patients, no one survived for long periods of time without a functioning gastrointestinal tract. To the psychologically oriented, this uncharted territory of experience tempts exploration. What is it like to gain weight and lose one's appetite without ever swallowing a morsel of food? The analytical aspects of oral deprivation are intriguing to theorize about, and some clinicians have begun this exploration already [12].

For our purposes, more practical considerations are relevant. There are elements of emotional support that seem basic and necessary to the person receiving total parenteral nutrition [10]. None of the following is presented as absolute fact, but is the experience of a nurse who has known more than 1200 patients receiving hyperalimentation therapy. The needs of these patients, as they have expressed them to their care-takers, make the following issues more than esoteric considerations; they point the way toward a plan of care which should decrease the patient's anxiety and allay sometimes terrifying fears.

Hallucinations of taste and smell have been reported by hyperalimentation patients. As the period of "nothing by mouth" becomes prolonged, this phenomenon seems to increase. Television commercials, daydreams, a roommate's tray, or even simple conversations about food have all been stimuli which triggered this experience. We noticed it so often that we began to tell the patients it is not unusual to imagine one tastes, smells, or even sees food while undergoing hyperalimentation therapy. Although it is unclear why this happens, we know that many patients breathe a sigh of relief after being told that somewhat bizarre perceptions are not unusual. Often they have already experienced this and were worried that something was terribly wrong with them.

Undue preoccupation with food is not relegated totally to unconscious stimuli. Patients think about all kinds of things: "Will I be able to eat again?" "If my appetite's gone, why do I still miss food?" "How can they really be sure they are giving me the right diet, with nothing missing?" We do not make intense drama of all of this, but we are ever alert to the mention of food. It is important to the patient receiving total parenteral nutrition that he be supported and reassured. He needs to know that hyperalimentation therapy is not irreversible; that in fact as soon as physical conditions permit, he may begin to eat while still undergoing therapy.

Many patients become angry or sleepy at mealtime. It is considerate to locate the patient's room away from the kitchen, if possible. The aroma and observation of dozens of meals is often frustrating to one who cannot eat! Some patients have related impulses to leap out of bed and grab another patient's meal. Again, this happened often enough that we now tell patients (in a calm, pleasant fashion) that others have felt this way and they might also.

When we began these reassurances, it was with trepidation. There is always the possibility that direct suggestion will put ideas into a person's head. It has been striking to us that we have not witnessed this. A spontaneous smile of relief and a sheepish admission have often told us that we were describing an ongoing experience within the patient as we chatted about this intriguing psychodynamic process.

Because the therapy is still new in many hospitals, a great deal of teaching occurs at the bedside. Patients become aware that something special is happening to them. Quite often a hyperalimentation team of hospital personnel visit them; this enhances their feelings of uniqueness. There is a tendency to be guarded and protective toward one's "lifeline," as the hyperalimentation catheter is often called. It is important to encourage as much ambulation as possible. As long as the tubing junctions are secured and the intravenous pole is freely mobile, patients may safely ambulate about the hospital. In fact, active exercise helps prevent the catabolic breakdown of lean tissue mass which often results from inactivity.

The absence of taste causes physical and psychological unpleasantness. Some of our patients have enjoyed flavored lip balms or a variety of mouth washes; this offers at least some experience of different taste sensations. One of our cancer patients had a pitcher of martinis at his bedside. He used this as a mouth rinse each afternoon and evening. This provided the man's family with an opportunity to mix their loved one his favorite cocktail, and it afforded the patient some semblance of his normal pleasurable routine.

In addition to considering the aesthetic gratification a variety of tastes will provide, the nurse should carefully plan for consistent, adequate mouth care. If the oral examination is overlooked or adequate mouth care is not provided, the NPO, often clinically starving patient is prone to suffer from parotitis; glossy tongue; inflamed, dry uncomfortable areas; and oral lesions.

Remember that these patients are already under a great deal of stress and that being deprived of food often adds to this stress. On the other hand, when the nurse has properly explained total nutrition by vein to the patient and his family, they are usually quite relieved to know that this aspect of care has not been ignored. In foreign countries and primitive societies, it is common practice for the family to carry food to a hospitalized relative. Here in the United States we often become so involved in highly technical therapy that we forget about this basic concern. It is quite usual, after a family teaching session, for a relative to remark, "Oh good, I couldn't figure out how he'd ever get well without getting enough food." This is so simple and logical, but until the 1960s and Dudrick's work, many patients did not get well, because they could not eat.

In summary, explanation, feedback for ascertaining whether one's message has been perceived as intended, reassurance, and careful planning help the patient receiving total parenteral nutrition enormously.

Burns

The hypermetabolic rate of a severely burned adult can exceed 10,000 calories per day just for basal metabolism. It is difficult for a healthy person to consume this many calories orally. Often the burned patient cannot ingest the caloric amount he needs to avoid catabolism. Complications of diarrhea often make tube feedings ineffective, and ileus makes use of the gastrointestinal tract impossible.

When it is necessary to hyperaliment the severely burned patient, stringent aseptic technique must be preserved [19]. These patients are acutely ill; normal host defenses are severely compromised. Sepsis is a dreaded complication of any burn patient's progress. Hyperalimentation is a calculated risk and should never be prescribed unless there is no alternative.

At the Massachusetts General Hospital each burn patient on total parenteral nutrition therapy receives a careful review by his primary physicians, his nurses, and the clinical pharmacologist. A personal care plan is devised specific to the individual patient's needs. This is necessary because quite often the total parenteral nutrition catheter must also be used for administering colloids, blood, antibiotics, and intravenous bolus drugs, and for monitoring central venous pressure. This practice is discouraged; but when it is necessary, the following considerations are relevant.

The choice of intravenous tubing for intermittent administration of solutions other than the nutrient infusion is determined by that which will stay fixed to the main-line intravenous line without constant insertion of needles into side-arm medication injection sites. The piggyback tubing should be inserted in a stringently sterile fashion and fixed permanently. Breaks in the system are made for bottle changes only. A Y-tube system is also advantageous because it affords two independent sources of infusion by a totally closed method.

Intravenous bolus drugs are administered through a side-arm medication injection site after vigorous scrubbing (of the injection site) with an antibacterial, antifungal solution which is allowed to air dry before needle penetration.

Compatibility of solutions and drugs should always be checked by the pharmacist. When incompatibilities prevent concurrent administration with total parenteral nutrition solution, the hyperalimentation fluid should be shut off, the tubing flushed, and the alternate infusion delivered. This is followed by another flush and resumption of the hyperalimentation. The hypertonic nutrient solution should never be shut off for greater than 1 hour in order to avoid rebound hypoglycemic shock; it is desirable to limit the shut-off time to a maximum of 30 minutes.

Central venous pressure monitoring may be done by the closed system described by Parsa [16]. This eliminates the need for an easily contaminated stopcock and does not require the open channel to room air seen with many manometers.

Because of the grave danger of sepsis in burn patients, frequent changes of intravenous catheters are necessary. Some clinicians experienced in the treatment of burn patients rotate lifeline catheter sites, removing the catheters as frequently as every 2 to 3 days. This decreases the chance of a catheter's seeding from circulating bacteria.

Hyperalimentation of burned patients presents a great challenge to the caretakers. When it is necessary, it is usually the difference between life and death for these patients, but it must be managed well.

Pediatrics

The highly specialized technique of total parenteral nutrition has fed many babies who were born prematurely and has supported others with intestinal anomalies or metabolic derangements from intractable diarrhea and malabsorption.

When infants and young children are hyperalimented, there are special considerations. Catheter placement is done in the operating room, where a jugular vein cut-down is performed. Silastic tubing is threaded into a central vessel, the opposite end is tunneled subcutaneously to a scalp exit site, and the initial cut-down is closed. An adapter that functions like a regular intracatheter hub is fed into the exposed catheter tubing.

A sterile iodophor ointment dressing is placed over the neck wound and changed daily until the wound heals. The scalp exit site is dressed much like that of the adult patient receiving total parenteral nutrition, although there are a few differences. After the skin is defatted with acetone, iodophor solution is applied for 2 minutes and left on. After the solution has dried completely, small gauze sponges are placed over the catheter exit site and a sterile plastic drape is applied to occlude the area totally.

The catheter tubing is also treated differently. A small amount, about 2 inches, is coiled beneath the gauze sponges at the scalp exit site and at least 2 inches of the distal catheter is left external to the occlusive dressing. Both of these manipulations reduce tension on the catheter: although it is sutured subcutaneously, it could become dislodged. The same amount of catheter length should always be left exposed, to avoid contamination [5].

Administration of hypertonic dextrose is a delicate matter with small babies. Initial solution flow rates are often administered half-strength, in minute amounts. Frequent serum glucose measurements are necessary until metabolic tolerance is demonstrated. The flow rate is gradually increased until the desired hourly volume may be administered full-strength.

Because fluid overload is life threatening to small children, a positive pressure, constant infusion pump should always be used for parenteral nutrition administration. The apparatus must employ a totally closed system (some syringe pumps are exposed to room air and easily contaminated during intravenous administration). Use of positive pressure also avoids blood back flow, which is possible when a baby cries, reproducing Valsalva's maneuver. When positive pressure is used, an airlock filter is mandatory. Without the filter, if the bottle empties accidentally, some pumps will keep operating, introducing air into the central veins. However, this devastating event will not happen if the intravenous line contains a filter which blocks the passage of all air.

Infants, often not on a routine feeding schedule, miss regular intervals of being held while fed. It is important that the nurse be cognizant of the baby's need to be held and touched. Contact comfort (by holding) should be maintained and normal sensory stimulation provided, both by talking to the infant and by providing him with mobiles or toys. Sucking needs may be met with a pacifier, which often yields extra pleasure when moistened with juices. The infant's parents, of course, need reassurance and explanation so that they understand the therapy and do not feel isolated from their child.

Children in the other developmental stages also require specific considerations related to this treatment. The toddler's biggest fear is separation from his parents; keeping parents in close contact and comfortable with the hyperalimentation apparatus is important. The toddler is also concerned about immobility; although he is restrained because of the intravenous equipment he should be given time to move about under careful supervision. All explanations to this child should be brief, concrete, and given in his individual vocabulary in order to respect his limited concept formation and cognitive ability.

The preschool child is especially prone to fears of body mutilation and needs reassurance that intrusive apparatus, such as the catheter, and painful procedures (e.g., catheterization and dressing change), are not jeopardizing the safety of his body. Simple, truthful reassurance which is clearly stated, often decreases his anxiety, e.g., "When the I.V. tube comes out, we'll put a Band-Aid on you and you'll be all fixed up, as good as new." At this age, dramatic play is a very useful form of activity; for example, in doll play, the nurse can demonstrate procedures and the child can express his fears.

By the time a child has reached school age, his understanding of things has grown because of developing intellectual abilities. The school-age child is often stimulated by the challenge of a new treatment and wants to understand the reason for the hyperalimentation. He has usually heard about nutrition, basic food groups, and such things and benefits from the realization that this is a substitute. He should be encouraged to discuss his ideas. The treatment procedures should be done in a way that respects the child's need for personal privacy.

Adolescents receiving hyperalimentation therapy generally require the same explanations and support that the adult does. Because it is usual at this stage to test one's environment and to exhibit strong needs for recognition, consistency of care, respect shown through explanation and discussion which fosters free expression, and regard for personal privacy are all important. They have special meaning to the adolescent as he experiences a developing sense of identity. Adolescents often enjoy participation in their own care; it gives them a sense of control over what is happening to them. Testing of urine for sugar and acetone is an example of a simple, easily taught skill. This aspect of care could then become the adolescent's responsibility, under nursing supervision, of course [15].

Future Trends

Tailor-made amino acid diets are administered to children with inborn metabolic disorders. For children who cannot utilize their gastrointestinal tract, this method of feeding is, indeed, sophisticated total parenteral nutrition. As more is learned about amino acid deficiencies and more solutions with highly specific amino acid distributions become available, we will see more of this type of treatment.

An investigational solution containing essential amino acids and hypertonic dextrose was studied at Massachusetts General Hospital, with gratifying results. Improved survival of patients with acute renal failure was demonstrated in a double-blind clinical trial [1]. This solution is called *Renal Failure I.V. Diet;* basically it is an intravenous version of the oral Giordano-Giovannetti diet, which has been used for years in the therapy of renal failure. It should be available as Freamine-E* in the future.

Central venous feeding of hypertonic glucose solutions with protein, vitamins, trace elements, and electrolytes is the crude beginning of a new era in medicine. However, it still carries the risks of sepsis and metabolic imbalance with it, especially when not performed by highly skilled teams of practitioners (physicians, nurses, and pharmacists).

There will be other ways to avoid starvation while bypassing the gastrointestinal tract. Currently, European physicians are infusing isotonic fat solutions† peripherally. These solutions are emulsified soybean oil, and this treatment has resulted in success, while avoiding the risks of sepsis and metabolic imbalance. Intravenous fat administration is still being investigated in the United States and is not yet available commercially. Another peripheral form that is currently being in-

* McGaw Laboratories, Glendale, Calif.; division of American Hospital Supply Corporation.
† Intralipid (Vitrum, Stockholm, Sweden); Lipofundin (Braun, Melsungen, Germany).

vestigated involves administration of amino acids mixed with other carbohydrate-free fluids [11]. Theoretically this method of alimentation provides very few calories per day, decreases insulin levels, and mobilizes the body's own fat as an energy source [3]. Blackburn and Flatt reported that this "peripheral protein-sparing therapy" results in positive nitrogen balance. It certainly deserves consideration for the catabolic patient who is obese or who may be too great an infectious risk for central venous nutrition, or both. Other physicians are testing this principle now [2].

Nutritional biochemistry will yield many exciting discoveries in the future. It is to be hoped that these findings will be applied to clinical practice as methods of intravenous feeding become more sophisticated.

References

1. Abel, R. M., Clyde, H. B., Abbott, W. M., Ryan, J. A., Jr., Barnett, G. O., and Fischer, J. E. Improved survival from acute renal failure after treatment with intravenous essential L-amino acids and glucose. Results of a prospective, double-blind study. *New England Journal of Medicine* 288:695, 1973.
2. Blackburn, G. L., Flatt, J. P., Clowes, G. H. A., and O'Donnel, T. E. Peripheral intravenous feeding with isotonic amino acid solutions. *American Journal of Surgery* 125:447, 1973.
3. Blackburn, G. L., Flatt, J. P., and Hensle, T. E. Peripheral Amino Acid Infusions. In J. E. Fischer (Ed.), *Total Parenteral Nutrition*. In press.
4. Block, P. C. Transvenous retrieval of foreign bodies in the cardiac circulation. *Journal of the American Medical Association* 224:241, 1973.
5. Colley, R., and Phillips, K. Helping with hyperalimentation. *Nursing '73* July, 1973.
6. Dudrick, S. J., and Rhoads, J. E. Total intravenous feeding. *Scientific American* 226:73, 1972.
7. Fischer, J. E. *Guidelines for Care of Hyperalimentation Patients at the Massachusetts General Hospital.* Boston: Massachusetts General Hospital, 1974.
8. Giovanoni, R. Insulin Radioimmune Assay of Standard Hyperalimentation Formulation. In *Pharmacy Service Technical Information Bulletin.* Boston: Massachusetts General Hospital, October 1971.
9. Giovanoni, R. A suggested profile for selected total parenteral nutrition additives. *Clinical Medicine* 81:28–31, 1974.
10. Grant, J. N. Patient care in parenteral hyperalimentation. *Nursing Clinics of North America* 8:165, 1973.
11. Hoover, H. C., Jr., Grant, J., and Gorshbach, K. *Protein Sparing Intravenous Fluids in Postoperative Surgical Patients.* Bethesda, Md.: Surgery Branch, National Cancer Institute, National Institutes of Health, 1974.
12. Jordan, H. A., Moses, H., MacFayden, B. V., Jr., and Dudrick, S. J. Hunger and satiety in humans during parenteral hyperalimentation. *Psychosomatic Medicine* 36:144, 1974.
13. Kaminski, M. V., Jr. *Total Parenteral Nutrition (Hyperalimentation).*

Prevention and Treatment of Complications. A Policy and Procedure Manual. Washington, D.C.: Hyperalimentation Registry, Walter Reed General Hospital, November, 1972. (Revised Sept. 1974.)

14. Massachusetts General Hospital. *Nursing Procedure Manual.* Boston: Little, Brown, 1974.

15. Massachusetts General Hospital. *Pediatric Nursing Service Policy and Procedure Manual, Massachusetts General Hospital, Dept. of Nursing, Section III, Publications: Standards of Care of the Hospitalized Infant, Toddler, Pre School Child, School-Aged Child and Adolescent.* Boston, 1974.

16. Parsa, M. H., Ferrer, J. M., and Habif, D. V. *Safe and Sterile Maintenance of Long-Term Central Venous Catheters* (monograph). Presented at the 58th Annual Clinical Congress of the American College of Surgeons, San Francisco, Oct., 1972.

17. Ryan, J. A., Jr. Complications of Total Parenteral Nutrition: Etiology, Prevention and Treatment. In J. E. Fischer (Ed.), *Total Parenteral Nutrition.* Boston: Little, Brown. In press.

18. Ryan, J. A., Jr., Abel, R. M., Abbott, W. M., Hopkins, C. C., Chesney, T. M., Colley, R., Phillips, K., and Fischer, J. E. Catheter complications in total parenteral nutrition. *New England Journal of Medicine* 290:757, 1974.

19. Wilmore, D. W., and Pruitt, B. A., Jr. Parenteral Nutrition in Burn Patients. In J. E. Fischer (Ed.), *Total Parenteral Nutrition.* Boston: Little, Brown. In press.

14. Intravenous Administration of Drugs

Not so long ago the subcutaneous and the intramuscular routes were the preferred routes for the parenteral administration of drugs. With the success of and increase in intravenous therapy, the practice grew of including drugs in infusions. Today intravenous therapy is used extensively for drug administration.

Advantages
The venous route for drug administration offers pronounced advantages which are given below.

1. Some drugs cannot be absorbed by any other route; the large molecular size of some drugs prevents absorption by the gastrointestinal route, while other drugs, unstable in the presence of gastric juices, are destroyed.
2. Certain drugs, because of their irritating properties, cause pain and trauma when given by the intramuscular or subcutaneous route and must be given intravenously.
3. The vascular system affords a method for providing instant drug action.
4. The intravenous route offers a better control over the rate of administration of drugs; prolonged action can be provided by administering a dilute infusion intermittently or over a prolonged period of time.
5. The vascular route affords a route of administration for the patient who cannot tolerate fluids and drugs by the gastrointestinal route.
6. Slow intravenous administration of the drug permits termination of the infusion if sensitivity occurs.

Hazards
In spite of the advantages offered by the venous route, there are certain hazards which are not found in other forms of drug therapy.

1. Possibility of incompatibilities when one or more drugs are added to the intravenous solution
2. Speed shock (a systemic reaction to a substance rapidly injected into the bloodstream)
3. Vascular irritations and subsequent hazards
4. Rapid onset of action with inability to recall drug once it has entered the bloodstream

Incompatibilities

The number of possible drug combinations, provided by the ever-increasing production of drugs and parenteral fluids, is astronomical. With the increase in drug combinations comes an increase in potential incompatibilities. How and why incompatibilities occur and how best to avoid them are problems confronting all those involved in compounding intravenous additives. However well we know the chemical action of one group of drugs, our knowledge falls short when many groups are combined into complex compounds. The nurse, confronted with these problems, faces increased responsibility.

Many hospitals have set up pharmacy-centralized intravenous additive programs. This places the responsibility for prescription compounding with the department best qualified to assume it. The pharmacist is best able to predict or to detect incompatibilities and is alert to prescribed errors. The greater opportunity for sterility and accuracy when drugs are prepared in the pharmacy is obviously an advantage.

However, if such a pharmacy-centralized intravenous additive program is lacking, the responsibility is often left with the nurse. The pharmacist must be directly available, alerting her to possible chemical incompatibilities, communicating with various manufacturers on specific pharmaceutical problems, and providing information on certain drugs. An in-service program should be instituted, supplying an approved list of drugs for administration and acquainting the nurse with reactions, contraindications, dosage, stability, and compatibilities.

The individual who mixes and compounds intravenous drugs must be alert to the hazards of drug therapy. Since incompatibilities are a complication of prime consideration in the preparation of solutions, the nurse should have an acquaintance with the concepts involved in this hazard.

Compatibility charts are available but generally show only physical incompatibilities. Even chemical compatibility charts may be useless because of differences in the drug formation from one manufacturer to another or because of changes made by one manufacturer. The order of mixing drugs, the quantity of the drug and the solution, room temperature, and light contribute to incompatibilities not noted on the chart. Incompatibilities are not always obvious, as chemical changes may occur which do not produce a visible change.

Precipitation may occur when one or more drugs are added to parenteral solution [12]. It does not always occur at the time the solution is prepared, which increases the problem of intravenous administration. Some drugs, stable for a limited period of time, degrade and may or may not precipitate as they become less therapeutically active. If administered intravenously, solutions containing insoluble matter carry potential danger of embolism, myocardial damage, and effect on other organs such as the liver and the kidneys.

Chemical Interactions

The most common incompatibilities are the result of certain chemical reactions [12].

1. *Hydrolysis* is the process in which water absorption causes decomposition of a compound. In preparing solutions of salt, the nurse should understand that certain salts, when placed in water, hydrolyze, forming a very strong acid and a weak base, or a weak acid and a strong base. Since pH is a significant factor in the solubility of drugs, the increased acidity or alkalinity from hydrolysis of a salt may result in an incompatibility if another drug is added. *Example:* The acid salt sodium bicarbonate when placed in water hydrolyzes to form a strong alkali (sodium hydroxide) and a weak and unstable acid (carbonic acid). Many organic acids are known as weak acids since they ionize only slightly [9].

2. *Reduction* is the process whereby one or more atoms gain electrons at the expense of some other part of the system [4].

3. *Oxidation* is the corresponding loss of electrons occurring when reduction takes place. Antioxidants are often used as a preservative to prevent oxidation of a compound [4].

4. *Double decomposition* is the chemical reaction in which ions of two compounds change places and two new compounds are thus formed [9]. A great many salts act by double decomposition to form other salts and probably represent the largest number of incompatibilities. *Example:* Calcium chloride is incompatible with sodium bicarbonate; the double decomposition results in the formation of the insoluble salt calcium carbonate.

Classification of Incompatibilities

Incompatibilities may be divided into three categories:

1. *Therapeutic.* An undesirable reaction resulting from overlapping effects of two drugs given together or close together.

2. *Physical.* According to Endicott [5], "The term 'physical incompatibility' is somewhat misleading but has come to be accepted as a physical or chemical interaction between two or more ingredients which leads to a visible change in the mixture which can be readily observed." A visible change may not occur with many chemical reactions. The physical change may be [12]:

   a. Gas formation, such as occurs when carbonates are placed in acid. (Sodium bicarbonate in acid forms carbon dioxide gas.)
   b. Color change, such as occurs when riboflavin in vitamin B complex and methylene blue form a green color.
   c. Precipitation, occurring when compounds are insoluble. (Acid salts in alkali cause free base to precipitate; base salts in acid cause free acid to precipitate.)

3. *Chemical.* A chemical change is classified here as a change in drug compounds which is not readily observed. Since it may go undetected it has a greater capacity for causing biological effects.

pH and Its Role in Stability of Drugs

Since pH plays an important role in the solubility of drugs it may be well to define it. pH is the symbol for the degree of concentration of hydrogen ions or the acidity of the solution. The weight of hydrogen ions in 1 liter of pure water is 0.0000001 gm, which is numerically equal to 10^{-7}. For convenience, the negative logarithm 7 is used. Since it is at this concentration that the hydrogen ions balance the hydroxyl ions, a pH of 7 is neutral. Each unit decrease in pH represents a tenfold increase in hydrogen ions [9].

It appears likely that the largest number of incompatibilities may be produced by changes in pH [11]. Precipitation occurs when a compound is insoluble in solution. The degree of solubility often varies with the pH. A drastic change in the pH of a drug when added to an intravenous solution suggests an incompatibility or a decrease in stability. Solutions of a high pH appear to be incompatible with solutions of a low pH and may form insoluble free acids or free bases. A chart denoting the pH of certain drugs and certain solutions to be used as a vehicle is helpful in warning of potential incompatibilities.

FACTORS AFFECTING STABILITY OR PH. Many factors may affect the stability or pH of drugs:

1. *Parenteral solutions.* Some commonly prescribed drugs precipitate when added to intravenous solutions. Over ninety different infusion solutions, along with their pH, are listed by one company alone. Differences in the physical and chemical properties of each of these

solutions may affect the stability of any drug introduced. A compound soluble in one solution may precipitate in another. Sodium ampicillin deteriorates in acid solutions. This drug, when added to isotonic sodium chloride at a concentration of 30 mg per milliliter, loses less than 10 percent activity in 8 hours. However, when it is added to 5 percent dextrose in water, usually a more acid solution, its stability is reduced to a 4-hour period.

Another factor affecting the stability of drugs is the broad pH range (3.5 to 6.5) of dextrose solutions allowed by the United States Pharmacopeia (U.S.P.) "A drug may be stable in one bottle of dextrose 5 percent in water and not in another" [6].

2. *Additional drugs.* One drug may be compatible in a solution, but a second additive may alter the established pH to such an extent as to make the drugs unstable [10].

3. *Buffering agents in drugs.* An important consideration in the stability of drugs is the presence of buffers or antioxidants which may cause two drugs, however compatible, to precipitate. For example, ascorbic acid, the buffering component of tetracycline, lowers the pH of the product and therefore may accelerate the decomposition of a drug susceptible to an acid environment.

4. *Preservatives in the diluent.* Sterile diluents for reconstitution of drugs are available with or without a bacteriostatic agent. The bacteriostatic agents usually consist of parabens or phenol preservatives. Certain drugs, including nitrofurantoin, amphotericin B, and erythromycin, are incompatible with these preservatives and should be reconstituted with sterile water for injection.

5. *Degree of dilution.* Solubility often varies with the volume of solution in which a drug is introduced. For example, tetracycline HCl, mixed in a small volume of fluid, maintains its pH range over 24 hours. However, when added to a large volume (1 liter), it degrades after 12 hours, becoming less therapeutically active.

6. *Period of time solution stands.* Decomposition of substances in solution is proportional to the length of time they stand. For example, dextrose solutions are unstable when maintained in a neutral or basic environment. Therefore it is recommended that when bicarbonate is to be added to dextrose solutions, it be added immediately prior to use [7].

7. *Order of mixing.* The order in which drugs are added to infusions often determines their compatibility.

8. *Light.* Light may provide energy for chemical reactions to occur. Therefore certain drugs, such as amphotericin B and nitrofurantoin, once diluted must be protected from light [10].

9. *Room temperature.* Heat also provides energy for reactions. After reconstitution or initial dilution, refrigeration prolongs the stability of many drugs.

219

Vascular Irritation

The hazards of intravenous therapy can be reduced by adequate precautions (see Chapter 8).

Vascular irritation is a significant hazard of drugs intravenously administered. Any irritation that inflames and roughens the endothelial cells of the venous wall allows platelets to adhere; a thrombus is formed. Thrombophlebitis is the result of the sterile inflammation. When a thrombus occurs, there is always the inherent danger of embolism.

If aseptic technique is not strictly adhered to, septic thrombophlebitis may result from bacteria introduced through the infusion needle and trapped in the thrombus. This is much more serious, as it carries with it the potential dangers of septicemia and acute bacterial endocarditis.

Preventive Measures

The following precautions must be observed to diminish the potential hazards of vascular irritation:

1. Veins with ample blood volume should be selected when infusing hypertonic solutions or solutions containing irritating compounds.
2. The needle should be appreciably smaller than the lumen of the vein. A large needle may occlude the lumen, obstructing the flow of blood; the solution then flows undiluted, irritating the wall of the vein.
3. The venipuncture should be performed at the distal end of the extremity to allow each successive puncture to be executed proximal to the previous. Hypertonic solutions, when allowed to flow through a traumatized vein, cause increased irritation and pain.
4. Veins in the lower extremities are prone to trauma and should be avoided.
5. Isotonic solutions should, when possible, follow hypertonic solutions to wash irritating substances from the veins.
6. The rate of infusion may contribute to the irritation. (1) In a large vein, slow administration permits greater dilution of the drug with the circulating blood. (2) In a small vein lacking ample circulating blood, a slow drip prolongs the irritation, increasing the inflammation.
7. Prolonged duration of an infusion increases the risk of phlebitis. After a 24-hour period the danger increases. Periodic inspection of the injection site to detect developing phlebitis is important. After 72 hours the injection site should be changed.
8. Precautions should be observed to avoid administering solutions containing particulate matter by

a. Proper reconstitution and dilution of additives.
b. Inspection of parenteral fluids before administration.
c. Use of freshly prepared solutions.
d. Use of a set with a filter when danger of precipitation exists.
e. Periodic inspection of solutions containing additives.
f. Avoidance of administration of cloudy solutions unless affirmed by the manufacturer.

Responsibility of Hospital Committee

The special committee which deals with problems concerning therapeutic procedures should

1. Provide the nurse with an approved list of medications that may be added to parenteral solutions.
2. Delineate the types of fluids she may administer.
3. Provide an in-service program to acquaint the nurse with reactions, contraindications, dosage, and effects.

Physician's Responsibility

The physician writes and signs all orders for intravenous fluids and drug solutions. In each case the doctor should specify the rate of flow either as milliliters per hour or the approximate length of time of administration of the infusion.

He is responsible for administering intravenously all medications not on the list approved for nurses. This usually consists of certain types of drugs such as

1. Those which may produce a severe immediate reaction [13]. *Example:* Nitrogen mustard, iron preparations, and other drugs in which the possibility of anaphylaxis is of prime concern.
2. Those whose dose is dependent upon the response of the patient and which are to be injected directly into the vein [13]. *Example:* Epinephrine—dilution permits slow infusion and minimizes occurrence of reactions.
3. Those whose extravasation may result in necrosis [13]. *Example:* Levarterenol bitartrate. Infiltration of this drug may lead to severe sloughing of the tissues. It increases the blood pressure by producing peripheral venous restriction, resulting in ischemia of the skin.

Intravenous Nurse's Responsibility

The following tasks are the responsibility of the intravenous nurse. She

1. Checks the doctor's book for all complete orders of intravenous ther-

apy. If a doubt exists regarding the compatibility or safety of a drug, the physician or pharmacist should be consulted.

2. Compounds only the drugs on the authorized list.
3. Labels solution, indicating patient's name, drug, amount, date, time prepared, and her signature.
4. Delivers compounded, labeled solution to patient's unit, substantiating identification of patient and compounded solution. The nurse is legally responsible for all drugs and solutions that she prepares and administers.
5. Initiates the infusion and adjusts the rate of flow. No coercion should be used on rational, adult patients. If the patient refuses the infusion, the nurse should notify the physician in charge of the patient.
6. Questions patient regarding sensitivity to drugs which may cause anaphylaxis. Observes patient for a short time following initial administration of such drugs. If a question of sensitivity exists, the drug should be administered by the physician.

Attending Nurse's Responsibility

The nurse in attendance is responsible for maintaining the infusion. Through periodic inspection she

1. Regulates and maintains the prescribed rate of flow.
2. Observes the injection site for any developing complications before serious damage occurs. If phlebitis or infiltration occurs, she removes the needle.
3. Hangs consecutive bottles of intravenous fluid, inspecting compounded solutions for precipitation.
4. Discontinues intravenous therapy, taking care to prevent hematomas from occurring by applying firm pressure over puncture site for at least 2 minutes, or longer if necessary.

Nurses' Intravenous Additive Station

A specially equipped additive unit creates an environment of safety for the preparation of parenteral admixtures. This unit should provide the following:

1. *Isolated clean area.* Medications should be prepared in an area that permits complete concentration, since distraction increases the potential risk of human error.

   As traffic generates airborne contamination, an isolated area provides a better opportunity for sterility. The air in the typical hospital includes tiny contaminating particles, such as dust, lint, medication, and spores, in constant motion. These particles provide lodgment on which airborne bacteria thrive. The increased activity of bed-making, sweeping, and other functions increases the number of airborne particles and provides an environment which interferes with aseptic technique and may contribute to contamination [1].

2. *Laminar flow hood.* Some additive stations are equipped with a laminar flow unit to provide a clean work area where aseptic techniques can be performed. The concept of such a unit was evolved in 1961 and defined by Federal Standard 209a [2] as "air flow in which the entire body of air within a confined area moves with uniform velocity along parallel flow lines, with a minimum of eddies." These units, available in small bench models, play an important role in eliminating the hazard of airborne contamination of intravenous solutions.

3. *Proper illumination.* Adequate light permits visualization of particulate matter. Black and white backgrounds aid in the visual detection of these foreign substances. Laminar flow units provide illumination by fluorescent light [3].

4. *Supplies.* A complete stock of equipment should be available, including

    a. Parenteral solutions and administration sets
    b. Syringes and needles
    c. Commonly used intravenous additives
    d. Diluents
        1) Sterile bacteriostatic water injection, U.S.P.
        2) Sterile water injection, U.S.P.
        3) Normal saline injection, U.S.P.
    e. Container for the proper disposal of needles and syringes

5. A list of drugs and drug combinations approved for intravenous administration by nurses should be posted.

Preparation of Intravenous Solutions and Additives

Extreme care in the preparation of solutions diminishes the risks associated with intravenous therapy.

1. *Aseptic technique is imperative.* Pyrogenic contamination of drug products and parenteral solutions must be avoided.

2. *Proper dilution of lyophilized drugs is essential.* Two special cautions to assure complete solubility in the reconstitution of drugs must be observed: (1) The specific diluent recommended by the manufacturer should be used. (2) The drug should be initially diluted in the volume recommended.

3. *Introduction of extraneous particles into parenteral solutions must*

be avoided. Fragments of rubber stoppers are frequently cut out by the needles used and accidentally injected into solutions [8]. Large-bore (15-gauge) needles are practical for use in the nurses' station and appear to provide less disadvantage than the smaller needles. (1) Smaller needles may encourage particles which may be difficult to see on inspection. (2) The small particles may be of a size capable of passing through the indwelling needle.

A solution which upon inspection contains fragments of rubber must be discarded or filtered.

Procedure in Compounding and Administering Parenteral Solutions
The following steps should be carried out in the preparation of solutions for infusion:

1. Inscribe order for drug additive directly from original order to medication label.
2. Substantiate drug orders with the drug product and the parenteral solution.
3. Inspect solution for extraneous particles.
4. Check drug product for

    a. Expiration date: Outdated drugs should not be used, as loss of potency or stability may have occurred.
    b. Method of administration: (1) Intramuscular preparations are not usually used for intravenous administration; they may contain certain components such as anesthetics or preservatives not meant for administration by the vascular route. (2) Some are packaged in multiple-dose vials which may contribute to contamination. (3) The dosage by the intramuscular route may not coincide with that for intravenous use.

5. With an accepted antiseptic, clean rubber injection site of both the drug product and the diluent.
6. Use sterile syringe and needle.
7. Reconstitute according to manufacturer's recommendation.
8. Check diluted drug for complete solubility before adding to parenteral solution.
9. After adding to solution, invert solution bottle to mix the additive completely.
10. Clearly and properly label solution bottle:

    a. Name of patient
    b. Drug and dosage
    c. Date and time
    d. Signature

11. As an added precaution to prevent errors, recheck label with used drug ampules before discarding ampules.
12. Inspect solution for precipitates; if necessary, use an administration set with a filter.
13. Deliver parenteral solutions to patient's unit; substantiate identity of patient with solution prepared.
14. Perform venipuncture (see Chapter 5).
15. Observe patient for a few minutes following the initial intravenous administration of any drug that may cause anaphylaxis.
16. Use added caution in administering drugs, the fast action of which could produce untoward reactions:

    a. Controlled volume set
    b. Micro drip
    c. Double clamp

PROCEDURE FOR USING A DOUBLE CLAMP. A Hoffman Clamp* is initially regulated to the prescribed rate of flow. The clamp included with the administration set is then regulated to the prescribed rate of flow. If the clamp lets go, the second clamp provides added protection against rapid infusion of fluid and subsequently, circulatory overload and cardiovascular disturbances.

General Safety Rules
The following safety rules for preparation and intravenous administration of drugs by nurses should be adhered to at all times:

1. Nurses will, upon written order, prepare and administer only those solutions, medications, and combinations of drugs approved in writing by the Pharmacy and the Therapeutics Committee.
2. No intravenous infusion should be given that is cloudy or contains a precipitate.
3. All intravenous infusions must be used or discarded within 24 hours of the time the container is opened.
4. Any question regarding chemical compatibility or the relative safety of any drug added to an intravenous infusion should be directed to the Director of the Pharmacy.

Table 15 was prepared by John Webb, Director of Pharmacy and Supplies at Massachusetts General Hospital. It lists authorized drugs along with their pH and preservatives.

Intermittent Infusion
"Piggyback" infusions have become popular as a result of the increase in the number of intravenous drugs requiring by-the-clock administra-

* Humboldt Manufacturing Company, Chicago, Ill.

Table 15. Solubility of Medications in Commonly Used Intravenous Fluids

Drug	Dextrose 5% or 10% in Water 3.5–6.5	Sodium Chloride 0.9% 5.0–6.0	Lactated Ringer's Injection 6.0–7.5	Remarks and "Product May also Contain"
pH Range→				
Aminophylline 8.5–9.0	S	S	S	Ethylenediamine
Ammonium Chloride 4.0–6.0	S	S	S	
Amphotericin B 7.0	S**	I	I	Sodium phosphates, sodium desoxycholate
Ascorbic Acid 5.5–7.0	S	S	S	As sodium ascorbate. Sodium sulfite, sodium bisulfite
Calcium Chloride 6.5–8.5	S	S	S	
Calcium Disodium Edetate 6.5–8.0	S	S	–	
Calcium Gluceptate 6.2	S	S	S	Monothioglycerol
Cephaloridine 5.2	S	S	–	
Corticotropin 3.0–7.0	S	S	S	Hydrolyzed gelatin
Diazepam 6.2–6.9	–	–	–	Benzyl alcohol, sodium benzoate, benzoic acid, propylene glycol, ethyl alcohol
Epinephrine HCl 2.5–5.0	S	S	I	Initial diluent should be water without preservative
Erythromycin Gluceptate 6.0–8.0	S	S	S	Glycine
Fibinolysin 8.0–8.1	S⁴	I	–	
Glucagon HCl 2.0	S	S	–	Glycerin, phenol
Insulin 2.5–3.5	S	S	–	
Isoproterenol HCl 3.3–5.0	S	S	S	Lactate ion, sodium bisulfite
Lincomycin HCl 3.0–5.5	S	S	S	Benzyl alcohol

Drug	pH				Additives
Magnesium Sulfate	6.0–7.0	S	S	S	
Mannitol	6.4–6.8	–	S	S	
Menadione Sodium Bisulfite	2.0–4.0	S	S	S	Sodium bisulfite
Metaraminol Bitartrate	3.5–4.5	S	S	–	Methylparaben, propylparaben, sodium bisulfite
Methoxamine HCl	3.0–5.0	S	S	–	Citric acid, sodium citrate, potassium metabisulfite, disodium versenate, calcium chloride, methylparaben
Methyldopate HCl	3.0–6.0	S	–	–	Disodium edetate, monothioglycerol, sodium bisulfite, citric acid, parabens
Methylene Blue	3.0–4.5	S	S	S	Acetic acid, sodium acetate, chlorobutanol, alcohol
Oxytocin	2.5–4.5	S	S	S	
Phenylephrine HCl	3.0–7.0	S**	S	S	Sodium citrate, citric acid, sodium bisulfite, sodium acetate, phenol
Phytonadione	5.0–7.0	S	S	–	Benzyl alcohol, polyoxyethylated fatty acid derivative, dextrose
Polymyxin B Sulfate	5.0–7.5	S	S	–	
Potassium Chloride	4.0–7.0	S	S	S	
Potassium Penicillin, Buffered	5.0–7.5	S	S	S	Citrates, parabens
Procainamide HCl	4.0–6.0	S	S	–	Benzyl alcohol, sodium bisulfite
Sodium Amobarbital	9.6–10.4	S^1	S^1	S^1	
Sodium Ampicillin	8.5–9.5	S^2	S^3	–	
Sodium Bicarbonate	7.0–8.5	S	S	S	
Sodium Cephalothin	5.2	S	S	S	
Sodium Chloramphenicol-Succinate	6.4–7.0	S	S	S	
Sodium Chloride	4.5–7.0	S	S	S	
Sodium Dexamethasone Phosphate	7.5–10.5	S	S	–	Sodium citrate, methylparaben, propylparaben, sodium bisulfite, creatinine
Sodium Edetate	7.2	S	S	S	
Sodium Heparin	6.0–7.5	S	S	S	Benzyl alcohol, phenol, parabens
Sodium Hydrocortisone Phosphate	7.0–8.0	S	S	S	Phenol, sodium citrate, sodium bisulfite

Table 15 (Continued)

Drug	pH Range	Dextrose 5% or 10% in Water (3.5–6.5)	Sodium Chloride 0.9% (5.0–6.0)	Lactated Ringer's Injection (6.0–7.5)	Remarks and "Product May also Contain"
Sodium Hydrocortisone-Succinate	6.0–8.0	S	S	S	Phosphates, parabens, sodium biphosphate, sodium phosphate, chlorobutanol
Sodium Menadiol Diphosphate	7.5–8.5	S	S	S	Sodium citrate, parabens
Sodium Methicillin, Buffered	7.0–8.0	S	S	S	Phosphates, parabens
Sodium Methylprednisolone-Succinate	7.0–8.0	S	S	–	Sodium citrate
Sodium Nafcillin	6.0–6.5	I	S	S	Niacinamide, N-N-dimethylacetamide, benzyl alcohol
Sodium Novobiocin	7.5–8.5	S	S	S	Dibasic sodium phosphate, parabens
Sodium Oxacillin	6.0–8.5	S	S	–	Alcohol, propylene glycol
Sodium Pentobarbital	10.0–10.5	S[5]	S[5]	S[5]	
Sodium Phenobarbital	8.5–10.0	S[5]	S[5]	S[5]	Sodium bisulfite
Sodium Prednisolone Phosphate	6.0–7.0	S	S	S	Polyethylene glycol, phenol
Sodium Secobarbital	9.7–10.5	S[5]	S[5]	S[5]	Sodium metabisulfite
Sulfisoxazole Diolamine	7.3–7.8	S	S	S	
Tetracycline HCl	1.8–2.8	S	S	S[6]	Contains 2.5–3 gm ascorbic acid/1 gm tetracycline HCl
Urea	7.2	S	S	–	Citric acid
Vancomycin HCl	5.8	S	S	–	
Vitamin B Complex with C	4.0–5.1	S	S	S	Phenol, benzyl alcohol

S = Soluble
I = Incompatible
* At pH above 4.2
** Not to be used in dextrose 10% in water.
[1] Requires at least 1.5 ml to dissolve each milligram of amobarbital.
[2] Use within 4 hours.
[3] Use within 8 hours.
[4] Use within 2 hours.
[5] Requires at least 1 ml to dissolve each milligram of pentobarbital, phenobarbital, and secobarbital, respectively.
[6] Use within 12 hours.

tion. This technique allows drugs to be given on an intermittent basis through a slow keep-open infusion. The secondary bottle, containing a single-dose additive, or a multiple-dose admixture connected to a controlled volume set, is piggybacked through the injection site of the primary infusion. At the desired time, the initial infusion is clamped off and the prescribed dose of medication administered. An in-line check-valve set, which automatically allows the primary infusion to flow when the secondary bottle empties and prevents air from entering the line, may be used.

EQUIPMENT. The following equipment is used:

Intravenous container with admixture
Intravenous administration set (controlled volume set, if desired)
1-inch 20-gauge needle
Antiseptic (isopropyl alcohol) swabs
Tape

PROCEDURE. The following steps should be adhered to in administering piggyback infusions:

1. Wash hands.
2. Substantiate the identity of the patient and the admixture.
3. Attach the sterile administration set to the fluid container.
4. Suspend the bottle and flush the tubing to clear the set of air.
5. Clamp off the infusion.
6. Scrub the injection site with an accepted antiseptic. Strict adherence to aseptic and antiseptic technique is imperative.
7. Attach a sterile 1-inch 20-gauge needle to adapter of administration set. A longer needle may accidentally puncture the tubing. Small-bore needles are susceptible to breakage, with risk of the needle shaft's entering the infusion.
8. Insert the needle, up to the hub, in the injection site.
9. Tape the needle securely. In-and-out motion of the needle potentially increases the risk of contamination.

The Heparin Lock

The heparin lock provides a ready route for the intermittent administration of medications. It consists of a scalp vein needle with a short length of plastic tubing to which is permanently attached a resealable injection site. To maintain patency of the needle when it is not in use, a dilute solution of heparin is injected in sufficient volume to fill the needle and the tubing.

The heparin lock saves the patient the trauma of multiple punctures, conserves veins, offers freedom of motion between infusions, and provides a minimal amount of fluid to the patient on restricted intake.

One of the disadvantages of the heparin lock is the necessity for constant vigilance in order to prevent the fluid container from running empty. Once the container runs dry, venous pressure causes the blood to back up in the needle and tubing and a clot forms. A clot is an excellent trap for bacteria, whether they enter through the needle or migrate from an infection in a remote area of the body. Irrigation may embolize small infected needle thrombi, providing a potential focus for septicemia. After each infusion the scalp vein needle must be *immediately* flushed with heparin to maintain its patency.

EQUIPMENT. The following equipment is used:

Antiseptic (isopropyl alcohol)
Scalp vein needle containing an adapter with a medication site
Syringe and needle for injecting heparin
Sodium heparin injection, U.S.P., 2-ml ampule (250 units per milliliter)

PROCEDURE. Prepare and insert the heparin lock as follows:

1. Wash hands.
2. With syringe and needle draw up prescribed dose of heparin.
3. Scrub the injection site of the scalp vein needle with an accepted antiseptic.
4. Inject the heparin, through the medication site of the scalp vein needle, in order to expel the air and fill the lumen of the heparin lock.
5. Leave syringe and needle attached to the heparin lock.
6. Select vein. Take special precaution to definitely differentiate the vein from an aberrant artery. Signs of a probable aberrant artery include pulse, thick tough wall, bright red blood, and excruciating pain on venipuncture or on injection of medication. Inadvertent arterial injections of some medications could result in arteriospasm with impairment of the circulation and gangrene.
7. Make venipuncture.

   a. Scrub the skin site with 70 percent isopropyl alcohol.
   b. Perform the venipuncture using the scalp vein needle which has been prepared as a heparin lock.
   c. With the syringe, already attached, aspirate slightly to check for a blood return. Inject the remaining dosage (prescribed) of heparin and remove the syringe and needle.
   d. Tape heparin lock securely.

e. Indicate the date of insertion and the size of the needle on the tape.

The following points should be emphasized:

1. The infusion set should be changed every 24 hours.
2. The needle on the set should be replaced for each intermittent infusion.
3. The heparin lock should be changed every 72 hours.
4. The heparin lock must be flushed *immediately* on termination of the infusion.

Intravenous "Push"

The intravenous push is the direct injection of a medication into the vein. It may be administered through the injection site in the intravenous tubing, the heparin lock, or a needle. Because the technique allows instant absorption of medications in the blood, it offers immediate relief to the critically ill patient. Frequently nurses in special care units are trained and authorized to administer specific intravenous pushes. A list of drugs with limitations and restrictions are provided by special care unit committees. The intravenous push is usually restricted to the intensive care unit, where the patient is monitored and where a potential crisis may arise requiring its immediate use in the absence of a physician.

Since the medication is instantly absorbed, the injection must be administered slowly. Rapid injection increases the drug concentration in the plasma, which may reach toxic proportions, flooding the organs rich in blood—the heart and the brain—and resulting in shock and cardiac arrest. The drug must be diluted sufficiently, according to the manufacturer's recommendations, to prevent trauma to the vessel wall.

References

1. Abbott Laboratories. *The Abbott Clean Air Center.* North Chicago, Ill., 1969.
2. General Services Administration. *Clean Room and Work Station Requirements: Controlled Environment* (Federal Standard 209a). Washington, D.C., 1963.
3. Davies, W. L., and Lamy, P. P. Laminar flow. *Lippincott's Hospital Pharmacy* 3:3, 1968.
4. Degering, E. F. *Organic Chemistry* (6th ed.). New York: Barnes & Noble, 1961. P. 331.
5. Endicott, C. J. Workshop on Parenteral Incompatibilities. Silver Spring, Md., June 1966. *American Journal of Hospital Pharmacy* 23: 599, 1966.
6. Edward, M. pH—An important factor in the compatibility of additives

in intravenous therapy. *American Journal of Hospital Pharmacy* 24:442, 1967.

7. Fonkalsrud, E. W., Pederson, B. M., Murphy, J., and Beckerman, J. H. Reduction of infusion thrombophlebitis with buffered glucose solutions. *Surgery* 63:280, 1968.
8. Ho, H. F. Particulate matter in parenteral solutions. *Drug Intelligence* 1:7–25, 1967.
9. Luros, G. O., and Oram, F. *Essentials of Chemistry* (7th ed.). Philadelphia: Lippincott, 1966. Pp. 32, 74.
10. Pelissier, N. A., and Burgee, S. L. Guide to incompatibilities. *Lippincott's Hospital Pharmacy* 3:15, 1968.
11. Provost, G. E. Prescription compounding by nurses in hospitals. *American Journal of Hospital Pharmacy* 23:595, 1966.
12. Webb, J. W. A pH pattern of I.V. additives. *American Journal of Hospital Pharmacy* 26:31–35, 1969.
13. Williams, J. T., and Moravec, D. F. *Intravenous Therapy.* Hammond, Ind.: Clissold Publishing, 1967. P. 53.

15. Venous Pressure

The management of hypotension continues to be one of the most urgent problems facing the surgeon. The parameters used in evaluating a patient in shock consist of the following [2]:

1. Blood pressure
2. Rate and quality of pulse
3. Skin temperature and color
4. Urinary output
5. Peripheral venous filling
6. Blood pH

Blood Volume Determination

New methods are increasingly available to assist in diagnosis and treatment. Of these, blood volume determination plays an important role. Maintenance of an optimal blood volume is essential for survival. Prolonged hypovolemia may cause poor tissue perfusion with the inherent risk of renal and myocardial complication; hypovolemia, uncorrected, can eventually lead to shock and death [8]. Blood volume is not necessarily reflected by the blood pressure. In cardiogenic shock the blood volume is increased and the blood pressure is low. In septic shock, hypotension accompanies a normal blood volume.

Various methods have been employed to detect change in a patient's blood volume: hematocrit, change in patient's weight, and blood volume computations before and after surgery. Blood volume determinations are an important guide during

1. *Surgery,* when the risk exists of overloading an anesthetized, traumatized patient who is continuously losing blood.
2. *Shock,* when origin is unknown.

3. *Massive fluid replacement* in open-heart surgery and in critical cases, such as the severely burned, where circulatory overload is a hazard.
4. *Anuria* or *oliguria*, when questionable cause is dehydration.

The Volemetron,* using radioactive isotopes, has proved extremely valuable in computing accurate blood volume determinations. Some disadvantages accompany this process: (1) the time involved, (2) the limited number of determinations that can be performed on one patient, (3) the fact that the determination quickly becomes obsolete with change produced by therapy, and (4) the expensive equipment and personnel that are needed.

Venous Pressure Determination

Venous pressure determination has overcome the disadvantages associated with the Volemetron. It requires no laboratory personnel, no expensive equipment, is simple in technique, and once set up may be monitored quickly and as often as required.

Venous pressure may be measured centrally or peripherally. *Central venous pressure* denotes the pressure in the right atrium of the venous blood as it returns from all parts of the body. The pressure varies among individuals, usually ranging between 5 and 12 cm of water (50 and 120 mm of water), but a low of 2 to 3 cm may be normal for some patients [2, 5]. The normal range has little significance since the true value lies in the change or lack of change following attempts to alter the blood volume or to improve cardiac action [2]. Since central venous pressure relates to a fully sufficient circulation, it facilitates assessment of both the blood volume and the ability of the heart to tolerate an increased volume, thereby providing a valuable guide for fluid administration.

Peripheral venous pressure is the pressure of the blood on the walls of the peripheral veins; to a certain extent it reflects the central venous pressure [4]. However, monitoring peripherally is less reliable: Accuracy can be affected by acute flexion of the extremity containing the catheter; thrombophlebitis or venous constriction by tumor can produce marked local elevations; poor circulation in a cold extremity may reflect only the local venous blood return, and sudden loss of blood may occur before compensatory vasoconstriction has time to take place. When accuracy is of utmost importance, caval position of the catheter is desirable.

* Ames Atomium Co., Elkhart, Ind.; division of Miles Laboratories, Inc.

Since central venous pressure relates to an adequate circulatory blood volume it is dependent upon [3, 8]:

1. Volume of blood
2. Status of the myocardium (heart muscle)
3. Tone of blood vessels

Circulatory failure may result from deficiency in any one or combination of these essential factors.

BLOOD VOLUME. Changes in blood volume alter the tone of the blood vessels and the ability of the heart to circulate the blood. A reduced blood volume results in less pressure at the right atrium, indicated by a drop in central venous pressure; an increased blood volume produces more pressure at the atrium, with a rise in central venous pressure [4].

In managing an inadequate circulation, one must first establish a normal blood volume. If the inadequate circulation is due to deficiency in the blood volume, manipulation is made by administering expanders; or in the case of increased volume, phlebotomy.

If the circulation still remains insufficient, it becomes necessary to look at the remaining two essential components—status of the myocardium and tone of the blood vessels.

STATUS OF THE MYOCARDIUM. The status of the myocardium may be affected by disease, drugs, fluids, or anesthesia. Because the central venous pressure is a measure of the capacity of the myocardium as well as the blood volume, it is invaluable in monitoring the effects of anesthesia and surgery on elderly patients with arteriosclerosis or patients with myocardial insufficiency. The central venous pressure rises if the heart muscle is impaired—the pressure of the volume of blood at the heart increases because the heart muscle is no longer able to pump an adequate flow of blood out of the right atrium [4]. An elevated central venous pressure of 15 to 20 cm suggests cardiac failure [8]. This is one of the commonest causes of an elevated central venous pressure in shock.

Drugs or chemicals are administered to improve myocardial response, thus increasing cardiac output and lowering the central venous pressure.

Temporary impairment of the myocardium may be due to electrolyte imbalance and cause an early rise in central venous pressure—not above the normal range. Acidosis affects the myocardial response; if it is due to pulmonary insufficiency, correction is made by increasing the excretion of carbon dioxide [8].

TONE OF THE BLOOD VESSELS. The third essential component, the tone of the blood vessels, is dependent upon the arterial pressure and upon external and internal pressures on the veins. The arterial pressure arises from the contractile force of the left ventricle and is transmitted through the capillaries to the veins.

The external pressures upon the vein result from (1) the muscular and fascial pumping action in the extremities, (2) the intra-abdominal pressure from straining and distension, and (3) the intrathoracic pressure due to contraction of the diaphragm and chest wall. Central venous pressure of patients on positive pressure respirators is usually increased by 4 cm, while patients on negative pressure show a decreased central venous pressure [5].

The internal pressure on the veins is due to blood volume, myocardial response, and sympathomimetic amines (epinephrine, norepinephrine). Vasopressors, by stimulating contraction of the venous wall, decrease the capacity of the venous system and improve vascular tone.

Central Venous Pressure Monitoring

Central venous pressure monitoring (see Figure 39) is achieved by attaching an intravenous set to a three-way stopcock and to an extension tube with a radiopaque catheter of approximately 24 inches. A vertical length of infusion tubing that serves as the manometer is connected to the stopcock and attached to the intravenous stand against a marked centimeter tape. Central venous pressure sets are available with disposable water manometers, graduated in units. The zero mark on the tape is adjusted to the level of the patient's right atrium. The pressure is measured at either the superior vena cava by introducing the catheter via the antecubital, jugular, or subclavian vein, or at the inferior vena cava via the femoral vein.

The superior vena cava is most commonly used. Complications have been associated with inferior vena caval catheters; Bansmer and associates [1] reported a 46 percent incidence in 24 cases. In each case, with one exception, the catheter had been in place over 4 days. Use of the femoral vein and the long duration of time the catheter is in the vein enhance the risk of thrombotic complications. A second disadvantage is the fact that abdominal distension interferes with monitoring an accurate right atrial pressure.

Equipment

The following equipment is needed for monitoring central venous pressure:

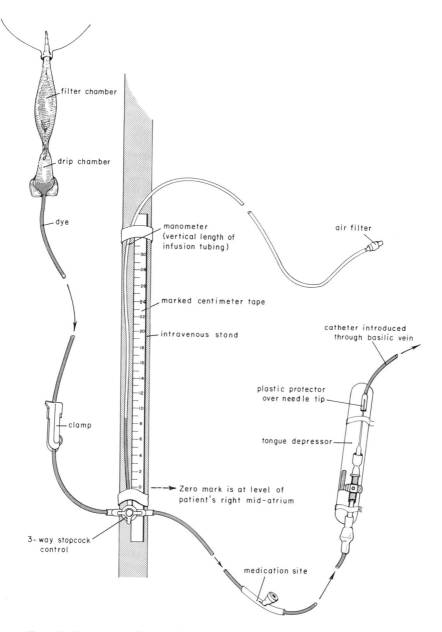

filter chamber

drip chamber

dye

manometer
(vertical length of
infusion tubing)

air filter

marked centimeter tape

intravenous stand

catheter introduced
through basilic vein

plastic protector
over needle tip

tongue depressor

clamp

Zero mark is at level of
patient's right mid-atrium

3-way stopcock
control

medication site

Fig. 39. Equipment for monitoring central venous pressure. Zero mark on the tape is level with the right atrium. Notice precautions taken to prevent cutting edge of the needle from severing catheter: the bevel shield is in place and the tongue depressor provides added protection.

Intravenous Equipment PLUS	Venous Pressure Equipment
Intravenous set	Local anesthetic (usually 1 per-
Intravenous stand	cent procaine)
Armboard	Central venous pressure set
Solution as ordered	Catheter approximately 24 inches
Tourniquet	in length
Antiseptic	Dye (methylene blue), if ordered
Adhesive tape	Heparin 1:1000, if ordered
	Antibiotic ointment
	Venous pressure level

Procedure

Monitoring the central venous pressure is carried out as follows:

1. Explain procedure to patient.

2. Wash hands thoroughly and dry.

3. Prepare solution bottles.

   Add dye (methylene blue) or vitamin B complex, if ordered.
   Facilitates reading of the manometer.

   Add heparin, if ordered.
   Reduces thrombus formation and provides catheter patency.

4. Prepare equipment.

   Close three-way stopcock.

   Squeeze and hold filter chamber and insert into solution bottle.

   Completely fill filter chamber.

   Fill drip chamber one-quarter full.
   Prefilling chambers prevents air bubbles from entering the manometer arm.

   Tape centimeter strip onto intravenous stand with zero point adjusted to the mid-atrial level.
   Patient should be in a supine position with the bed flat.
   Use venous pressure level for accuracy.

Mid-atrial level is at a point approximately equidistant from the sternum and back.

Tape stopcock to pole at a level below patient's right atrium.
Do not tape directly on the stopcock (see Figure 39).

Tape upper end of manometer tube taut to intravenous stand.

Adjust stopcock to allow solution to flow into manometer arm, filling it halfway.

Adjust three-way clamp to fill remaining intravenous tubing.

5. Select vein.

Basilic. The basilic vein provides the most readily accessible route (see Figure 40). The catheter is introduced into the basilic vein and through the axillary vein, which is a continuation of the basilic. The axillary vein ends in the subclavian vein and the catheter is threaded into the right innominate to the junction of the superior vena cava.

Cephalic. Difficulties are frequently encountered when introducing the catheter through the cephalic vein. The cephalic vein enters the axillary vein at its termination; this junction may offer resistance when the catheter is inserted. Positioning the patient's arm at right angle to the body may facilitate introduction of the catheter.

6. Approximate catheter length to be introduced.

With the catheter, measure the distance from the suprasternal notch to the anticipated puncture point.

7. Prepare site with an accepted antiseptic. (Iodine-containing disinfectants have been recommended.)

8. Inject 1 percent procaine subdermally to raise a small wheal.

9. After applying a tourniquet, puncture the skin and fascia using a needle with a 15-gauge bore.

Avoid puncturing the vein.
The prepuncture prevents the sharp cutting edge of the can-

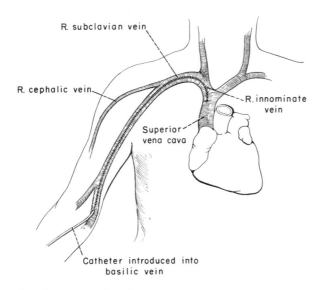

R. subclavian vein

R. cephalic vein

R. innominate vein

Superior vena cava

Catheter introduced into basilic vein

Fig. 40. Course that the central venous catheter takes when introduced into the basilic vein. Notice the smooth, uninterrupted route of the catheter as it passes from the basilic vein, through the axillary vein, and into the subclavian.

nula from boring a plug of skin or subcutaneous tissue that may plug the catheter or form an embolus.

10. Perform venipuncture with cannula which comes connected to the catheter.

11. Thread catheter short distance through the cannula.
    Grasp the catheter lightly with one hand while threading with the other: this is an important precautionary measure to prevent the catheter from being accidentally withdrawn and possibly severed by the cutting edge of the cannula.

12. Release tourniquet.

13. Thread catheter to the premeasured distance.

14. If the venipuncture is unsuccessful, remove the needle and catheter together.

    Never manipulate catheter by withdrawing it through the cannula.

The catheter is presumed to be in the thoracic cavity when (1) manometer fluid fluctuates 3 to 5 cm during breathing, and (2) coughing and straining cause the column of water to rise [2]. It may be necessary to advance the catheter slightly farther than suggested by superficial measurement. If the catheter is inserted too far and reaches the heart, higher pressure waves synchronous with the pulse will be seen [6].

15. Withdraw cannula.

16. Slide cannula into its adapter.

17. Slide bevel protector from base of cannula to cover cutting edge.

18. Connect intravenous assembly and start the infusion.

19. Apply antibiotic ointment to puncture site.

20. Apply pressure dressing.

21. Secure the catheter.

> Place a ½-inch strip of tape—adhesive up—under catheter. Cross one end tightly and diagonally over catheter. Repeat with the other end, crossing the first.
>
> A tongue depressor placed under needle and catheter and taped over shield, independent of the arm, protects the catheter. Tape to arm.
>
> Tape intravenous tubing securely to arm.
>
> Secure arm to armboard.
> Motion of catheter upon flexion of the arm increases the potential risk of phlebitis; a kinked catheter results in unreliable readings and leads to clogging of the lumen.

22. Inscribe on tape the date of catheter insertion.
    This will help ensure removal of catheter within a safe period of time—usually 48 to 72 hours.

Central Venous Pressure Measurement

The pressure is usually read at half-hour or hourly intervals. The patient must be quiet, not coughing or straining, and in a supine position with the zero reading at the mid-axillary level. The procedure is as follows:

1. Turn stopcock so the central venous pressure solution flows from bottle to manometer arm.
2. When manometer level reaches 30 cm turn stopcock to stop flow from the solution bottle and direct manometer flow to the patient.
3. The fluid level will drop rapidly, reaching the reading level in about 15 seconds. The central venous pressure is measured at the high point of the fluctuation.
4. Readjust the stopcock so the infusion resumes.
5. Record measurements on Vital Signs Record.

When 5 percent dextrose in water is used for monitoring venous pressure, it may be necessary to open and flush 5 ml of the solution through the catheter at 3-hour intervals to maintain patency; dextrose may cause a rouleau to form at the catheter tip as it mixes with blood, contributing to catheter plugging.

Complications

Awareness of the serious complications associated with caval catheterization and the exercising of particular caution contribute to greater safety for the patient.

CATHETER EMBOLISM. One of the serious complications is catheter embolism. In 1968 Wellman and associates [7] published a review of 37 cases of catheter embolism, in 13 of which death followed the embolism. They tabulated the causes of catheter embolism, as shown in Table 16.

Special precautions should be observed to prevent catheter embolism:

1. Anchor catheter securely; if accidentally severed or separated from the adapter the catheter is then anchored rather than liberated.
2. Cover the needle point with the bevel shield to prevent severing the catheter.
3. Since the shield may be dislodged, tape in place on a tongue depressor.
4. Never withdraw the catheter through the needle.
5. Know the exact length of the catheter; after removal, measure to detect immediately any lost fragments.

Table 16. Causes of Catheter Embolism in 37 Patients

Number of Patients	Cause of Embolism
15	Catheter severed by cutting edge of needle
6	Catheter broke, independent of the needle
4	Catheter separated from the adapter
2	Catheter severed during dressings
10	Unknown

Source: Adapted from Wellman et al. [7].

OTHER COMPLICATIONS. Other complications of central venous pressure measurement include the following:

1. Local thrombosis
2. Thrombosis with embolism
3. Septic thrombophlebitis with septicemia and acute bacterial endo-carditis.

The polyethylene catheter, because it remains flexible and elastic without the use of plasticizers, is comparatively tissue inert. After a period of time, however, local thrombosis may occur. Clot formation in the vein may be due to mechanical trauma from insertion of the catheter, from motion of the catheter within the vein, or from the chemical irritation of hypertonic solutions. Thrombosis of the vena cava and the larger veins has been known to result from sclerosing agents.

Precautions to observe are these:

1. Immobilize the arm whenever a catheter is inserted over an area of joint flexion.
2. Limit duration of time to 72 hours.
3. Maintain sterility in technique.
4. Maintain asepsis by topical application of antibiotic ointment.
5. Avoid catheterization of the inferior vena cava via the femoral vein.

References

1. Bansmer, G., Keith, D., and Tesluk, H. Complications following use of indwelling catheter of IVC. *Journal of the American Medical Association* 167:1606, 1958.
2. Hallin, R. W. Continuous venous pressure monitoring as a guide to fluid administration in hypotensive patient. *American Journal of Surgery* 106:164, 1963.

3. Landis, E. M., and Hortenstine, J. C. Functional significance of venous blood pressure. *Physiological Reviews* 30:1, 1950.
4. Metheny, N. M., and Snively, W. D., Jr. *Nurses' Handbook of Fluid Balance.* Philadelphia: Lippincott, 1967. Pp. 145, 210.
5. Russell, M. V., and Maier, W. P. The ABCs of C.V.P. measurement. *R.N.* 32:34, 1969.
6. Ryan, G. M., and Howland, W. S. An evaluation of central venous pressure monitoring. *Anesthesia and Analgesia: Current Researches* 45: 754–759, 1966.
7. Wellman, K. F., Reinhard, A., and Salazar, E. P. Polyethylene catheter embolism. *Circulation* 37:380, 1968.
8. Wilson, J. N., and Owens, J. C. Continuous monitoring of venous pressure in optimal blood volume maintenance. *Archives of Surgery* (Chicago) 85:563, 1962.

16. Transfusion Therapy

With the increasing use of blood and its components, transfusion therapy has become an integral part of the daily treatment of patients. Administration of blood should be performed by competent, experienced, well-qualified personnel. This specialized group should be familiar with the disadvantages as well as the advantages that accompany a transfusion.

Vast improvement in methods of blood collection and storage, together with growing knowledge in the field of immunohematology, has increased the safety level of transfusion therapy; however, there is still an inherent risk with every unit of transfused blood. Both the therapist and the attending nurse should be aware of this fact and be alert to symptoms of untoward reaction.

Proper handling of the blood is vital. Contamination must be avoided; hemolysis must be prevented. The therapist must be familiar with the large variety of available blood products—their advantages, disadvantages, and the proper procedures for their safe administration.

Knowledge of the fundamental principles of immunohematology provides the nurse with a better understanding of the problems associated with blood administration. Recognition of the factors that govern red cell destruction contributes to safe transfusion therapy. This information instills in the therapist an awareness of the possibility that patients may become sensitized to the many blood factors, and of the danger which this incurs. These facts bring out clearly the necessity for screening patients for antibodies which they may develop from infused blood. Through an understanding of why bloods react unfavorably with other bloods, the therapist is keenly alert to the early symptoms of transfusion reactions.

Basic Immunohematology

Immunohematology is the science that deals with antigens of the blood and their antibodies. *Antibodies* (or agglutinins) are proteins in the plasma which react with specific *antigens*. They may occur naturally or may be the result of immunization against an antigen (an agglutinogen). The most important antigens in the blood transfusion are situated on the surface of the red cells.

In vitro (in a test tube) antibodies first react with their antigens by being adsorbed onto the red cells (coating). The reaction may stop there or may proceed to their agglutination, in which the red cells are stuck together in clumps, or hemolysis, in which the cells burst, releasing their hemoglobin [4]. Which of these processes occurs depends upon the particular antibody involved. Coating or agglutination in the test tube is associated in vivo (in the body) with sequestration of the affected cells in the liver or spleen prior to destruction (extravascular destruction). Hemolysis in the test tube is associated with in vivo destruction of red cells in the circulation (intravascular hemolysis).

An antibody bears the same designation as the antigen with which it reacts. For instance, anti-A reacts with antigen A. A red cell antigen and its corresponding antibody are not produced in the same individual; i.e., anti-A antibody is not produced by an individual whose red cells bear the A antigen.

Blood Group Systems

The best-known blood group system is the ABO system, discovered by Karl Landsteiner in 1901. He demonstrated a classification of human blood based on antigens on the red cells and antibodies in the serum [4] (see Table 17).

In 1940 Landsteiner and Wiener discovered the Rhesus (Rh) system, so called because of its relationship to the substance in the red cells of the rhesus monkey. The antigens belonging to the Rh system are C, D, E, c, and e. Because of the ease with which antibody D is built up, typing is done to ensure that D-negative recipients receive D-negative blood. If a person is found to be D-negative, a complete Rh typing should be done to check for the presence of C and E antigens. A person whose blood contains a D antigen is classified as Rh-positive; lacking the D, C, and E antigens, Rh-negative.

Occasionally weak variants of the $Rh_o(D)$ factor exist and are identified by means of an indirect Coombs test. These individuals, called D^u variants, are considered Rh-positive but should as recipients receive Rh-negative blood.

The serum of an Rh-negative individual differs from the main groups in that the anti-Rh antibodies are not usually present in significant quantities until the individual is exposed to an Rh positive factor, through either transfusion or pregnancy.

Nine main blood group systems have been defined on the basis of reaction of cells with antibodies: ABO, Rh, Kell, Duffy, Kidd, Lewis,

Table 17. ABO Classification of Human Blood

Group	Cell Antigens		Plasma Antibodies		% U.S. Populace
	A	B	A	B	
O	−	−	+	+	45
A	+	−	−	+	40
B	−	+	+	−	10
AB	+	+	−	−	5

MNS, P, and Lutheran. Others are under investigation. Corresponding antibodies to the blood group antigens in most of these systems are found so infrequently that they do not cause an everyday problem. When present, these antibodies may produce hemolytic reactions; once discovered, precautions must be taken to ensure that the patient receives compatible blood. When difficulty arises in cross-matching, or when a transfusion reaction occurs, these systems take on a special significance. The American Association of Blood Banks (A.A.B.B.) requires that a patient once transfused must be screened for irregular antibodies in the 48 hours preceding any further transfusions.

The term *hemolytic transfusion reaction* denotes the clinical symptoms caused when the red cells of either the recipient or the donor are destroyed in the recipient during a transfusion. Of prime importance in transfusion therapy is the assurance of ABO compatibility between donor and recipient. Since serious transfusion reactions have been reported due to transfused anti-A or anti-B antibodies, type O blood should not be used for A, B, or AB recipients. According to A.A.B.B. Standards [2], when a delay in blood transfusion may jeopardize life, uncross-matched type O blood may be given to recipients whose ABO type is not known, providing certain requirements are met:

1. Levels of anti-A and anti-B are reduced by removal of at least 70 percent of the plasma from whole blood. This is the preferred method.
2. Type O whole blood is free of hemolytic anti-A and anti-B when administered to other than type O recipients.

The same requirements apply when type A or type B blood is used for type AB recipient: 70 percent plasma removed from whole blood, or whole blood free of hemolytic antibodies.

Objectives of Transfusion Therapy
There are three main objectives of transfusion therapy:

1. Maintenance of blood volume
2. Maintenance of oxygen-carrying capacity of the blood by supplying red cells
3. Maintenance of coagulation properties by supplying the clotting factors found in platelets and plasma

Transfusion therapy is also vital when blood exchange is imperative, as in the treatment of newborn infants with hemolytic anemia. In cardiac surgery blood is needed to prime the oxygenating pump and maintain circulation.

Whole Blood

Acid-citrate-dextrose (ACD) solution is commonly used for blood preservation and storage. Sodium citrate, by combining with ionized calcium, inhibits clotting and serves as an anticoagulant. Dextrose prolongs the life of the red cells. Acid prevents caramel formation of dextrose after autoclaving. Under controlled refrigeration of $1°$ to $6°$ C, ACD blood can be safely stored up to 21 days. This time duration is based on the standard that 70 percent of the red cells of such blood (21 days old) must be present in the bloodstream of the recipient for more than 24 hours after transfusion [5].

Whole blood transfusions are indicated when an acute blood loss has occurred. The volume expanders, plasma, dextran, and albumin, are useful only as a temporary measure. They lack the oxygen-carrying red cells necessary in treating hypoxia, associated with hypovolemic shock. Frequently acute blood loss requires massive transfusion.

Definite changes take place in stored blood which make age a problem for consideration when a large quantity of blood (over 6 pints) is infused in a short period of time. With the continuous metabolic changes of red cells occurring during blood storage, the potassium content of the plasma increases; potassium leaks out of the cells into the plasma. This potassium, plus that released from the intact cells, causes the plasma potassium level to rise from 7 mEq per liter the first day to 23 mEq per liter by the twenty-first day [5]. This is an important factor in the event of massive transfusions and in blood exchange of the newborn infant.

In major surgery when rapid transfusion of large quantities of blood is indicated, whole blood—as fresh as possible—is used. When the patient's plasma potassium level reaches 10 to 15 mEq per liter, cardiac arrest and death occur [8].

Coagulation factors of the plasma and platelets are also affected by the age of the blood. In hemorrhage, when viable platelets are a consideration, fresh blood must be used. Fresh blood is also used in blood exchange in the newborn infant.

Blood stored for transfusion is known to contain increasing amounts of cellular degradation debris such as microaggregates of leukocytes, platelets, and other amorphous material [11]. Studies suggest that the pulmonary insufficiency following massive transfusion may be due to this debris. Since the standard 170-micron filter has been found inadequate, several blood filters with small pore size (40 microns and under) have been designed to protect the lung against this particulate matter when several units of stored blood are infused (see Chapter 9).

The anticoagulant can present problems. Rapid administration of citrated blood can cause calcium deficit. A damaged liver may be unable to keep up with rapid administration of sodium citrated blood, unable to metabolize the citrate ions; the citrate ions combine with ionized calcium in the bloodstream, causing a calcium deficit [8].

In conjunction with cardiac surgery, massive amounts of whole blood are required to prime the oxygenating pumps, maintain circulation, and replace blood loss. ACD blood, preferably less than 5 days old, is used for the priming of the pump. Freshly collected blood may be needed if the patient is bleeding after operation.

Packed Red Cells

Packed red cells are prepared by the removal of approximately 200 to 225 ml of plasma from whole blood, either by centrifuge or by sedimentation. Packed cells with a hematocrit of about 70 percent are readily transfusable; the National Institutes of Health standard is for a hematocrit reading of 60 to 70 percent. With the removal of greater amounts of plasma, difficulty is encountered upon infusion owing to the dense packing of the cells.

There are definite advantages in the use of packed red cells: reduced volume, reduced chemical content, and reduced agglutinins.

REDUCED VOLUME. Because of its reduced volume, a unit of packed cells can supply red cells without overloading the circulation—a definite advantage in patients with normal or increased blood volume and those with heart disease. Packed red cells are used for patients not in need of plasma. One unit of packed cells, in a much reduced volume, provides the same amount of oxygen-carrying red cells as one unit of whole blood.

REDUCED CHEMICAL CONTENT. The excess plasma potassium content in stored blood is reduced by the removal of plasma. Red cells can be provided for a patient with kidney or heart disease without adding to the patient's hyperkalemia.

Packed cells have an advantage for patients on sodium restriction, since the sodium excess in the plasma (increased by the anticoagulant sodium citrate) is thus avoided. Packed cells also reduce hazards associated with sodium citrate, such as citrate intoxication caused by the inability of the liver to metabolize citrate.

REDUCED AGGLUTININS. Packed cells provide relatively safe, low-titer type O blood. Most of the plasma is removed, thereby reducing the amount of anti-A and anti-B agglutinins.

Frozen Blood

The storage time for donated blood has been increased to 3 years or better by the process of freezing blood. This processing is accomplished through a machine, the Cytoglomerator,* invented by Charles E. Huggins. Early attempts at freezing blood proved unsuccessful because of the ice crystals which damaged the red cells. Several techniques have been developed in the past fifteen to twenty-one years, but Huggins's method has proved the simplest and quickest.

Plasma is extracted from the whole blood. The red cells are then coated with glycerol to prevent damage from freezing and packed in disposable plastic bags. They are then frozen at −85° C, labeled, and stored until used.

Just prior to use, the plastic bag with the frozen cells is thawed in a water bath of about 40° C. The thawing time is about 3 minutes. The bag is then inserted into the Cytoglomerator for a glycerol washout of about 20 minutes. Sugar solutions are used to cause a rapid sediment of the red cells. The machine takes its name from *cyto* (cell) and *glomerator* (cluster). Three dilutions are necessary. Five pints of blood can be processed every 20 minutes by one machine.

Frozen blood offers advantages other than the long storage period. (1) It is believed that the possibility of transmitting hepatitis by transfusion of frozen blood is negligible. (2) Owing to the selection of donors, frozen blood may be given to patients sensitized from previous transfusions. Type O frozen blood can safely be used as a universal donor because anti-A and anti-B antibodies are removed during washings. (3) Some surgeons believe that frozen blood plays a big part in improving results in kidney transplantations; fewer of the white blood cell antigens remain to trigger the body's rejection to foreign tissue [7].

The hematocrit of frozen blood is 80 percent—a little more than that of packed cells, but because of the lack of any plasma, the viscosity is less, making it easily transfusable. It may be administered rapidly to most patients.

* International Equipment Co., Needham Heights, Mass.

Plasma

Plasma is the liquid content remaining after the red cells have been removed from whole blood by centrifuge. Commercially it is available in the liquid and the dried state. The storage of plasma presents less of a problem than that of blood. When stored according to A.A.B.B. Standards [2], the shelf life of single-donor liquid plasma in a glass container is no more than 3 years, freeze-dried plasma no more than 7 years, frozen plasma no more than 5 years, and fresh-frozen plasma no more than 1 year.

Liquid stored plasma is prepared from ACD blood. Special precaution must be taken to avoid contamination in the preparation of plasma. A closed system under sterile conditions is used to separate plasma from red cells. Further precautions include culture of the plasma plus visual inspection.

Plasma is prepared as single-donor plasma, and labeled with the specific blood group. Because plasma is a vehicle for transmitting hepatitis, the single-donor plasma carries fewer risks. Many donors are involved in the preparation of pooled plasma, thereby increasing the likelihood of viral contamination. The use of pooled plasma is to be discouraged.

Every precaution is used to reduce the risk of hepatitis. Donors are questioned for any possible history of hepatitis; this in itself is helpful, but there is no sure way to eliminate donors who may transmit hepatitis. It was thought that storage of plasma for 6 months at 30° to 34° C would inactivate the virus, but cases of hepatitis have continued to appear after the use of commercially pooled plasma so stored, raising doubts as to the effectiveness of this procedure. The use of single-donor plasma, which carries less risk, or the use of a substitute such as 5 percent albumin, is preferable.

Plasma plays an important role in the treatment of burns. It supplies plasma protein and prevents shock without overloading the circulation with red cells. It may be used in emergency to correct hypovolemia. Most of the clotting factors are lost during storage, making it of little use in patients with coagulation problems.

Under ordinary circumstances when single-donor plasma is used, it should be compatible with the recipient's red cells. AB plasma, because it lacks anti-A and anti-B agglutinins, may be used for all ABO groups. The group O patient may receive plasma of any group. For the group A patient, only plasma taken from blood group A or AB may be used. For the group B patient, only plasma taken from blood group B or AB may be used. For the group AB patient, plasma from group AB blood only is used. In an emergency when the patient's blood group has not been determined, AB plasma is used.

Freeze-dried plasma is dried plasma that has been stored in a liquid state at 32° C for 6 months before being dried [5]. It may be made from pooled plasma and used for patients of any blood type. It must be reconstituted with sterile water before use. The sterile water is packaged in a kit with the plasma. A sterile pyrogen-free filter must always be used in the administration of all plasma. Once reconstituted, freeze-dried plasma should be used immediately.

Fresh-frozen plasma is beneficial to patients with inherited or acquired disorders of coagulation. Special donors with blood high in certain clotting factors are desirable. The plasma is separated from the cells and frozen within 4 hours of collection. Freezing preserves the various clotting factors, in particular factors V and VIII, to control hemorrhage in the presurgical hemophiliac.

Fresh-frozen plasma must be stored at −20° to −30° C and kept frozen until transfusion time. It is thawed in a water bath of 37° C. The fresh-frozen plasma must be administered immediately upon thawing; any delay causing a rise in the temperature of the plasma results in loss of factor VIII (antihemophiliac factor, AHF).

PLASMA COMPONENTS. *Cryoprecipitate* is a concentrate containing factor VIII (AHF) extracted from cold-thawed plasma. It was discovered by Judith G. Pool, Stanford University Medical Center, who began work on it in 1959. Since 1965 it has been used for treatment of hemophilia, this being the only coagulation deficiency for which it is therapeutically valuable [10].

The potency of AHF in cryoprecipitate far exceeds that in fresh-frozen plasma. Pool [10] stated that approximately 6 units, or 1600 ml, of plasma would be necessary to raise the patient's AHF level from less than 1 percent of normal to 50 percent of normal, whereas only 55 ml or less of the concentrate produces the same results. It would take 2 hours or more to infuse the plasma but only 5 minutes to infuse the precipitate. This small volume avoids the risk of overloading circulation in patients who are not able to tolerate an increase in blood volume.

The blood from which the precipitate is taken can be reconstituted and used as whole blood or separated into components for patients other than the hemophiliac.

In the preparation of AHF, the plasma goes through a quick-freeze process. When frozen solid it is thawed at 4° C, which takes about 24 hours. The precipitate is then removed from the cold-thawed plasma.

Studies indicate that AHF levels in cryoprecipitate remain after 3 months of storage in frozen packs.

Fibrinogen, a concentrate of the fibrinogen factor, is useful in the treatment of hemorrhage resulting from a deficiency of this protein. This deficiency is most frequently seen in the obstetrical patient and at times in patients with fibrinolysin undergoing major surgery. Approximately 12 units of blood are needed to supply the amount of fibrinogen in a 2-gm unit [3]. It is stored at a temperature of 2° to 10° C in the lyophilized state.

Because the hepatitis virus and fibrinogen combine during fractionation, there is increased risk of hepatitis to the patient infused with this product.

Fibrinogen is reconstituted with sterile distilled water—the sterile water is supplied in a kit with the fibrinogen. Care in preparation is important. Rapid shaking traps the fibrinogen particles, increasing the difficulty in reconstitution; hot water must not be used, and the fibrinogen itself must not be warmed. Administration requires a filter, preferably the set in which the filter is supplied with the product. Dosage varies from 2 to 8 gm, the amount depending upon individual need. Fibrinogen must be administered within 1 hour of reconstitution.

The disadvantages in the use of fibrinogen are the increased risk of hepatitis [3] and the large volume of blood needed to prepare this product.

Human albumin is prepared in a 25 percent solution containing the protein of albumin in concentrated form. Because of its low salt content, it is indicated in cases of hypoalbuminemia caused by liver and kidney disease. Albumin serves the same function as plasma. It is useful in the treatment of shock and burns without the added risk of transmitting serum hepatitis; processing by heating at 60° C for 10 hours destroys the hepatitis virus [3]. One hundred milliliters containing 25 gm of albumin require 3000 ml of blood for processing [5]. Albumin increases the osmolality of the plasma and draws fluid into the circulation, relieving hypovolemia. One hundred milliliters is osmotically equivalent to 500 ml of citrated plasma and produces a plasma volume increase of about 450 ml.

Human albumin is also available as a 5 percent solution in saline. Preparations contain 5 gm of normal serum albumin in each 100 ml, with the sodium content approximately that of isotonic sodium chloride solution. It is osmotically equivalent to an approximately equal volume of citrated plasma and may be used as a substitute for plasma; special processing destroys the hepatitis virus. Maximal osmotic effect is obtained with no additional fluid, while the 25 percent albumin depends for its maximal osmotic effect on additional fluids either drawn from the tissues or administered separately.

Concentrated albumin (25 percent) is sometimes diluted in parenteral solutions of dextrose, saline, or sodium lactate to obtain a less concentrated solution for patients with edema unable to tolerate large, concentrated doses. Once mixed it must be used immediately and not stored in a refrigerator for further use. To do so could cause serious reactions from bacterial contamination. Albumin contains no preservative; once the vial is entered with a needle, it must be used immediately or discarded. The set supplied with the albumin contains a small, concealed mesh filter. *Plasma protein fraction (human)* is plasma from which the fibrinogen and much of the globulin have been removed. The preparation Plasmanate* contains 88 percent normal human albumin, 12 percent globulin, and a minimal concentration of electrolytes. It provides a substitute for plasma with minimal risk of viral hepatitis; processing by heating to 60° C for 10 hours inactivates the virus [5]. It is indicated as a plasma expander in treatment of shock and burns.

Administration is by intravenous route, using the set provided in the package. Rate of administration and dosage are gauged to the individual and his needs. The minimal dose is usually 250 to 500 ml; rates up to 1 liter per hour have been well tolerated. Untoward reactions are rare. Plasmanate should not be mixed with protein hydrolysate solution or solutions containing ethyl alcohol or administered through the same administration sets.

Plasma Substitute

Dextran is a plasma volume expander used for the treatment of hypovolemic shock. When introduced into the bloodstream, dextran increases the osmotic pressure, draws interstitial fluid into the vessels, and increases the blood volume. It is a synthetic product with two advantages: (1) no storage problem and (2) no danger of hepatitis [8].

It is available as dextran 6 percent in normal saline solution or dextran 5 percent in water for patients requiring low sodium intake. The usual dose is 500 ml. Military hospitals and Massachusetts General Hospital use no more than 1 liter per 24 hours.

Allergic reactions to dextran are rare, but precautions should be taken. The first few milliliters of dextran should be administered slowly and the patient observed for possible reactions. These may include mild urticaria, tightness of the chest, and hypotension [8]. If any such symptoms occur, the dextran must be discontinued.

The rate of flow should be ordered by the physician. Caution must be observed when dextran is administered to patients with heart or kidney disease; a rapid rate may cause congestive heart failure and pulmonary edema.

Rho(D) Immune Globulin†

The successful prevention of maternal sensitization to the Rh factor by an anti-Rh immunoglobulin was first announced by Freda, Gorman,

* Cutter Laboratories, Inc., Berkeley, Calif.
† Gamulin Rh (Dow Pharmaceuticals, Indianapolis, Ind.); Hypo Rho-D (Cutter Laboratories, Inc., Berkeley, Calif.); RhoGAM (Ortho Diagnostics, Inc., Raritan, N.J.); Rho-Immune (Lederle Laboratories, Pearl River, N.Y.).

and Pollack in 1965, and RhoGAM was approved for distribution to physicians in 1968 [9].

The $Rh_o(D)$ antibody produced by the Rh-negative mother after delivery of an Rh-positive infant is the cause of Rh hemolytic disease of the newborn in subsequent pregnancies. $Rh_o(D)$ immune globulin administered within 72 hours after delivery suppresses the development of this antibody in the mother.

To be considered a candidate for $Rh_o(D)$ immune globulin the postpartum mother must (1) be $Rh_o(D)$-negative, D^u-negative, (2) not be already immunized to the $Rh_o(D)$ factor, and (3) have delivered a baby who is either $Rh_o(D)$-positive or D^u-positive [9]. The same conditions apply in an abortion or miscarriage. Since the fetal blood type may be unknown, the mother should receive $Rh_o(D)$ immune globulin if the father is $Rh_o(D)$-positive or D^u-positive. Rh immunoglobulin is also used to protect the Rh-negative patient not already sensitized to the $Rh_o(D)$ factor against immunization from infused Rh-positive blood components.

A cross-match must be performed with the recipient's fresh red cells and the anti-Rh immunoglobulin being used. It is important to substantiate the identity of the patient and verify the cross-match with the vial to be used.

One vial of RhoGAM will completely suppress immunity to 15 ml of Rh-positive red blood cells and is sufficient to suppress immunity to the Rh antigen in the usual full-term delivery. The volume of Rh-positive blood which enters the bloodstream determines the dose of Rho-GAM, which is administered intramuscularly. Reactions to Rh immunoglobulin are infrequent and mild and usually confined to the area of injection.

Blood Administration

With the rapid advancement in transfusion therapy, responsibility for administering this vital fluid increases. Only those well versed in every phase of therapy should hold this responsibility. The patient's safety depends upon adherence to specific rules regarding safe administration. The therapist is responsible for the following:

1. Patient-blood identification. The avoidance of mistaken identity is imperative.
2. Inspection of blood prior to administration to avoid infusing the patient with hemolyzed, clotted, or contaminated blood.
3. Proper technique.
4. Close observation of the patient. Early detection of symptoms of a reaction is important.

Patient-Blood Identification

Patient-blood identification is of paramount importance in preventing reactions from incompatible blood. The risk of identification errors occurring from copying information onto requisitions has been reduced by the use of the photocopier. The use of triplicate requisitions also reduces the danger of identification errors. This requisition, identifying the patient, indicating amount and kind of blood and time needed, is sent to the blood bank with the blood sample. One copy is retained at Dispatch or on the ward for demand of the processed blood. The upper portion is returned with the cross-matched blood to the floor.

All personnel handling blood are responsible for checking patient–bottle identification: name and unit number of the patient, blood groups of donor and recipient with blood groups on blood container, blood numbers and expiration date. The nurse on the ward is responsible for the first check when accepting the blood.

The intravenous nurse is responsible for a repeat check. In addition the requisition is checked with the patient's chart and then with the patient himself.

The patient receiving the blood must identify himself by complete name. Identity should never be made by addressing the patient by name and awaiting his response. Errors can occur from faulty response of medicated patients.

Hospital numbers on the identification bracelet must match unit numbers on the tag to prevent errors in case of like names. Any discrepancy must be investigated and corrected before the blood is administered.

Blood must never be administered to a patient who is unable to identify himself without some form of identification bracelet. An attending nurse may supply the identification.

Handling of Blood

Blood should be administered within 30 minutes of the time it leaves the bank. The National Institutes of Health and Massachusetts state regulations require controlled refrigeration (1° to 6° C). Ward refrigeration is not controlled and contains no alarm in case of fluctuation of temperature; therefore it must *not* be used for blood storage. Present regulations require that the temperature for storing blood must not vary more than 2°. Red blood cells deteriorate rapidly when blood remains at room temperature over 2 hours. If warm blood is indicated, a special set containing a heat exchange coil should be used (see Chapter 3). Hot water must never be used to heat blood.

Blood Inspections

Just prior to use, the transfusion therapist should carefully inspect the blood for abnormal color or gas bubbles which may indicate bacterial growth, and for abnormal appearance which may denote hemolysis or clotting.

Administration

Before the blood is administered, the red cells should be resuspended by repeated inversion. A sterile pyrogen-free filter must be used for any blood administration. The filter should be changed often enough to prevent clogging of the filter by accumulation.

When possible, isotonic saline should be used to initiate the transfusion. Whole blood should not be hooked up in series with 5 percent dextrose in water, or run simultaneously with 5 percent dextrose in water via the Y tube; hemolysis may result. (Hemolysis does not occur when 5 percent dextrose in water solution is infused into the bloodstream, because of its rapid dilution with the blood [8].)

Hypotonic or hypertonic solutions should not be used to dilute blood. Extreme hypotonicity causes water to invade the red cells until they swell and burst, causing hemolysis. Hypertonic solutions diluting blood result in reversal of this process, with shrinkage of the red cells. Solutions containing calcium should not be used to start citrated blood; to do so could cause clotting of the blood in the infusion set.

The administration set, with a filter, may contain a chamber for compressing to expedite the flow of blood. When whole blood is needed with such rapidity that positive pressure is necessary, it should be the physician's responsibility. Great caution is necessary. Certain risks may be involved when the blood is rapidly infused: circulatory overloading with pulmonary edema, citrate toxicity, cardiac arrest, and air embolism.

Once the transfusion is initiated, the therapist should observe the patient for at least the first 5 minutes of the infusion. Many of the fatal incompatible transfusion reactions produce symptoms early in the course of the infusion. The therapist and the attending nurse share a responsibility for safe transfusion administration. They must be familiar with the various transfusion reactions, recognize adverse reactions, and know what procedure to follow.

Transfusion Reactions

The following are adverse reactions which are hazards of transfusion administration.

FEBRILE REACTIONS. Chills, rapid rise of temperature, and headache are associated with leukocyte agglutinins. They appear more frequently in women who have had multiple pregnancies and in repeatedly transfused patients, i.e., patients who have had ± 40 units of blood. The infrequency of the development of leukocyte antibodies may be explained by the fact that leukocytes are not well preserved in stored blood [6]. Frozen blood is an answer to the problem; white cells have been removed by the repeated washings. In addition to the symptoms indicated, when the reaction is more severe, backache, nausea, vomiting, and hypotension may develop. The nurse, on observing the symptoms of a febrile reaction, should stop the transfusion immediately, note vital signs, and notify the physician and the Blood Bank.

CONTAMINATED BLOOD. Reactions from contaminated blood are rare. Improved techniques in blood collection, innovation of disposable equipment, and rules governing controlled refrigeration in storage of blood have reduced the risks of contaminated blood. Careful inspection of blood prior to use may alert the therapist to contamination. Reactions are severe and may be fatal. Severe shock usually occurs at the onset. Vasopressors and antibiotics have been used to treat such reactions.

PYROGENIC REACTIONS. Chills and fever occur when substances of nonpathogenic bacterial origin are infused into a patient. They occur during or after a transfusion and recovery is usually uneventful. Pyrogen-free solutions and disposable equipment have reduced such reactions.

ALLERGIC REACTIONS. Allergic reactions are manifested by urticaria or hives and occasionally are accompanied by chills and fever. Severe reactions may occur with asthmatic symptoms, fever, and anaphylactic shock. The appearance of any of these symptoms is an indication for immediate interruption of the transfusion.

Donors with allergies or hypersensitivity to certain drugs may be responsible for some of these reactions. A donor hypersensitive to a drug may have developed antibodies against the drug; blood from the donor infused into a patient who is receiving the drug may cause allergic reactions [5].

Elimination of donors with allergies and hypersensitivity to drugs reduces the incidence of allergic reactions, but reactions still occur. Treatment consists of administration of antihistaminics. Epinephrine or steroids are used in the most severe cases.

HEMOLYTIC TRANSFUSION REACTIONS. Hemolytic transfusion reactions are the most serious and may be fatal. These reactions are caused by intravascular hemolysis (rupture of red cells within the bloodstream) from an infusion of incompatible blood. Blood accidentally hemolyzed from improper handling may also produce hemolytic reactions when infused. Symptoms usually occur early in the course of the transfusion and include pain in the lower back and legs and tightness of the chest with breathlessness and shock. Fever may develop later and then hemoglobinuria, owing to the accumulation of free hemoglobin in the bloodstream.

The transfusion must be stopped at the first sign of a reaction, vital signs taken, and the physician and Blood Bank notified. A blood sample of 10 ml should be sent to the Blood Bank with the blood container. A sample of urine should be collected for detection of hemoglobin and urobilinogen, and all urine saved for observation of discoloration.

Treatment of hemolytic transfusion reactions usually consists first of combating shock by infusion of plasma and other fluids. Pressor agents may be used to treat hypotension. When kidney function is adequate, fluid and electrolytes may be necessary to maintain balance.

DANGERS FROM OVERTRANSFUSION. If the blood is infused too rapidly, a rise in the venous pressure may result. This is especially true in the aged and in patients on the verge of cardiac failure. Pulmonary edema, congestive failure, or hemorrhage into the lungs and the gastrointestinal tract may occur.

Monitoring the venous pressure guards against overtransfusion. The use of packed cells to infuse patients with normal blood volume may prevent overloading of the circulation.

The patient may complain of pounding headache, constriction of the chest, flushed feeling, back pain, chills, or fever. The nurse should stop the transfusion and notify the physician.

CITRATE TOXICITY. Citrate toxicity may be the result of an accumulation of citrate from infused ACD blood. It occurs from rapid administration of large volumes of citrated blood or from massive transfusion to patients with liver or renal impairment. The liver, unable to keep up with the rapid administration, is not able to metabolize the citrate ions; the citrate ions combine with calcium in the bloodstream, causing a calcium deficit. The normal plasma citrate level for a healthy person is 3 mg per 100 ml. When the level exceeds 50 mg per 100 ml, symptoms of toxicity may occur. Citrate administered at the rate of 1 mg per minute increases the plasma level to 12.5 mg per 100 ml; blood pumped in at the rate of 500 ml in 5 minutes would increase citrate to this dangerous level [5].

Symptoms of excess citrate include tingling of fingers, muscular cramps, convulsions, hypotension, and cardiac arrest. Most of these symptoms are absent in the anesthetized patient, making detection of toxicity difficult.

Treatment consists of slow administration by a physician of ionized calcium such as calcium chloride.

AIR EMBOLISM. Air embolism is a hazard of intravenous and transfusion therapy. It may result from

1. Rapid emptying of the blood container by application of positive pressure in a vented set.
2. Emptying of the blood container when negative pressure exists in the vein.
3. Introduction of air in the process of changing bottles.
4. Careless use of the Y-type administration set.

The risk of air embolism has been reduced by the closed system, using the collapsible plastic container. Air pressure should not be used for rapid blood infusion; air emboli may result from tenacious bubbles in the blood becoming lodged in the pulmonary capillaries [1].

If a vented blood container is allowed to go dry and a negative venous pressure exists, air will be sucked into the recipient's circulation [5]. The arm should never be elevated above the chest level; this causes a negative venous pressure in the arm.

Care should be taken in changing bottles. If the fluid level had dropped in the administration set, the trapped air will be forced into the circulation when a fresh solution is hung. The pressure pump in an administration set should be kept filled at all times.

Air emboli can result from careless use of a Y-type administration set, or an intravenous set piggybacked onto an initial intravenous setup. If the clamps on both sets are left open and the vented bottle is allowed to go dry, air is sucked into the circulation; the atmospheric pressure, being greater in the empty bottle, will cause the empty bottle to become the source of air for the air vent. Although a less obvious source of air emboli, this may cause large quantities of air to be introduced into the tubing and circulation [12].

References
1. Adriani, J. Venipuncture. *American Journal of Nursing* 62:66, 1962.
2. American Association of Blood Banks. *Standards for Blood Banks and Transfusion Services* (5th ed.). Chicago: Twentieth Century Press, 1970. Pp. 12, 13.
3. Crouch, M. L., and Gibson, S. T. Blood therapy. *American Journal of Nursing* 62:71, 1962.
4. Fisk, R. T. *A Manual of Blood Grouping and Rh Typing Serums* (3d ed.). Los Angeles: Hyland Laboratories, 1956. Pp. 5, 8.
5. Grove-Rasmussen, M., Lesses, M. F., and Anstall, H. B. Medical progress: Transfusion therapy. *New England Journal of Medicine* 264:1034–1044, 1088–1095, 1961.
6. Hyland Laboratories. *Hyland Reference Manual of Immunohematology* (3d ed.). Los Angeles, 1965. Pp. 3–7, 36, 85–87.
7. Machine Extends Blood Storage Time. *Hospital Formulary Management*. Chicago: Clissold Publishing, 1966. P. 44.
8. Metheny, N. M., and Snively, W. D., Jr. *Nurses' Handbook of Fluid Balance*. Philadelphia: Lippincott, 1967. P. 139.

9. Ortho Diagnostics. *RhoGAM One Year Later* (Proceedings of Symposium on RhoGAM, $RH_0[D]$ Immune Globulin [Human], New York, April 17, 1969). Raritan, N.J., 1969. Pp. 11, 14, 59.
10. Pool, J. G. Precipitate from cold thawed plasma potent in therapy for hemophiliacs. *Journal of the American Medical Association* 193:27, 1965.
11. Solis, R. T., and Gibbs, M. B. Filtration of the microaggregates in stored blood. *Transfusion* 12:245, 1972.
12. Tarail, R. Practice of fluid therapy. *Journal of the American Medical Association* 171:45–49, 1950.

17. The Therapeutic Phlebotomy

The purpose of this chapter is to acquaint the physician or nurse who may be called upon to perform a phlebotomy outside the confines of the blood bank with the equipment, the procedure, and the technique recommended for the protection of the donor and the recipient. The phlebotomy, a bleeding of usually 400 to 500 ml of blood, is performed for transfusion purposes and therapeutically for acute pulmonary congestion, polycythemia vera, hemochromatosis, and porphyria cutanea tarda.

Blood for Transfusion Purposes

Routine Blood Bank Blood
When the bleeding is performed for routine bank blood, donor selection is based on the medical history and the physical examination (weight, temperature, pulse, blood pressure, and hemoglobin). The technique is according to the standards of the American Association of Blood Banks (A.A.B.B.) [1].

Autotransfusion
Autotransfusion is used to return the patient's own blood to the circulation. The phlebotomy may be a:

1. *Blood bank procedure.* When the phlebotomy is performed in the blood bank, the usual blood bank procedure is followed. The blood can be stored at 4° C or the red cells can be frozen.
2. *Non-blood bank procedure.* When the bleeding is performed outside the confines of the blood bank, the same technique (according to the standards of the A.A.B.B.) is used. However, the donor criteria can be modified; for example, a person with a history of cancer cannot make a routine donation but may donate for himself. Blood which is suitable only for the donor must be labeled with his name, hospital number, or social security number and segregated from

other donor bloods. The ABO type is confirmed just prior to transfusion.

An important fact to bear in mind is the possibility of sepsis; clinically undetected bacteremia may exist in the patient with a catheter, a tracheostomy, or a disease process.

Therapeutic Purposes

The therapeutic phlebotomy is a valuable therapeutic means by which a quantity of blood is removed to promote the health of the donor. It requires a written order by the physician specifying the date and the amount of blood to be drawn. If the recipient's physician approves and if the diagnosis is conspicuously labeled, the blood may be used for transfusion.

Acute Pulmonary Congestion (Inpatient)

The phlebotomy is performed to reduce venous pressure and to relieve the work load on the heart of a patient suffering from acute pulmonary edema of cardiac failure or overtransfusion. Overtransfusion is much less likely to occur today since central venous pressure monitoring provides a valuable guide for fluid administration and drugs are available to increase cardiac output and lower the central venous pressure. Since the patient with acute pulmonary congestion is critically ill, the phlebotomy should probably be done by, or in the presence of, the patient's physician.

Polycythemia Vera (Inpatient or Outpatient)

The therapeutic phlebotomy is most frequently performed on the hospital patient for the production of remissions in the treatment of polycythemia vera, a disease characterized by a striking absolute increase in the number of circulating red blood corpuscles. It is used to reduce the red cell mass, either alone or in combination with radioactive phosphorus (^{32}P), lowering the blood volume, reducing blood viscosity, and improving circulatory efficiency. The number of and interval between phlebotomies should be specified by the physician and the hematocrit value determined after the blood donation.

Hemochromatosis (Usually Outpatient)

Hemochromatosis is characterized by excessive body stores of iron. The phlebotomy is performed to reduce the total body iron. Since these patients usually have a hematocrit value in the normal range, periodic checks on the hematocrit value are desirable.

Porphyria Cutanea Tarda (Usually Outpatient)
The mechanism of relief of these skin lesions by phlebotomy is not clear. Since these patients have a normal hematocrit reading they are most likely to be bled too much; periodic hematocrit checks are desirable.

Procedure for Bleeding
To allay apprehension and to avoid a vasovagal reaction (an undesirable autonomic nervous system response), the procedure should be explained, and the patient reassured and put at ease.

Donor Arm Preparation
Adequate preparation of the skin is vital in providing an aseptic site for venipuncture which will protect both the donor and the recipient. In preparing the area always start at the venipuncture site and move outward in concentric spirals for at least 1½ inches.

1. Using a surgical soap, scrub vigorously for at least 30 seconds with gauze, or 60 seconds with cotton balls.
2. Apply 10 percent acetone in 70 percent alcohol to remove the soap; let dry.
3. Apply tincture of iodine (3 percent in 70 percent alcohol) and allow to dry.
4. Use 10 percent acetone in 70 percent alcohol to remove the iodine.
5. Place a dry sterile gauze over the site until ready to perform the venipuncture.

Alternative procedure:
1. Use 0.75 percent aqueous scrub solution of iodophor compound (povidone-iodine or poloxamer iodine complex), scrubbing the area for 2 minutes. Remove the foam; it is not necessary to dry the arm.
2. Prepare with iodophor complex solution (e.g., 10 percent povidone-iodine); allow to stand 1 minute.
3. Place a dry sterile gauze sponge over the site until ready to perform the venipuncture.

Collection of Blood
The following procedure for the collection of blood (see Figure 41) using both the plastic bag and the vacuum bottle, together with the instructions for the treatment of reactions, is reproduced from the A.A.B.B.'s *Technical Methods and Procedures* [1]. Modification to this procedure may be made when the blood is to be discarded.

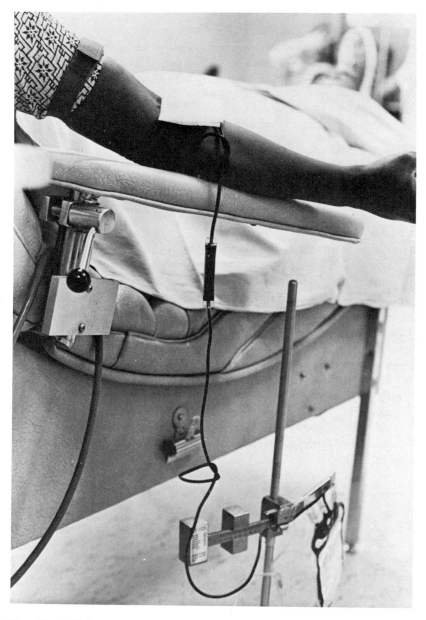

Fig. 41. A phlebotomy. Note the sterile sponge placed over the venipuncture site during bleeding.

1. Plastic bags

   Blood may be collected either by gravity or with a vacuum assist device. These devices also mix the blood and automatically stop the collection at the proper time. When they are used, certain modifications of the collection procedure are necessary and the manufacturer's directions should be consulted. Most bags have an integral needle and donor set, but some are available with a separate donor set (procedures must be modified accordingly). Before starting, make sure that the numbers on the container, pilot tubes, and donor record are in agreement.

   a. If a balance system is used, be sure that the counter-balance is properly adjusted for the amount of blood to be collected. Hang the bag and route the plastic donor tubing through the pinch clamp after making a *very loose* overhand knot in the tubing.

      If a balance system is not used, position the bag low enough to permit gravity collection.

      It may be hung from the loops at the bottom so that the blood is collected through the solution. A spring scale may be used to measure the collection, after adjusting it to allow for the weight of the bag and attached pilot tubes.

   b. After adjusting the tourniquet, or inflating the blood pressure cuff (50–60 mm of mercury), instruct the donor to open and close his hand several times, then to keep his hand closed tightly.

   c. Uncover the donor needle, being careful not to contaminate it. If there is any question that it has touched an unsterile surface, the plastic bag must be discarded. Do the venipuncture at once.

   d. Plastic bags have a temporary closure between the interior of the bag and the integral donor tubing. Open this closure (following manufacturer's directions) to permit the flow of blood into the bag. Be careful not to puncture the bag with sharp fingernails or metal objects.

   e. Tape the tubing to the arm of the donor to hold the needle in place. The phlebotomy site and needle should be covered with sterile gauze. Ask the donor to open and close his fist continuously. A resilient ball, roll of cloth, or other object for the donor to squeeze will help.

   f. Mix the blood and anticoagulant solution gently, frequently enough to prevent coagulation. This is done automatically by most vacuum-assisted devices.

   g. If a balance system is used, blood flow will stop when the proper amount of blood has been collected. If spring scales are used, collection must be stopped manually.

   h. Seal the donor tubing approximately 12 inches from the needle by making a "white knot" or by metal clips and a hand-sealer. The white knot is one that is pulled tightly until white and free of blood. This is easier to do if the tubing is slightly wet with alcohol. It is accepted as a hermetic seal.

   i. Strip the blood in the donor tubing from the knot into the donor bag, mix, and allow the tubing to refill. Repeat at least once.

   j. Grasping the tubing on the donor side of the knot between thumb and forefinger, press to remove the blood for a distance of not more than one inch. Using a hemostat, clamp the tubing close to the thumb. *Caution: Do not* strip for a greater distance because, in the unlikely event that the blood in the needle has already clotted, pressure may dislodge the clot into the donor's vein.

k. Cut the tubing between the hemostat and the seal.
l. Samples to be used for blood processing, or pilot samples, may be collected from the cut end of donor tubing by releasing the hemostat and allowing blood to flow into the tube. Such samples are not sterile.
m. Reapply the hemostat, deflate and remove tourniquet. Remove the tape, withdraw the needle from the donor's arm, and immediately apply pressure to the gauze over the venipuncture site. Tell the donor to raise his arm, keeping his elbow straight, and to hold the gauze firmly onto the phlebotomy site with his other hand. Discard the needle assembly.
n. The donor tubing may be sealed into segments, using knots, clips, or a heat sealer. Leave the segments attached to the bag. They constitute sterile pilot samples, suitable for crossmatching. A final seal should be within two inches of the bag.
Note: The foregoing procedure provides nonsterile blood samples and pilot samples consisting of segments of tubing containing ACD blood. If sterile pilot samples are needed, other technics will be required. Some plastic bags are equipped with another needle, either at the bag end or in the integral donor tubing. At the completion of blood collection, and before removing the needle from the donor's arm, this extra needle may be exposed and used to fill sterile pilot tubes with blood direct from the donor (consult manufacturer's detailed directions). If clotted blood is desired for pilot tubes, the technic should include precautions not to allow the entry of anticoagulated blood from the container.
o. Initial the Donor Record and record the amount of blood drawn.
p. Refrigerate the unit of blood as soon as possible.
2. Bottles—vacuum
Bottles for the collection of blood should not be cooled before use, since this may cause hemolysis. If there is any doubt that either of the two donor set needles has touched an unsterile surface, *the set must not be used.* Before blood is collected, the container and pilot tube or tubes must be properly numbered and firmly attached to the bottle, in such a manner that removal of them will be clearly evident.
a. Inspect the bottle to be sure the anticoagulant is clear, that the numbers on the pilot tubes, bottle and history card agree and that the vacuum is intact. (Shake the bottle and listen for sound. Splashy sound indicates loss of vacuum; no sound indicates vacuum present.)
b. Remove protective cap from bottle.
c. Clamp donor set near bottle needle.
d. Uncover and insert needle into "inlet" of bottle. The parts marked "outlet" and "air" or "vent" do not provide proper sealing.
e. Invert the bottle at once to check for bubbles rising in the anticoagulant solution. These indicate that air is entering the bottle, usually around the needle. Such a bottle and donor set must be discarded and another of each used. If no air enters, leave the bottle inverted and hang it in this position.
f. Uncover the donor needle and do the venipuncture at once.
g. Open the tubing clamp. Blood should be collected with the bottle *inverted* so that the blood passes up through the anticoagulant and foaming is minimal. The bottle should be gently rotated throughout the phlebotomy to ensure adequate mixing. The bottle must be below the level of the donor's arm throughout the bleeding to guard against air embolism.

h. After blood collection, clamp the tubing, remove the needle from the *bottle,* insert it into the attached pre-numbered pilot tubes and fill them with blood.

i. Release the tourniquet or blood pressure cuff and quickly remove the needle from the donor's arm. Apply pressure over the phlebotomy site with sterile gauze. Tell the donor to raise his arm, keeping his elbow straight, and to hold the gauze firmly over the phlebotomy site with his other hand.

j. After the collection of blood, the bottle should be *gently* inverted several times to ensure thorough mixing of the contents. Paint the rubber stopper with iodine. Replace the metal cap and seal. Promptly refrigerate the unit of blood.

Instructions for the treatment of donor reactions are provided by the American Association of Blood Banks [1] as follows:

1. General
   a. At the first sign of reaction during the phlebotomy, remove the tourniquet and withdraw the needle from the arm.
   b. If the treatment listed in the items below does not result in a rapid recovery, call the Blood Bank Medical Director or the physician designated by him for such purposes. If this person is not available, call the nearest physician.
2. Syncope (fainting)
   a. Place the donor on his back, and raise his feet above the level of his head.
   b. Loosen tight clothing.
   c. Administer aromatic spirits of ammonia by inhalation. Test the ammonia on yourself before passing it under the donor's nose, as it may be too strong or too weak. Strong ammonia may injure the nasal membranes; weak ammonia is not effective. The donor should respond by coughing.
   d. Be sure the donor has an ADEQUATE AIRWAY.
   e. Check and record the blood pressure, pulse and respiration periodically until the donor recovers.
   f. Cold compresses may be applied to the donor's forehead or the back of his neck.
3. Nausea and vomiting
   a. Make the donor as comfortable as possible.
   b. If the donor is only nauseated, instruct him to breathe deeply and slowly.
   c. Apply cold compresses to the donor's forehead.
   d. If the donor vomits, provide an emesis basin and have cleansing tissues or a damp towel ready.
   e. Give the donor a *paper* cup of water to rinse out his mouth.
4. Convulsions
   a. Prevent the donor from injuring himself. Call someone to help you. During seizures, some people exhibit great muscular power.
      (1) Place tongue blades wrapped with gauze between the teeth of the donor to prevent him from chewing his tongue. Keep the blades in place until the donor recovers.
      (2) If possible, hold the donor on the chair or bed; if not possible, place the donor on the floor. Do not restrain the movements of

the donor's extremities completely, but try to prevent him from injuring himself or you.

    b. Be sure the donor has an ADEQUATE AIRWAY.

    c. In case of convulsions, call for medical aid.

5. Cardiac or respiratory difficulties

    Call for medical aid. If there is any suspicion of air embolism, turn donor on his left side, head down.

6. Hyperventilation

    Extremely anxious donors sometimes hyperventilate, causing a faint, muscular twitching, or tetanic spasms of their hands. If this syndrome is recognized, having the donor re-breathe into a paper bag will usually produce prompt relief.

7. Hematoma

    a. Remove the tourniquet.

    b. Place three or four sterile gauze squares over the hematoma and apply firm digital pressure for 7 to 10 minutes with the donor's arm held above the heart level.

The following is a suggested list of drugs . . . that may be considered desirable for immediate use by the physician called to treat donor reactions:

    a. Vasopressors

        Aramine (Metaraminol—ampules, 10 mg/ml)

        Wyamine (Mephentermine—ampules, 30 mg/ml)

        Levophed (Levarterenol—ampules, 2 mg/ml, 4 ml)

    b. Cardiac stimulants

        Adrenaline (Epinephrine—1:1,000, 1 ml ampules)

    c. Coronary vasodilators

        Nitroglycerine tablets, 0.3 mg for sublingual use

    d. Anticonvulsants and sedatives

        Dilantin Sodium (Diphenylhydantoin sodium—250 mg)

        Sodium Amytal (Sodium Amobarbital—ampules, 250 mg)

    e. Bronchodilators

        Aminophyllin—ampules, 250 mg

        Isuprel (Isoproterenol—10 mg tablets for sublingual use)

Suggested Procedure for Therapeutic Phlebotomy

The blood must be discarded. This procedure is not adequate for recipient protection.

Equipment

Phlebotomy pack (obtained from Blood Bank); if only double pack is available, ignore the satellite pack.

Counterbalance stand (obtained from Blood Bank) or small spring scale.

Blood pressure cuff or tourniquet

Tincture of iodine (3 percent in 70 percent alcohol) or iodophor complex solution (10 percent povidone-iodine)

10 percent acetone in 70 percent isopropyl alcohol for use with tincture of iodine

Sterile sponges

Technique

PREPARATION

1. Select the most suitable vein. Apply a tourniquet or a blood pressure cuff inflated to 50 to 60 mm of mercury. Opening and closing the fist will make the vein more prominent. Remove tourniquet.
2. Prepare venipuncture site. Always start at puncture site and move out in concentric spirals for 1½ inches.

   a. Apply tincture of iodine; allow to dry. *Question patient before applying; some patients may be allergic to iodine.*

   b. Apply 10 percent acetone in 70 percent alcohol to remove iodine. Allow to dry. Iodophor complex (10 percent povidone-iodine) may be substituted for iodine. It does not cause skin reactions even in iodine-sensitive individuals. Do not wash off iodophor complex. Cover site with dry sterile gauze to prevent contamination until phlebotomy is begun.

COLLECTION OF BLOOD

1. Suspend bag from donor scale as far below donor's arm as possible.
2. If counterbalance scales are used, adjust the balance for amount of blood to be drawn.
3. Make loose overhand knot in donor tube near needle.
4. Apply tourniquet (do not impair arterial circulation).
5. *Do not touch or repalpate vein.*
6. Perform phlebotomy.
7. Tape needle in place and cover with sterile sponge.
8. Pinch bead into bag from junction of donor tube and bag to open lumen and allow blood to flow.
9. Instruct patient to open and close fist slowly.
10. Collect blood until bag falls on scale. If spring scales are used, collect until prescribed amount has been withdrawn.
11. Pull knot tight.
12. Release tourniquet, withdraw needle, and apply pressure with gauze pad until bleeding has stopped. *Do not flex arm.* The arm may be elevated while applying pressure.

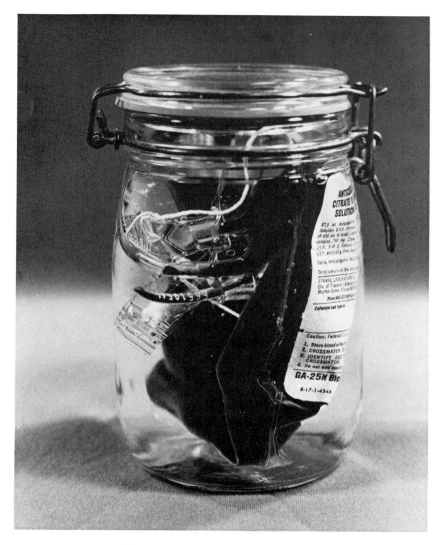

Fig. 42. During autoclaving to decontaminate a unit of blood, bag is protected by a water bath in a sealed glass container. (Specimen bottle, Wheaton Scientific, Millville, N.J.)

13. Dispose of blood and equipment as directed by hospital procedure. *Caution:* blood infected with the hepatitis virus should be decontaminated before disposal. The bag of blood, protected by a water bath in a sealed glass container (see Figure 42), is autoclaved at 120° C at 15 pounds of pressure per square inch for 60 minutes.

14. Record procedure in patient's record.

Reference

1. American Association of Blood Banks. *Technical Methods and Procedures of the American Association of Blood Banks* (5th ed.). Chicago, Ill., 1970. Pp. 12–13, 18–22, 25–28.

18. Hypodermoclysis

On January 26, 1966, the Massachusetts Board of Registration in Nursing passed a ruling currently in effect which states that "Hypodermoclysis administration is not a nursing function." The hospital may assume responsibility, however, and delegate the procedure to a special group of professional registered nurses whom they have certified.

Hypodermoclysis is a term used to denote an injection of fluid into the subcutaneous tissue. In recent years there has been a decrease in this method of fluid administration. Problems which once justified the hypodermoclysis have been resolved by new innovations in intravenous equipment. Controlled volume sets and precision pumps have reduced the risk of speed shock which once made slow absorption by subcutaneous tissues essential. The use of the intracatheter has reduced the frequency of infiltrations, a problem which increased the use of the clysis.

Disadvantages
Definite disadvantages and hazards are associated with the subcutaneous route.

1. Fluids are not readily absorbed when infused into the subcutaneous tissues of patients with a severely reduced blood volume because of the accompanying peripheral collapse.
2. Many types of fluids required by patients cannot be given subcutaneously. Fluids must resemble plasma in tonicity and electrolyte composition if subcutaneous absorption is to occur. Hypertonic solutions, not absorbed, draw body fluid and electrolyte into the tissues in the infused area; this may result in a reduced fluid volume, with the threat of circulatory collapse. These solutions increase swelling and edema, which may cause ischemia of the skin's blood vessels with subsequent sloughing of the tissues.
3. Nonelectrolyte sugar solutions are contraindicated since they may

produce circulatory difficulties such as hypotension and anuria when infused into patients with a sodium deficit, a low blood volume, or renal impairment [2]. Dextrose in water attracts body fluid and electrolyte, increasing edema in the injection area and reducing the plasma volume [3].

4. Solutions such as the gastric replacement solutions, containing a pH significantly different from the blood pH, are contraindicated for subcutaneous infusion [3]. Solutions containing alcohol are irritating and may cause sloughing of the tissues. Solutions of high molecular weight, such as albumin, are not absorbed.

Suitable Solutions

The solutions considered suitable for subcutaneous administration include

0.9 percent sodium chloride injection, U.S.P.
2½ percent dextrose in 0.45 percent sodium chloride, U.S.P.
2½ percent dextrose in half-strength Ringer's solution
Ringer's solution
Lactated Ringer's injection
2½ percent dextrose in half-strength lactated Ringer's injection

Procedure for Administration

The fluid may be administered through an intravenous administration set, but to hasten the infusion the hypodermoclysis set is usually used. This is a Y-type set employing two needles. Each arm of the Y contains a clamp to control the rate of flow.

The area most commonly used is the outer front of the thighs between the knee and the hip [1]. A generous area of skin is thoroughly prepared with iodine and alcohol. If local anesthesia is required, 0.5 ml of 1 percent procaine may be used, provided the patient has never demonstrated a sensitivity to the drug.

The following steps should be carried out:

1. Expel all air from tubing.
2. To provide sterile dressings at injection site during infusion, pierce the center of sterile gauze sponges with each needle.
3. Prepare skin thoroughly.
4. If desired, inject procaine intradermally to raise a wheal through which the needle can be inserted.
5. Hold tissues firmly in the left hand. The needle should be inserted at about a 30-degree angle with a quick motion.

6. Check for backflow of blood to ascertain that a blood vessel has not been entered. If a blood return is obtained relocate needle in subcutaneous tissue.
7. Start fluid and regulate flow.
8. Tape needle securely.

The *rate of administration* depends upon the individual's ability to absorb the fluid and should be regulated accordingly. If necessary the flow can be completely stopped until the fluid has been absorbed. To accelerate absorption, an enzyme, hyaluronidase, is sometimes injected into the tissues or added to the infusion [3].

Cautions
The following precautions should be observed:

1. The solution should be checked carefully to prevent hypertonic solution from being administered in error.
2. The rate of flow should be checked frequently to prevent any increased pressure that may impair the circulation and cause sloughing.
3. Aseptic technique must be adhered to in order to prevent abscesses due to infection. Unlike the blood, the tissues lack the abundance of antibodies necessary to combat infection, and infection in the subcutaneous tissue spreads rapidly.
4. As edematous fluid is an excellent culture medium for bacteria, a sterile dressing should be applied following removal of the needles.

References
1. McGaw Laboratories. *Parenteral Fluid Therapy by the Subcutaneous Route*. Technical Information Bulletin. Glendale, Calif., 1966. Pp. 1–2.
2. McGaw Laboratories. *Guide to Parenteral Fluid Therapy*. Glendale, Calif., 1963. P. 27.
3. Metheny, N. M., and Snively, W. D., Jr. *Nurses' Handbook of Fluid Balance*. Philadelphia: Lippincott, 1967. P. 116.

19. Laboratory Tests

Many intravenous departments are now including as one of their functions the collection of venous blood samples. Definite advantages are gained when this function is allocated to the intravenous nurse. (1) The nurse, understanding the importance of the preservation of veins for infusion therapy, is cautious in her choice of veins and in her technique in drawing blood. (2) Frequently one venipuncture permits both the withdrawal of blood and the initiation of the infusion, thereby preserving veins, reducing discomfort, and avoiding undue distress of the patient. (3) The patient-blood identification is of paramount importance in preventing the error of infusing incompatible blood. Because the department assumes responsibility in patient-blood identification in administering bloods and is aware of existing hazards, its personnel are well qualified and trained in the collection of samples for typing and cross-matching.

The nurse is often faced with the problem of collecting blood with little or no knowledge of the tests other than the amount of blood needed and the type of tube required. This chapter is primarily for the purpose of providing the nurse with information concerning the most commonly performed laboratory tests—their purpose, normal values, and the collection and proper handling of the specimens. No attempt is made to explain laboratory procedures.

Collection of Venous Blood Samples

Proper Collection and Handling of Specimens

The collection of blood samples for certain tests must meet special requirements. Some tests call for whole blood, while others require components such as plasma, serum, or cells. The proper requirement must be met to prevent erroneous or misleading laboratory analysis.

Serum "contains all the stable constituents of plasma except fibrinogen" [3] and is obtained by drawing blood in a dry tube and allowing it to coagulate. Serum is required by the majority of laboratory tests in common use.

Plasma "contains all the stable components of blood except the cells" [3] and is obtained by using an anticoagulant to prevent the blood from clotting. Several anticoagulants are available in color-coded tubes. Choice of the anticoagulant depends upon the test to be performed. Most of the anticoagulants, including sodium or potassium oxalate, citrate, and ethylenediaminetetraacetic acid (EDTA), prevent coagulation by binding the serum calcium. Other anticoagulants, such as heparin, are valuable in specific tests but not commonly used. Heparin prevents coagulation for only limited periods of time.

Whole blood is required for many tests, including blood counts and bleeding time. Potassium oxalate is commonly used to preserve whole blood.

Fasting. As absorption of food may alter the blood, some tests depend upon the patient's fasting. Blood glucose and serum lipid levels are increased by ingestion of food. Serum inorganic phosphorous values are depressed after meals.

Intravenous solutions may contribute to misleading laboratory interpretations. Blood samples should never be drawn proximal to an infusion but preferably from the other extremity. If the solution contains a substance which may affect the analysis, an indication of its presence should be made on the requisition—for example, potassium determination during an infusion of electrolyte solution.

Hemoconcentration through venous stasis should be avoided or inaccurate results will occur in some tests. Hemoconcentration increases proportionally with the length of time the tourniquet is applied. Once the venipuncture has been made, the tourniquet should be removed. This is a simple but important precaution, ignored by many. Carbon dioxide and pH are examples of tests affected by hemoconcentration. If the tourniquet is required to withdraw the blood, it should be noted on the requisition that the blood was drawn with stasis.

Promptness of examination. Immediate dispatch of blood samples to the laboratory is vital to the accurate determination of some blood tests; promptness in examining blood samples is necessary in the analysis of labile constituents of blood. In certain tests, such as potassium, the substance being measured diffuses out of the cells into the serum being examined and gives a false measurement. To prevent this rise in serum concentration, the cells must be separated from the serum promptly.

Special handling is required with some samples when a delay is unavoidable. Some determinations, such as the pH, must be done within 10 minutes after the blood is drawn. When a delay is inevitable, the sample is placed in ice, which partially inhibits glycolysis. Glycolysis is the production of lactic acid by the glycolytic enzymes of the blood cells and results in a rapid lowering of pH on standing.

Blood gases also require special handling and must be analyzed as soon as collected. When the carbon dioxide content of serum is to be determined, the blood is placed in a tube with mineral oil to prevent the escape of carbon dioxide. Any disturbance in the interface between the blood and the oil will permit carbon dioxide to escape.

Hemolysis causes serious errors in many tests in which lysis of the red cells permits the substance being measured to escape into the serum. When red cells rich in potassium rupture, the serum potassium level rises, giving a false measurement. To avoid hemolysis, special precautions should be observed:

1. Dry syringes and dry tubes must be used.
2. Excess pressure on the plunger of the syringe should be avoided; such pressure collapses the vein and may cause air bubbles to be sucked from around the hub of the needle into the blood.
3. Clotted blood specimens should not be shaken unnecessarily.
4. Force should be avoided in transferring blood to a container or tube; force of the blood against the tube results in rupture of the cells. In transferring blood to a vacuum tube, no needle larger than 20 gauge should be used.

Infected samples. Special caution must be observed in the care of blood specimens suspected of harboring microorganisms that cause infectious disease. Specimens should not be allowed to spill on the outside of the containers and should be placed in a paper bag or plastic container and well labeled.

Emergency tests. Blood tests ordered as emergency must be sent directly to the laboratory. Red cellophane tape is helpful in indicating a state of emergency. Tests most likely to be designated as emergencies include amylase, blood urea nitrogen (BUN), carbon dioxide, potassium, prothrombin, sodium, sugar, and blood typing.

Venipuncture for Withdrawing Blood

A venipuncture when skillfully executed subjects the patient to little discomfort. The numerous blood determinations necessary for diagnosis and treatment make good technique imperative.

The stab technique should be avoided as it too often results in through-and-through punctures, contributing to hematoma formation. The needle should be inserted under the skin and then, after relocation of the vein, into the vessel.

The veins most commonly used are those in the antecubital fossa. The median antecubital vein, though not always visible, is usually large and palpable. Since it is well supported by subcutaneous tissue and least apt to roll, it is often the best choice for venipuncture. Second choice is the cephalic vein. The basilic vein, though often times the most prominent, is apt to be the least desirable. This vein rolls easily, making the venipuncture difficult, and a hematoma may readily occur if the patient is allowed to flex his arm; flexing the arm squeezes the blood from the engorged vein into the tissues.

Sufficient time should be spent in locating the vein before attempting venipuncture. Whenever the veins are difficult to see or palpate, the patient should lie down. If the patient is seated the arm should be well supported on a pillow.

Complications

Hematomas are the most common complication of routine venipuncture for withdrawing blood, and they contribute more to the limitation of available veins than any other complication. They may result from through-and-through puncture to the vein or from incomplete insertion of the needle into the lumen of the vein, which allows the blood to leak into the tissues by way of the bevel of the needle. In the latter case, correction may be made by advancing the needle into the vein. At the first sign of uncontrolled bleeding, the tourniquet should be released and the needle withdrawn.

Hematomas also result from the application of the tourniquet after an unsuccessful attempt has been made to draw blood. The tourniquet should never be applied to the extremity immediately after a venipuncture.

Hematomas most frequently result from insufficient time spent in applying pressure and from the bad habit of flexing the arm to stop the bleeding. Once the venipuncture is completed, the patient should be instructed to elevate his arm; elevation causes a negative pressure in the vein, collapsing it and facilitating clotting. With cardiac patients, elevation of the arm should be avoided. Constant pressure is maintained until the bleeding has stopped. Pressure is applied with a dry sterile sponge; a wet sponge encourages bleeding. Band-Aids do not take the place of pressure and, if ordered, are not applied until the bleeding has stopped. Ecchymoses on the arm indicate poor technique or haphazard manner.

Other complications of venipuncture include syncope, continued bleeding, and thrombosis of the vein. Serum hepatitis may occur if the same syringes or needle holders are used for multiple punctures.

Syncope is rarely encountered when the therapist is confident, skillful, and reassures the patient.

Continued bleeding is a complication which may affect the patient receiving anticoagulants or the patient with a blood dyscrasia. To prevent bleeding and to preserve the vein, pressure to the site may be required for an extended period of time. The therapist should remain with the patient until the bleeding has stopped.

Thrombosis in routine venipuncture occurs from injury to the endothelial lining of the vein during the venipuncture. Antecubital veins may be used indefinitely if the therapist is skillful in her technique.

Hepatitis. Special caution must be exercised in the care of needles used to draw blood from patients suspected of harboring microorganisms. Contaminated needles should be placed immediately in a separate container for disposal. A vacuum tube with stopper provides adequate protection against accidental puncture from the contaminated needle until proper disposal can be made. Any needle puncture should be reported at once.

The Vacuum System

The vacuum system, which is replacing the syringe for withdrawing blood, has done much to increase the efficiency of the program. It consists of a plastic holder into which screws a sterile disposable double-ended needle. A rubber-stoppered vacuum tube slips into the barrel. The barrel has a measured line denoting the distance the tube is inserted into the barrel; at this point the needle becomes embedded in the stopper. The stopper is not punctured until the needle has been introduced into the vein.

After entry into the vein, the rubber-stoppered tube is pushed the remaining distance into the barrel. This forces the needle into the vacuum tube which automatically draws the blood. The tourniquet is released and several specimens may be obtained by simply removing the tube containing the sample and replacing with another tube. To avoid excess blood from dripping into the needle holder during the process of changing tubes, the finger is pressed against the vein, stopping the flow until the new tube is inserted (see Figure 43).

If there is failure in locating the vein, removal of the tube before the needle is withdrawn will preserve the vacuum in the tube.

At times it becomes necessary to draw blood from small veins. If suction from the vacuum tube collapses the vein, difficulty will be encountered in drawing the blood. By pressing the finger against the vein beyond the point of the needle or by placing the bevel of the needle lightly against the wall of the vein, suction is reduced and the vein allowed to fill. In the latter process, particular caution should be exercised to prevent injury to the endothelial lining of the vein. The pressure is intermittently applied and released, filling and emptying the vein. A 22-gauge needle is available and often used successfully when small amounts of blood are needed; the smaller needle reduces the amount of suction and may prevent collapse of the vein. A syringe is

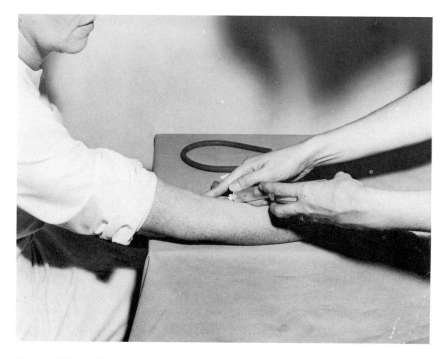

Fig. 43. When the needle holder with a vacuum tube is used for collecting multiple blood samples, pressure on the vein prevents blood from leaking into the barrel. (Becton, Dickinson and Co., Rutherford, N.J.)

often used to draw blood from small veins as the amount of suction can be more easily controlled.

Needle holders, when used with needles that are not designed to prevent leakage, should be disposed of after use with each patient. There is potential danger of transmitting hepatitis when holders are reused without gas sterilization. A needle holder free of blood gives no assurance of safety; the shaft of the needle may be contaminated by the blood sample in which it was contained. It is virtually impossible to remove the needle without touching the holder.

Special needles are available for use in drawing multiple blood samples. They prevent blood spills and reduce the risk of hepatitis. A rubber sheath covers the shaft of the needle. As the needle enters the rubber-stoppered tube, the sheath is pushed back allowing the blood to flow. As the tube is removed, the rubber sheath slips back over the needle, preventing blood from dripping into the holder.

Drawing Blood via the Central Venous Catheter
Occasionally it becomes desirable to draw blood samples via the central venous catheter. Such occasions include difficulty in obtaining

an adequate vein, cases in which the avoidance of stress is imperative, and situations in which blood tests are ordered frequently and repeatedly.

Aseptic technique is vital in preventing the introduction of bacteria into the catheter. A sterile I.V. Catheter Plug,* placed in the stopcock outlet at the time the catheter is inserted, reduces the risk of bacterial invasion.

PROCEDURE. Follow this procedure in drawing blood by way of the central venous catheter from a patient not on drug therapy:

1. Clamp off the infusion.
2. Remove catheter plug, protecting stopcock outlet, and with a sterile syringe withdraw 4 ml of blood; discard it.
3. Using a sterile syringe, withdraw the required amount of blood. If difficulty is encountered in drawing blood samples, raise the patient's arm to shoulder level or higher. This reduces axillary pressure on the catheter.
4. Recap stopcock with a sterile plug.
5. Open clamp and flush catheter with about 5 ml of infusion fluid to maintain patency of catheter.
6. Adjust flow to prescribed flow rate.

If the patient is receiving drug therapy, follow the same procedure, except *use a hemostat* to stop the infusion temporarily; after the blood is drawn, the control clamp maintains the prescribed rate of flow without readjustment.

PRECAUTION. Patients receiving vasopressors may not tolerate an interruption of medication. Check with the charge nurse before stopping the infusion; extra caution may be required, with a standby nurse to watch the monitor.

Withdrawing Blood and Initiating an Infusion
Drawing blood samples and initiating an infusion can be efficiently accomplished by a single venipuncture in the following way:

1. Fill intravenous set with solution.
2. Regulate the flow to a minimum rate.
3. Clamp tubing manually by kinking between third and little fingers (see Figure 44).
4. Hold adapter between the forefinger and second finger, leaving the

* McGaw Laboratories, Inc., Glendale, Calif.; division of American Hospital Supply Corporation.

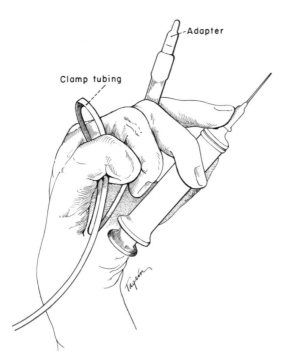

Fig. 44. Infusion tubing is kinked and held by the little finger; adapter is held between the forefinger and second finger, leaving the hand free for drawing blood sample.

hand free for holding the syringe and needle and collecting blood.

5. Draw blood.
6. Remove syringe; attach the infusion set to the needle, releasing little finger; solution will flow at the previously adjusted rate.
7. Secure needle with a piece of tape.
8. Attach syringe to needle, previously imbedded in stopper of vacuum tube, and transfer blood. Vacuum will cause tube to fill—never apply force. Use no larger needle than 20 gauge; lysis of cells could occur.

Commonly Used Laboratory Tests

Laboratory tests are performed (1) routinely, because they point out disorders which are relatively common; (2) for diagnostic purposes; (3) for following the course of a disease; (4) in regulating therapy. (See Table 18.)

Blood Cultures

In cases of suspected bacteremia, blood cultures are performed to identify the causative microorganisms. Isolation of the organism is necessary to enable the physician to direct proper antimicrobial therapy. Blood cultures are performed during febrile illnesses or when the patient is having chills with spiking fever. Intermittent bacteremia accompanies such infections as pyelonephritis, brucellosis, cholangitis, and other infections. In such cases repeated blood cultures are usually ordered to be performed when the fever spikes. In other infections, such as subacute bacterial endocarditis, the bacteremia is more constant during the 4 or 5 febrile days. Usually four or five cultures are obtained over a span of 1 or 2 days, and antimicrobial therapy is initiated with the realization that the majority of cultures will be found to harbor the offending microorganism. If antimicrobial therapy is administered prior to the blood culture or prior to the patient's admittance to the hospital, the bacteremia may be suppressed, rendering isolation difficult [3].

Penicillinase is often ordered to be added to the blood culture medium to neutralize the existing penicillinemia and to recover the organism. Usually antimicrobial therapy must be withheld to await report of culture in order to make a precise diagnosis. The penicillinase is added to the culture medium before or immediately after the blood sample is drawn.

Some bacteriology laboratories routinely culture blood under both aerobic and anaerobic conditions. If this is not done routinely and bacteremia with strict anaerobes is suspected, the laboratory should be notified, as a special culture broth is necessary.

Extreme care must be observed in preparing the area for venipuncture as the skin affords a fertile field for bacterial growth. *Staphylococcus albus*, diphtheroids, and yeast (common skin or environment contaminants) usually indicate contamination, whereas *S. aureus* presents a greater problem by indicating either a contaminant or the presence of a serious pathogen [3].

PROCEDURE. Specimens for blood cultures are obtained as follows:

1. Prepare the skin at proposed puncture site: Cleanse a wide area with iodine. Cleanse again with 70 percent isopropanol.
2. Perform venipuncture using sterile syringe and needle.
3. Draw approximately 8 ml of blood.
4. Remove needle and transfer blood to culture bottle, using care not to touch neck of bottle.
5. Do not shake bottle or disturb interface on the broth of cultures drawn for anaerobic bacteria.
6. Label specimens with name of patient, date, time, and number of culture.

Table 18. Blood, Plasma or Serum Values

Determination	Normal Value[a]	Material Analyzed	Minimal Ml of Blood Required	Note	Method
Acetoacetate plus acetone	0.3–2.0 mg per 100 ml	Serum	2		Behre: *J. Lab. Clin. Med.* 13: 770, 1928 (modified)
Aldolase	0.7–4.5 mU per ml	Serum	4	Use fresh, unhemolyzed serum	Beisenherz et al.: *Z. Natur-forsch.* 8b:555, 1953
Alpha amino nitrogen	3.0–5.5 mg per 100 ml	Plasma	5	Collect with heparin	Szentirmai et al.: *Clin. Chim. Acta* 7:459, 1962
Ammonia	80–110 μg per 100 ml	Blood	2	Collect in heparinized tube; deliver *immediately* packed in ice.	Seligson, Hirahara: *J. Lab. Clin. Med.* 49:962, 1957
Amylase	4–25 U per ml	Serum	3		Huggins, Russell: *Ann. Surg.* 128:668, 1948
Ascorbic acid	0.4–1.5 mg per 100 ml	Blood	7	Collect in heparin tube before any food is given	Roe, Kuether: *J. Biol. Chem.* 147:399, 1943
Barbiturate	0 Coma level: phenobarbital, approximately 11 mg per 100 ml; most other drugs, 2–4 mg per 100 ml	Serum	5		Goldbaum: *Anal. Chem.* 24: 1604, 1952
Bilirubin (van den Bergh test)	One minute: 0.4 mg per 100 ml Direct: 0.4 mg per 100 ml. Total: 0.7 mg per 100 ml. Indirect is total minus direct	Serum	3		Malloy, Evelyn: *J. Biol. Chem.* 119:481, 1937
Blood volume	8.5–9.0 percent of body weight in kg				Isotope dilution technic with 131I albumin
Bromide	0 Toxic level: 17 mEq per liter	Serum	3		Adapted from Wuth: *J.A.M.A.* 82:2013, 1927

Test	Normal Value	Specimen	ml	Special Instructions	Reference
Bromsulfalein (BSP)	Less than 5 percent retention	Serum	3	Inject intravenously 5 mg of dye per kg of body weight; draw blood 45 min later.	Goebler: *Am. J. Clin. Pathol.* 15:452, 1945
Calcium	8.5–10.5 mg per 100 ml (slightly higher in children)	Serum	3	BSP dye interferes	Bett, Fraser: *Clin. Chim. Acta* 4:346, 1959 Kessler, Wolfman: *Clin. Chem.* 10:686, 1964 (modified)
Carbon dioxide content	24–30 mEq per liter, 20–26 mEq per liter in infants (as HCO_3)	Serum	3	Draw without stasis under oil or in heparinized syringe	Van Slyke, Neill: *J. Biol. Chem.* 61:523, 1924 Tech. AutoAnalyzer Meth.
Carbon monoxide	Symptoms with over 20 percent saturation	Blood	5	Fill tube to top; tightly stopper; use anticoagulant.	Bruchner, Desmond: *Clin. Chim. Acta* 3:173, 1958
Carotenoids	0.8–4.0 µg per ml	Serum	3	Vitamin A may be done on same specimen	Natelson: *Microtechniques of Clin. Chem.* 2nd ed., 1961 p. 454
Ceruloplasmin	27–37 mg per 100 ml	Serum	2		Ravin: *J. Lab. Clin. Med.* 58:161, 1961
Chloride	100–106 mEq per liter	Serum	1		Modification of Schales, Schales: *J. Biol. Chem.* 140:879, 1941 Tech. AutoAnalyzer Meth.
Cholinesterase (pseudocholinesterase)	0.5 pH U or more per hr 0.7 pH U or more per hr for packed cells	Serum Packed cells	1 1		Michel: *J. Lab. Clin. Med.* 34:1564, 1949
Congo-red test	More than 60 percent retention in serum	Serum	5	Inject 10 ml of 1 percent Congo-red solution intravenously; draw blood from arm not injected 4 and 60 min. later.	Unger, et al.: *J. Clin. Invest.* 27:111, 1948
Copper	Total: 100–200 µg per 100 ml	Serum	3		MGH Methodology
Creatine phosphokinase (CPK)	Female 5–25 mU per ml Male 5–35 mU per ml	Serum	3	Immediately separate & freeze serum	Rosalki: *J. Lab. Med.* 69:696, 1967 (modified)

Table 18 (*Continued*)

Determination	Normal Value[a]	Material Analyzed	Minimal Ml of Blood Required	Note	Method
Creatinine	0.7–1.5 mg per 100 ml	Serum	3		Tech. AutoAnalyzer Meth.
Cryoglobulins	0	Serum	8	Collect and transport at 37° C	Barr, et al.: *Ann. Intern. Med.* 32:6, 1950 (modified)
Dilantin (diphenylhydantoin)	Therapeutic level, 5–20 μg per ml	Serum	5		Gas Liquid Chromatography
Doriden (glutethimide)	0	Serum	5		Rieder, Zervas: *Am. J. Clin. Pathol.* 44:520, 1965
Ethanol	0.3–0.4 percent, marked intoxication; 0.4–0.5 percent, alcoholic stupor; 0.5 percent or over, alcoholic coma.	Blood	2	Collect in oxalate & refrigerate	Natelson: *Microtechniques of Clin. Chem.* 2d ed., 1961, p. 208
Gastrin	0–200 pg per ml	Serum	2		Dent et al.: *Ann. Surg.* 176: 360, 1972
Glucose	Fasting: 70–100 mg per 100 ml	Blood	2	Collect with oxalate-fluoride mixture. Micromethod: add 0.1 ml of blood to 1.9 ml of 0.01 percent sodium fluoride solution	Tech. AutoAnalyzer Meth. Huggett, Nixon: *Lancet* 2: 368, 1957 (modified)
Iron	50–150 μg per 100 ml (higher in males)	Serum	5	Shows diurnal variation higher in A.M.	Tech. AutoAnalyzer Meth. (modified)
Iron-binding capacity	250–410 μg per 100 ml	Serum	5		Scalata, Moore: *Clin. Chem.* 8:360, 1962 Tech. AutoAnalyzer Meth.
Lactic acid	0.6–1.8 mEq per liter	Blood	2	Collect with oxalate-fluoride mixture; deliver immediately packed in ice.	Hadjivassiliou, Rieder: *Clin. Chim. Acta.* 19:357, 1968
Lactic dehydrogenase	60–120 U per ml	Serum	2	Unsuitable if hemolyzed	Wacker, et al.: *N. Engl. J. Med.* 255:449, 1956

Test	Value	Specimen	No.	Instructions	Reference
Lead	50 μg per 100 ml or less	Blood	2	Collect with oxalate-fluoride mixture	Berman: *Atom Absorp. Newsl.* 3:9, 1964 (modified)
Lipase	2 U per ml or less	Serum	3		Comfort, Osterberg: *J. Lab. Clin. Med.* 20:271, 1934
Lipids (cholesterol)	150–280 mg per 100 ml	Serum	2	Fasting	Tech. AutoAnalyzer Meth.
Cholesterol esters	60–75 percent of cholesterol	Serum	2	Fasting	Creech, Sewell: *Anal. Biochem.* 3:119, 1962 Tech. AutoAnalyzer Meth.
Phospholipids	9–16 mg per 100 ml as lipid phosphorus	Serum	5	Fasting	Fiske, SubbaRow: *J. Biol. Chem.* 66:2, 1925
Total fatty acids	190–420 mg per 100 ml	Serum	10	Fasting	Stoddard, Drury: *J. Biol. Chem.* 84:741, 1929
Total lipids	450–1000 mg per 100 ml	Serum	5	Fasting	Freedman: *Clin. Chim. Acta* 19:291, 1968
Triglycerides	40–150 mg per 100 ml	Serum	2	Fasting	Tech. AutoAnalyzer Meth.
Lipoprotein electrophoresis (LEP)		Serum	2	Fasting; do not freeze serum.	Lees, Hatch: *J. Lab. Clin. Med.* 61:518, 1963
Lithium	Toxic level 2 mEq per liter	Serum	1		Flame photometry
Magnesium	1.5–2.5 mEq per liter	Serum	1		Willis: *Clin. Chem.* 11:251, 1965 (modified)
Methanol	0	Blood	5	May be fatal as low as 115 mg per 100 ml; collect in oxalate.	Natelson: *Microtechniques of Clin. Chem.* 2d ed., 1961, p. 298
Mysoline (primidone)	Therapeutic level 4–12 μg per ml	Serum			Gas Liquid Chromatography
5' Nucleotidase	0.3–3.2 Bodansky U	Serum	1		Rieder, Otero: *Clin. Chem.* 8:727, 1969
Osmolality	285–295 mOsm per kg water	Serum	5		Crawford, Nicosia: *J. Lab. Clin. Med.* 40:907, 1952
Oxygen saturation (arterial)	96–100 percent	Arterial blood	3	Deliver in sealed heparinized syringe packed in ice	Gordy, Drabkin: *J. Biol. Chem.* 227:285, 1957
Pco2	35–45 mm of mercury	Arterial blood	2	Collect and deliver in sealed heparinized syringe	By CO_2 electrode

Table 18 (*Continued*)

Determination	Normal Value[a]	Material Analyzed	Minimal Ml of Blood Required	Note	Method
pH	7.35–7.45	Arterial blood	2	Collect without stasis in sealed heparinized syringe; deliver packed in ice	Glass electrode
P_{O_2}	75–100 mm of mercury (dependent on age) while breathing room air Above 500 mm of mercury while on 100% O_2	Arterial blood	2		Oxygen electrode
Phenylalanine	0–2 mg per 100 ml	Serum	0.4		Cullay, et al.: *Clin. Chem.* 8: 266, 1962 (modified)
Phosphatase (acid)	Male—Total: 0.13–0.63 Sigma U per ml Female—Total: 0.01–0.56 Sigma U per ml Prostatic: 0–0.7 Fishman-Lerner U per 100 ml	Serum	1	Must always be drawn just before analysis or stored as frozen serum; avoid hemolysis.	Bessey, et al.: *J. Biol. Chem.* 164:321, 1946 Babson, et al.: *Clin. Chim. Acta* 13:264, 1966
Phosphatase (alkaline)	2.0–4.5 Bodansky U (infants to 14 U; adolescents to 5 U)	Serum	1	BSP dye interferes	Bessey, et al.: *J. Biol. Chem.* 164:321, 1946
Phosphorus (inorganic)	3.0–4.5 mg per 100 ml (infants in 1st year up to 6.0 mg per 100 ml)	Serum	2	Obtain blood in fasting state; serum must be separated promptly from cells.	Fiske, SubbaRow: *J. Biol. Chem.* 66:375, 1925, Adapted for Tech. Auto-Analyzer Meth.
Potassium	3.5–5.0 mEq per liter	Serum	2	Serum must be separated promptly from cells (within 1 hr)	Flame photometry
Protein: Total	6.0–8.4 gm per 100 ml	Serum	1	Patient should be fasting; avoid BSP dye.	Refractometry (American Optical Co.)

Test	Normal value	Specimen	No.	Notes	Reference
Albumin	3.5–5.0 gm per 100 ml	Serum	1		Doumas et al.: *Clin. Chim. Acta* 31:87, 1971
Globulin	2.0–3.0 gm per 100 ml			Globulin calculated	Gornall, et al.: *J. Biol. Chem.* 177:751, 1949 (modified)
Paper electrophoresis	Percent of total protein	Serum	1	Quantitation by densitometry	Kunkel, Tiselius: *J. Gen. Physiol.* 35:89, 1951; Durrum: *J. Am. Chem. Soc.* 72:2943, 1950
Albumin	52–68				
Globulin:					
Alpha$_1$	4.2–7.2				
Alpha$_2$	6.8–12				
Beta	9.3–15				
Gamma	13–23				
Pyruvic acid	0–0.11 mEq per liter	Blood	2	Collect with oxalate fluoride. Deliver immediately packed in ice.	Hadjivassiliou, Rieder: *Clin. Chim. Acta* 19:357, 1968
Quinidine	Therapeutic: 4–6 µg per ml. Toxic: 10 µg per ml	Serum	1	Fluorometry	Cramer, Isakson: *Scand. J. Clin. Invest.* 15:553, 1963
Salicylate	0	Plasma	5	Collect in heparin or oxalate	Keller: *Am. J. Clin. Pathol.* 17:415, 1947
Therapeutic	20–25 mg per 100 ml; 25–30 mg per 100 ml to age 10 yrs. Over 30 mg per 100 ml; over 20 mg per 100 ml after age 60.				
Toxic					
Sodium	135–145 mEq per liter	Serum	2	Flame photometry	Letonoff, Reinhold: *J. Biol. Chem.* 114:147, 1936
Sulfate	0.5–1.5 mg per 100 ml	Serum	3	Avoid hemolysis	
Sulfonamide	0	Blood or serum	2	Value given as unconjugated unless total is requested	Bratton, Marshall: *J. Biol. Chem.* 128:537, 1939
Thymol Flocculation	Up to 1 + in 24 hr	Serum	1	Checked with phosphate buffer of higher molarity to rule out false-positive reaction	Maclagen: *Nature* 154:670, 1944
Turbidity	0–4 U				

Table 18 (*Continued*)

Determination	Normal Value[a]	Material Analyzed	Minimal Ml of Blood Required	Note	Method
Thyroxine					
Total	4–11 µg per 100 ml	Serum	3		Murphy: *J. Lab. Clin. Med.* 66:161, 1965 (modified)
Free	0.8–2.4 ng per 100 ml	Serum	6		Sterling, Bremner: *J. Clin. Invest.* 45:153, 1966 (modified)
Transaminase (SGOT)	10–40 U per ml	Serum	1		Karmen, et al.: *J. Clin Invest.* 34:126, 1955
Urea nitrogen (BUN)	8–25 mg per 100 ml	Blood or serum	1	Urea = BUN × 2.14. Use oxalate as anticoagulant.	Skeggs: *Am. J. Clin. Pathol.* 28:311, 1957 (modified)
Uric acid	3.0–7.0 mg per 100 ml	Serum	2	Serum must be separated from cells at once and refrigerated	Folin: *J. Biol. Chem.* 101:111, 1933, Adapted for Tech. AutoAnalyzer Meth.
Vitamin A	0.15–0.6 µg per ml	Serum	3		Natelson: *Microtechniques of Clin. Chem.* 2d ed., 1961, p. 451
Vitamin A tolerance test	Rise to twice fasting level in 3 to 5 hr	Serum	3	Samples taken fasting and at intervals up to 8 hr after test dose	Josephs: *Bull. Johns Hopkins Hosp.* 65:112, 1939

[a] Normal Laboratory Values. *New Eng. J. Med.* 234:24-28, 1946; 243:748-753, 1950; 254:29-35, 1956; 262:84-91, 1960; 268:1462-1469, 1963; 276:167-174, 1967; and 283:1276-1285, 1970.

Source: Prepared by Mary Zervas, B.S., H. George Hamacher, M.S., and Olive Holmes, B.S., Supervisors, and Sidney V. Rieder, Ph.D., Chief of Chemistry Laboratory; Bernard Kliman, M.D., Director of Endocrine-Steroid Laboratory; Gretchen Williams, Chief Technologist, Clinical Laboratories; William S. Beck, M.D., Director of Clinical Laboratories, and Robert W. Colman, M.D., in charge of Special Clotting Laboratory, Massachusetts General Hospital.

For values in newborn infants refer to Smith, C. A. *The Physiology of the Newborn Infant.* 3d ed., Springfield, Ill.: Charles C Thomas, 1959.

Reprinted with permission from the *New England Journal of Medicine* (290:39–42, Jan. 3, 1974) with revisions by the Chemical Laboratory of Massachusetts General Hospital.

Measurements of Electrolyte Concentration

Electrolyte imbalances are serious complications in the critically ill. Such imbalances must be recognized and corrected at once. Frequently electrolyte determinations are ordered on an emergency basis. Accurate measurement is essential and to a large degree depends upon the proper collection and handling of blood specimens.

POTASSIUM. Potassium is an electrolyte essential to body function. Approximately 98 percent of all body potassium is found in the cells; only small amounts are contained in the serum.

The kidneys normally do not conserve potassium. When large quantities of body fluid are lost without potassium replacement, a severe deficiency occurs. Chronic kidney disease and the use of diuretics may cause a potassium deficit. Adrenal steroids play a major role in controlling the concentration of potassium: hyperadrenalism causes increased potassium loss, with deficiency resulting; steroid therapy promotes potassium excretion.

An elevated potassium level results from potassium retention in renal failure or in adrenal cortical deficiency. Hypoventilation and cellular damage also result in an elevated potassium level.

Because intracellular ions are not accessible for measurement, determination must be made on the serum. As the concentration of potassium in the cells is roughly 15 times greater than that in the serum, the blood for potassium determination must be carefully drawn to prevent hemolysis.

Blood collection. Blood (2 ml) is drawn in a dry tube and allowed to clot or, preferably, placed under oil; oil minimizes friction and hemolysis of the red blood cells. The blood should be sent to the laboratory immediately as potassium diffuses out of the cells and gives a falsely high reading.

Normal serum range is 4 to 5 mEq per liter [2].

SODIUM. The main role of sodium is the control of the distribution of water throughout the body and the maintenance of a normal fluid balance.

The excretion of sodium is regulated to a large degree by the adrenocortical hormone aldosterone. The regulation of water excretion is regulated by ADH (antidiuretic hormone), and as long as these two systems are in harmony, the sodium and water remain in isosmotic proportion. Any change in the normal sodium concentration indicates that the loss or gain of water and sodium are in other than isosmotic proportion [3]. Increased sodium levels may be caused by excessive infusions of sodium, insufficient water intake, or excess loss of fluid without a sodium loss, as in tracheobronchitis. Decreased sodium levels may be caused by excessive sweating accompanied by intake of large amounts of water by mouth, adrenal insufficiency, excessive infusions of nonelectrolyte fluids, or gastrointestinal suction accompanied with water by mouth.

Blood collection. Blood (2 ml) is drawn carefully to prevent hemolysis and placed in a dry tube or a tube with oil.

Normal serum range is 138 to 145 mEq per liter.

CHLORIDES. Chlorides are usually measured along with other electrolytes of the blood. The measurement of chlorides is helpful in diagnosing disorders of acid–base balance and water balance of the body. Chloride has a reciprocal power of increasing or decreasing in concentration whenever changes in concentration of other anions occur. In metabolic acidosis there is a reciprocal rise in chloride concentration when the bicarbonate concentration drops.

Elevation in blood chlorides occurs in such conditions as Cushing's syndrome, hyperventilation, and some kidney disorders. A decrease in blood chlorides may occur in diabetic acidosis, heat exhaustion, and following vomiting and diarrhea.

Blood collection. Venous blood (1 ml) is withdrawn and placed in a dry tube to clot.

Normal serum range is 100 to 106 mEq per liter.

CALCIUM. Calcium, an essential electrolyte of the body, is required for blood clotting, muscular contraction, and nerve transmission. Only ionized calcium is useful but, since it cannot be satisfactorily measured, the total amount of body calcium is determined; 50 percent of the total is believed to be ionized [2]. In acidosis there is a higher level of ionized calcium; in alkalosis, a lower level.

Hypocalcemia (decrease in normal blood calcium) occurs whenever impairment of the gastrointestinal tract, such as sprue or celiac disease, prevents absorption. Deficiency also occurs in hypoparathyroidism and in some kidney diseases and is characterized by muscular twitching and tetanic convulsions.

Hypercalcemia (excess of calcium in the blood) occurs in hyperparathyroidism and in respiratory disturbance where carbon dioxide blood content is increased, such as in respiratory acidosis.

Blood collection. Venous blood (5 ml) is placed in a dry tube and allowed to clot. Analysis is performed on the serum.

Normal serum range is 8.5 to 10.5 mg per 100 ml [1].

PHOSPHORUS. Phosphorus metabolism is related to calcium metabolism and the serum level varies inversely with calcium.

Increased concentration of phosphorus may occur in such conditions as hypoparathyroidism, kidney disease, or excessive intake of vitamin D. Decreased concentrations may occur in hyperparathyroidism, rickets, and some kidney diseases.

Blood collection. Since red cells are rich in phosphorus, hemolysis of the blood must be avoided. Analysis is performed on the serum; 4 ml of blood is placed in a dry tube to clot.

Normal serum range is 3.0 to 4.5 mg per 100 ml.

Venous Blood Measurements of Acid–Base Balance

Acid–base balance is maintained by the buffer system, carbonic acid–base bicarbonate at a 1 to 20 ratio. When deviations occur in the normal ratio, a change in pH results and is accompanied by a change in bicarbonate concentration.

CARBON DIOXIDE CONTENT. Carbon dioxide content is the measurement of the free carbon dioxide and the bicarbonate content of the serum, which provides a general measure of acidity or alkalinity. An increase in carbon dioxide content usually indicates alkalosis; a decrease indicates acidosis. This test, along with clinical findings, is helpful in surmising the severity and nature of the disorder. Measurement of pH is necessary for accuracy—a change in carbon dioxide does not always signify a change in pH, as pH depends on the ratio and not the carbon dioxide content. When the carbon dioxide and pH are known, the buffer ratio can be determined.

An elevated carbon dioxide content is present in metabolic alkalosis, hypoventilation, loss of acid secretions such as occurs in persistent vomiting or drainage of the stomach, and excessive administration of ACTH or cortisone. A low carbon dioxide content usually occurs in loss of alkaline secretions such as in severe diarrhea, certain kidney diseases, diabetic acidosis, and hyperventilation.

Blood collection. Blood (4 ml) is drawn without stasis; hemoconcentration may result in an erroneous report. The blood is placed in a tube under oil as contact with air permits the escape of carbon dioxide.

Normal serum range is 24 to 30 mEq per liter.

ACIDITY (pH) CONTENT. pH, a symbol for acidity, indicates the serum concentration of hydrogen ions. The pH becomes lower in acid conditions such as hypoventilation, diarrhea, and diabetic acidosis. The pH rises in alkaline conditions such as hyperventilation and excessive vomiting.

Blood collection. The blood is collected *without stasis* in a heparinized 2-cc syringe; the syringe is then capped. The blood may be drawn with a scalp vein needle, the needle discarded, and the tubing tied off.

The specimen is left in the syringe and packed in ice. Loss of carbon dioxide from contact with the air is thus avoided and excess production of lactic acid by enzymic reaction reduced.

Normal blood range is 7.35 to 7.45.

Enzymes

AMYLASE. Amylase determination is helpful in the diagnosis of acute pancreatitis or the acute recurrence of chronic pancreatitis. Amylase is secreted by the pancreas; a rise in the serum level occurs when outflow of pancreatic juice is restricted. This test is usually performed on patients with acute abdominal pain, or on surgical patients in whom questionable injury may have occurred to the pancreas. Amylase levels usually remain elevated for only a short time—3 to 6 days.

Blood collection. Venous blood (6 ml) is allowed to clot in a dry tube.

Normal serum range is 4 to 25 units per milliliter. The range may depend upon the normal values established by clinical laboratories, as the method may be modified.

LIPASE. Lipase determination is used for detecting damage to the pancreas and is valuable when too much time has elapsed for the amylase level to remain elevated. When secretions of the pancreas are blocked, the serum lipase level rises.

Blood collection. The test is performed on serum from 6 ml of clotted blood.

Normal serum range is 2 units per milliter or less.

PHOSPHATASE, ACID. Acid phosphatase is useful in determining metastasizing tumors of the prostate. The prostate gland and carcinoma of the gland are rich in phosphatase but do not normally release the enzyme into the serum. Once the carcinoma has spread, it starts to release acid phosphatase, increasing the serum concentration [2].

Blood collection. Blood (10 ml) is allowed to clot in a dry tube. Hemolysis should be avoided. Analysis should be done immediately or the serum frozen.

Normal serum range. (1) Male: Total, 0.13 to 0.63 Sigma unit per milliliter. (2) Female: Total, 0.01 to 0.56 Sigma unit per milliliter. (3) Prostatic: 0 to 0.7 Fishman-Lerner unit per 100 ml [1].

PHOSPHATASE, ALKALINE. Alkaline phosphatase is a useful test in diagnosing bone diseases and obstructive jaundice. In bone diseases the small amount of alkaline usually present in the serum rises in proportion to the new-bone cells. When excretion of alkaline phosphatase is impaired as in some disorders of the liver and biliary tract, the serum level rises and may give some evidence of the degree of blockage in the biliary tract [2].

Blood collection. Blood (5 ml) is drawn and the test is performed on the serum. Sodium sulfobromophthalein dye should be avoided.

Normal serum range is 2.0 to 4.5 Bodansky units per milliliter.

Transaminase

The transaminases are enzymes found in large quantities in the heart, liver, muscle, kidney, and pancreas cells. Any disease that causes damage to these cells will result in an elevated serum transaminase level; clinical signs and other tests are used in diagnosis.

SGOT (SERUM GLUTAMIC OXALOACETIC TRANSAMINASE). SGOT is used to distinguish between myocardial infarction and acute coronary insufficiency without infarction. It is also useful as a liver function test in following the progression of liver damage or in ascertaining when the liver has recovered.

Blood collection. The test is performed on serum from 5 ml of clotted blood.

Normal serum range is 10 to 40 units per milliliter. In myocardial infarction, the level is increased 4 to 10 times, whereas in liver involvement a high of 10 to 100 times normal may occur. The serum level remains elevated for about 5 days.

SGPT (SERUM GLUTAMIC PYRUVATE TRANSAMINASE). SGPT is another transaminase that is more specific for hepatic malfunction than SGOT.

Blood collection. The test is performed on serum from 5 ml of blood.

Normal serum range is 7 to 25 units per milliliter [4].

SLD (SERUM LACTIC DEHYDROGENASE). The transaminase SLD is present in all tissues and in large quantities in the kidney, heart, and skeletal muscles. Elevated serum levels usually parallel the SGOT levels. Elevation occurs in myocardial infarction and may continue through the sixth day. Elevations have been found in lymphoma, disseminated carcinoma, and some cases of leukemia.

Blood collection. Blood (3 ml) is collected and allowed to coagulate. Care must be taken to avoid hemolysis, as only a slight degree may give an incorrect reading. "At room temperature, hemolysis may increase the SLD activity by as much as 25 percent in 1 hour" [4].

Normal serum range is 60 to 100 units per milliliter.

Liver Function Tests

ALBUMIN, GLOBULIN, TOTAL PROTEIN, AND A/G RATIO. These tests may be useful in diagnosing kidney and liver disease or in judging the effectiveness of treatment. The chief role of serum albumin is to maintain osmotic pressure of the blood; globulin assists. The globulin molecule, being larger than the albumin, is less efficient in maintaining osmotic pressure and does not leak out of the blood. With the loss of albumin through the capillary wall, the body compensates by producing more globulin. The osmotic pressure is reduced and may result in some edema. A shift in the albumin–globulin (A/G) ratio assists the physician in diagnosis. The ratio is lowered in liver disease and in chronic nephritis [2].

Blood collection. The test is performed on serum from 6 ml of clotted blood.

Normal serum range. (1) Total protein, 6 to 8.4 gm per 100 ml. (2) Albumin, 3.5 to 5.0 gm per 100 ml. (3) Globulin, 2.0 to 3.0 gm per 100 ml. (4) A/G ratio, 1.5:1 to 2.5:1.

BILIRUBIN (DIRECT AND INDIRECT). The bilirubin test differentiates between impairment of the liver by obstruction and hemolysis. Bilirubin arises from the hemoglobin liberated from broken-down red cells. It is the chief pigment of the bile, excreted by the liver. If the excretory power of the liver is impaired by obstruction, there is an excess of circulatory bilirubin and it is free of any attached protein. Measurement of free bilirubin (direct) usually indicates obstruction.

When increased red cell destruction (hemolysis) occurs, the increased bilirubin is believed to be bound to protein (indirect).

A *total bilirubin* determination detects increased concentration of bilirubin before jaundice is seen.

Blood collection. The test is performed on serum from 5 ml of clotted blood.

Normal serum range is 0.1 to 1.0 mg per 100 ml [2].

CEPHALIN FLOCCULATION. This is a useful test in diagnosing liver damage, frequently detecting damage before jaundice becomes evident. It is also useful in following the course of liver disease such as cirrhosis. The serum of patients with damaged liver cells flocculates a colloidal suspension of cephalin and cholesterol, while the serum of normal patients does not clump the suspension. Abscesses and neoplasms do not damage liver cells and therefore give negative results [2].

Blood collection. The test is performed on serum from 5 ml of clotted blood.

Normal serum range is either negative or 1+. Reports are delayed 24 to 48 hours.

CHOLESTEROL. Cholesterol, a normal constituent of the blood, is present in all body cells. In various disease states the cholesterol concentration in the serum may be raised or lowered. Elevation of the cholesterol level may be helpful in indicating certain liver diseases, hypothyroidism, and xanthomatosis [2].

Blood collection. The test is performed on serum from 5 ml of clotted blood.

Normal serum range is 120 to 260 mg per 100 ml.

CHOLESTEROL ESTERS. This test is helpful in estimating the amount of cellular damage in the liver and is of prognostic value in some patients with jaundice.

Blood collection. The test is performed on serum from 7 ml of clotted blood.

Normal serum range is up to 210 mg per 100 ml.

PROTHROMBIN TIME. The prothrombin time, considered one of the most important screening tests in coagulation studies, indirectly measures the ability of the blood to clot. It is an important guide in controlling drug therapy and is commonly used when anticoagulants are prescribed. The prothrombin content is reduced in liver diseases.

Blood collection. Venous blood (4 ml) is collected, added to the coagulant, and quickly mixed. It is important to avoid clot formation and hemolysis. The blood should be examined as soon as possible.

The *normal value* is between 11 and 18 seconds, depending on the type of thromboplastin used.

THYMOL TURBIDITY. Thymol turbidity detects damaged liver cells and differentiates between liver disease and biliary obstruction. Turbidity is usually increased when the serum of patients with liver damage is mixed with a saturated solution of thymol. Turbidity is usually normal in biliary obstruction without liver damage.

Blood collection. The test is performed on serum from 5 ml of clotted blood.

Normal serum range is 0 to 4 units.

Kidney Function Tests

CREATININE. The creatinine test measures kidney function. Creatinine, the result of a breakdown of muscle creatine phosphate, is produced daily in a constant amount in each individual. A disorder of kidney function prevents excretion and an elevated creatinine value gives a reliable indication of impaired kidney function. A normal serum creatinine value does not indicate unimpaired renal function, however.

Blood collection. The test is performed on serum from 6 ml of clotted blood.

Normal serum range is 0.6 to 1.3 mg per 100 ml.

BLOOD UREA NITROGEN (BUN). The BUN is a measure of kidney function. Urea, the end product of protein metabolism, is excreted by the kidneys. Impairment in kidney function results in an elevated concentration of urea nitrogen in the blood. Rapid protein catabolism may also increase the urea nitrogen above normal limits. The *nonprotein nitrogen* (NPN) is a similar test for measuring kidney function.

Blood collection. The test is performed on blood or serum. Blood (5 ml) is added to an oxalate tube and shaken or placed in a dry tube to clot.

Normal ranges are 9 to 20 mg per 100 ml.

Blood Sugar

The test for blood sugar is used to detect a disorder of glucose metabolism, which may be the result of any one of several factors, including (1) inability of pancreas islet cells to produce insulin, (2) inability of intestines to absorb glucose, (3) inability of liver to accumulate and break down glycogen, and (4) presence of increased amounts of certain hormones [4].

An elevated blood sugar level may indicate diabetes, chronic liver disease, or overactivity of the endocrine glands. A decrease in blood sugar may result from an overdose of insulin, tumors of the pancreas, or insufficiency of various endocrine glands.

FASTING BLOOD SUGAR (FBS). A fasting blood sugar test requires that the patient fast for 8 hours.

Blood collection. Venous blood (3 to 5 ml) is collected in an oxalate tube and shaken to prevent microscopic clots.

Normal range is 70 to 100 mg per 100 ml (true blood sugar method). The normal value depends upon the method of determination. Values over 120 mg per 100 ml on several occasions may indicate diabetes mellitus.

POSTPRANDIAL BLOOD SUGAR DETERMINATIONS. The postprandial sugar test is helpful in diagnosing diabetes mellitus. Blood is drawn 2 hours after the patient has begun to eat. If the blood sugar value is above the upper limits of normal for fasting, a glucose tolerance test is performed.

GLUCOSE TOLERANCE. The glucose tolerance test is indicated

1. When patient shows glycosuria.
2. When fasting or 2-hour blood sugar concentration is only slightly elevated.
3. When Cushing's syndrome or acromegaly is a questionable diagnosis.
4. To establish cause of hypoglycemia.

Blood collection. A fasting blood sugar sample is drawn. The patient drinks 100 gm of glucose in lemon-flavored water (some laboratories use 1.75 gm of glucose per kg of ideal body weight). Blood and urine samples are collected at 30, 60, 90, 120, and 180 minutes after ingestion of glucose.

Normal (true blood sugar) values. (1) FBS below 100 mg per 100 ml. (2) Peak below 160 mg per 100 ml in 30 or 60 minutes. (3) Two-hour value below 12 mg per 100 ml. The values depend upon the standards used.

Blood Typing

Blood typing is one of the commonest tests performed on blood, being required by all donors and by all patients who may need blood. The ABO system denotes four main groups, O, A, B, and AB. The designations refer to the particular antigen present on the red cells: group A contains red cells with the A antigen, B with B antigen, AB with A and B antigens, and O red cells contain neither A nor B antigens.

When red cells containing antigens are placed with serum containing corresponding antibodies under favorable conditions, agglutination (clumping) occurs. Therefore an antigen is known as an agglutinogen, and an antibody as an agglutinin [4].

An individual's serum contains antibodies that will react to corresponding antigens not usually found on the individual's own cells. For instance, serum of group O contains antibodies A and B, which will react with the corresponding antigens A and B found on the red cells of group AB.

Although agglutination occurs in antigen–antibody reaction in the laboratory, hemolysis occurs in vivo; antibody attacks red cells, causing rupture with liberation of hemoglobin. Hemolysis results from infusing incompatible blood and may lead to fatal consequences [4].

Rh FACTOR. The antigens belonging to the Rh system are D, C, E, c, and e; they are found in conjunction with the ABO group. The strongest of these factors is the $Rh_o(D)$ factor, found in about 85 percent of the white population. Therefore the $Rh_o(D)$ factor is often the only factor identified in Rh typing. When not present, further typing is done to identify any of the less common Rh factors before identifying an individual as Rh-negative.

BLOOD COLLECTION. Venous blood is collected and allowed to clot. Usually one tube (10 ml) will set up 4 to 5 units of blood. Positive patient identification must be made before the blood is drawn; the name and number on the identification bracelet must correspond to that on the requisition and label. Identity should never be made by addressing the patient by name and awaiting his response. The label is placed on the blood tube at the patient's bedside. Once a patient has received a blood transfusion, a new specimen must be obtained on the day of transfusion to detect antibodies that may appear in the patient's circulation in response to blood previously transfused.

BLOOD GROUPING. Various methods are used in typing blood, but all involve the same general principle: The patient's cells are mixed in standard saline serum samples of anti-A and of anti-B. The type of serum, A or B, which agglutinates the patient's cells indicates the blood group. As a double check, the patient's serum is mixed with saline suspensions of A and of B red cells. The ABO group is determined on the basis of agglutination or absence of agglutination of A and of B cells.

COOMBS' TEST. Not all antibodies cause agglutination in saline; some merely coat the red cells by combining with the antigen, which is not a visible reaction. The Coombs test is performed to detect antibodies that cannot cause agglutination in saline; these are known as *incomplete antibodies*. Antihuman globulin serum is used. This serum is obtained by the immunization of various animals, usually rabbits, against human gamma globulin by the injection of human serum, plasma, or isolated globulin. This antiserum, when added to sensitized red cells (red cells coated with incomplete antibody), causes visible agglutination (see Figure 45).

The Coombs test is performed in two ways. The *direct Coombs test* is performed when the patient's red cells have become coated in vivo. This test is a valuable procedure in

1. Diagnosis of erythroblastosis fetalis. The red cells of the baby are tested for sensitization.
2. Acquired hemolytic anemia. The patient may have produced an antibody that coats his own cells.
3. Investigation of reactions. The patient may have received incompatible blood that has sensitized his red cells.

The *indirect Coombs test* detects incomplete antibodies in the serum of patients sensitized to blood antigens. It involves use of the patient's serum, in contrast to the use of the patient's red cells in the direct Coombs test. When pooled, normal red cells containing the most important antigens are exposed in a test tube to the patient's serum and to Coombs' serum, agglutination of the red cells occurs and indicates the incomplete antibody present. This test is valuable in

1. Detecting incompatibilities not found by other methods.
2. Detecting weak or variant antigens.

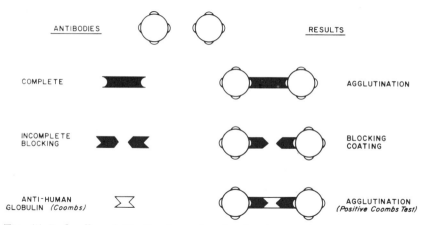

ANTIBODIES   RESULTS

COMPLETE   AGGLUTINATION

INCOMPLETE BLOCKING   BLOCKING COATING

ANTI-HUMAN GLOBULIN *(Coombs)*   AGGLUTINATION *(Positive Coombs Test)*

Fig. 45. Red cell agglutination is produced either by complete antibodies or indirectly by coating of the red cell antigens by incomplete (blocking) antibodies followed by exposure to antihuman globulin (Coombs') antibodies, which form the final bridge between the red cells. (Reprinted with permission from the *New England Journal of Medicine* 264:1089, 1961 [3]).

3. Typing with certain antiserums, such as anti-Duffy or anti-Kidd, which require Coombs' serum to produce agglutination.
4. Detecting antiagglutinins produced by exposure during pregnancy.

Blood Volume Determination

Blood volume determinations are extremely valuable in (1) hypotension, when the origin is unknown; (2) massive fluid replacement, when circulatory overload is a hazard; and (3) anuria or oliguria, when questionable cause is dehydration.

The patient is injected with radioactive isotopes and the computation is done by the Volemetron*—a precise automatic instrument that gives blood volume determinations within 15 minutes to an accuracy of 5 percent or better.

The Volemetron switch is set for adult, or for child if the blood volume is suspected to be less than 2.5 liters. The dose, 1 ml of radioiodinated serum albumin, prepackaged in its own disposable syringe, is placed in the center well of the Volemetron. When the switch is turned the machine automatically measures and stores the value of the total dose in its memory. If the dose is incorrect, a yellow light indicates a weak or outdated dose; a red light, too strong a dose.

Venous blood is drawn for a control (8 ml for adult, 2 ml for child). The syringe is removed from the needle and replaced by the dosage syringe, utilizing one venipuncture. The isotopes are injected, the needle removed, aspirated, and discarded. The cap is replaced on the

* Ames Atomium Co., Elkhart, Ind.; division of Miles Laboratories, Inc.

syringe. The sample of blood is transferred to a special tube marked "premixed."

The empty dose syringe is returned to the instrument for a measurement of the residual. The machine automatically counts the residual isotopes, subtracts them from the dose given, and stores in memory the amount received by the patient.

After a 10-minute interval the second blood specimen is drawn from a different vein and placed in the "postmix" tube.

The premix and postmix samples are placed in the appropriate wells. The machine automatically computes the volume, having subtracted any activity due to previous isotope administration in the premix sample. The premix sample may also be used for hematocrit determination, if desired.

References

1. Castleman, B., and McNeely, B.   Case records of the Massachusetts General Hospital: Normal laboratory values. *New England Journal of Medicine* 240:39–42, 1974.
2. Garb, S.   *Laboratory Tests in Common Use* (5th ed.). New York: Springer, 1971. Pp. 29–123.
3. Grove-Rasmussen, M., Lesses, M. F., and Anstall, H. B.   Transfusion therapy. *New England Journal of Medicine* 264:1089, 1961.
4. Page, L., and Culver, P.   *A Syllabus of Laboratory Examinations in Clinical Diagnosis*. Cambridge, Mass.: Harvard University Press, 1960. Pp. 22–24, 217, 260, 423, 447, 469, 550.

20. Levin Tubes

Legal Status of the Nurse

On December 23, 1964, the Massachusetts Board of Registration in Nursing passed a ruling currently in effect that states, "Insertion of Levin tube is a medical function that cannot be performed by a nurse." Each state may have its own rulings, and in some states the nurse practice acts relating to the definition of nursing are broad in wording and do not refer to specific procedures.

If the policy of a hospital is contrary to the ruling of the state, the hospital usually assumes responsibility and delegates the procedure to a special group of professional registered nurses whose competence has been established. The insertion of Levin tubes is becoming an added function of many intravenous departments. However, insertion of Levin tubes on patients with esophageal varices, aortic aneurysms, or severe hypertension should not be the responsibility of the nurse [2].

Importance of the Stomach Tube

Although the passage of a Levin tube is an uncomfortable procedure for the patient, it plays a major role in the diagnosis of certain conditions and aids in the medical and surgical management of some diseases of the stomach.

Diagnostic Tests

The following diagnostic tests require the use of the Levin tube:

1. *Gastric analysis* determines the degree of acidity of gastric contents.
2. *Cytological examination* aids in the diagnosis of gastric carcinoma.
3. *Acid-fast test* detects tubercle bacilli by aspirating stomach contents to recover swallowed sputum.
4. *Hollander test* demonstrates the integrity of the vagus nerve—usually after vagotomy.

Aid to Treatment

Gastric aspiration is carried out by means of the Levin tube

1. To relieve dilatation of the stomach in conditions of intestinal obstruction or diabetic coma.
2. To relieve distension and dilatation postoperatively.
3. To empty stomach completely before surgery or gastric radiography.
4. For removal of ingested toxic substances.

For patients unable to take nourishment by mouth, the Levin tube is used as a method of feeding.

Use of the Levin Tube

The Levin tube usually has a catheter tip and is available in rubber or plastic in sizes from 12 to 18, French scale. Markings on the tube indicate 18, 22, 26, and 30 inches from the catheter tip. The tube may be introduced through the nose or the mouth, but the nasal route is preferable. Introduction through the mouth causes the tube to come in contact with the soft palate, inducing considerable gagging [2].

Equipment

Before entering the patient's room, the nurse should assemble complete equipment. The tray should be covered so as not to upset the patient. Necessary equipment consists of

1. Levin tube in good condition, clean and with the lumen patent

    a. If the tube is rubber, immerse in ice water to achieve a proper degree of coldness to make it more comfortable for the patient to swallow.
    b. Do not immerse plastic tube in ice, as ice will make it stiff and nonpliable.

2. Lubricant
3. Glass of water with drinking tube
4. Aspirating syringe, preferably barrel-plunger type, large 50-cc size
5. Two emesis basins
6. Rubber sheet with a clean sheet to cover it
7. Adhesive tape
8. If a large fluid return is expected, a measured pitcher
9. If the stomach is to be lavaged, a large pitcher of warm water

Procedure

The patient should be told the necessity of the procedure. Explicit explanations should be given as to (1) what is to be done and (2) what the patient should expect. In this procedure the patient is sitting upright in bed with head resting on a pillow. Explain that

1. The tube will be introduced through the nose to the back of the throat.
2. He will be given a glass of water with a drinking tube.
3. When the nasal tube is felt in the back of the throat, the water should be swallowed.

Carry out the procedure in the following steps:

1. Lubricate 5 to 10 cm (2 to 4 inches) of the tube with water-soluble lubricant.
2. Gently insert the catheter tip into a patent nostril.
3. Introduce the tube until it touches the posterior nasopharynx.
4. Ask patient to swallow.
   Move tube slowly so that its motion coincides with swallowing. In this way it is introduced through the esophagus without kinking back of the uvula and without causing retching and vomiting.
5. Advance tube to the second marking (about 55 cm). This usually places the tip within the stomach.
6. Tape tube to nose to hold in place and prevent discomfort of a back-and-forth motion.
7. Aspirate contents completely.
   Often a nasal tube becomes obstructed during aspiration. This may give the false indication that the stomach is empty, whereas the openings in the tube may be up against the stomach wall or small particles of food may be plugging the lumen. A small amount (20 ml) of warm water will clear the obstruction for further aspirating; aspiration of more fluid than that introduced will show that the stomach is not completely empty.
8. Note the quantity and quality of the residual (color, odor, presence of mucus, food, blood, or bile) and record in patient's chart.

Insertion of Levin Tube in Unconscious Patients

Because the unconscious patient cannot cooperate in swallowing the tube, special care is required to prevent the tube from entering the trachea and bronchi.

PROCEDURE. Carry out the procedure as follows:

1. If possible, raise the patient to a near-sitting position.
2. Insert tube into nostril and advance tube cautiously. Sometimes stroking the throat will incite the reflex of swallowing.
3. If patient starts choking, the tube could be entering the trachea. Immerse the end of the tube in water: if air bubbles arise at each expiration the tube should be removed and another attempt made.

4. Make positive proof of the tube's position in the stomach before introducing fluid or before leaving the patient:

   a. Aspirate for stomach contents.
   b. Place a stethoscope on the stomach and introduce 20 cc of air into the tube; a loud pop will be heard if the tube is within the stomach.

Gastric Analysis

Gastric analysis is a diagnostic test performed to determine the degree of acidity of the stomach contents. If an ulcer is present, the degree of acidity may be greater than normal. In cases of gastric carcinoma or pernicious anemia, the degree of acidity may be decreased or acidity may be absent altogether [1].

Gastric analysis requires the stomach to be in a fasting state. The patient receives nothing by mouth after the evening meal; the procedure is usually carried out the following morning. As water dilutes the stomach contents, only a minimal amount should be swallowed with the tube. Since the degree of acidity of the gastric contents will be affected by contamination by saliva and duodenal contents, it is important that the tube be within the stomach [2]. Gastric juice that is bile-stained indicates that alkaline duodenal contents have flowed back into the stomach. After the tube has been introduced into the stomach, the patient should expectorate all saliva to prevent contamination of gastric secretion [2].

Use gentle suction when aspirating stomach contents. Vigorous suction may cause bleeding or cause the tube to be sucked against the gastric mucosa, obstructing the lumen of the tube.

FASTING GASTRIC CONTENTS. Aspirate entire stomach contents. Two or three drops of Töpfer's reagent may be added to the specimen to demonstrate free hydrochloric acid. Red color indicates the presence of free acid. If this screening test indicates no acid, the physician may order test meals or 7 percent alcohol to produce mild stimulation [2].

If ordered, 50 ml of 7 percent alcohol (ethanol) is instilled in the tube. A second specimen is taken about one-half hour later.

If maximal stimulation of the parietal cells is necessary, the physician will usually order parenteral administration of histamine. Usually 0.01 mg of histamine base per kilogram of body weight is injected subcutaneously [2]. A specimen is taken about one-half hour after the histamine injection. The tube is removed.

Histamine is contraindicated in paroxysmal hypertension and in patients who have a history of asthma. As histamine stimulates gastric secretion, it should not be given before gastric radiography, which requires an empty stomach.

Acid-Fast Test

The acid-fast test is performed on fasting patients, usually on 3 consecutive days, to detect the presence of tubercle bacilli. In handling specimens care should be taken to prevent the spread of infectious material. The entire contents of the stomach are aspirated and placed in a container—usually a glass jar with a screw top. The specimen is then placed in a paper bag, labeled to alert personnel of possible infectious material, and sent to the bacteriology laboratory.

Cytological Examination

Cytological studies are performed by specially trained personnel to detect the presence of carcinoma cells. The fasting specimen, free of food contamination, is analyzed shortly after recovery to prevent digestion of cells.

References

1. Garb, S. *Laboratory Tests in Common Use* (4th ed.). New York: Springer Publishing, 1966. Pp. 142–144.
2. Page, L., and Culver, P. *A Syllabus of Laboratory Examinations in Clinical Diagnosis.* Cambridge, Mass.: Harvard University Press, 1960. Pp. 386–389.

21. Organization of an Intravenous Department and Guide to Teaching

The Value of Parenteral Teams

An intravenous department plays an important role in the services of a hospital. The quality of patient care is improved because specialized nurses, freed from other responsibilities, are able to focus attention on developing standards of performance; programs relevant to intravenous therapy are easier to maintain. These nurses, cognizant of potential dangers, are vigilant and meticulous in performing and maintaining intravenous therapy. Their continuous experience contributes to the performance of atraumatic venipunctures, conservation of veins, and reduction of complications. The knowledge, skill, and experience of these specialized nurses add to the safety of the blood bank program. The simultaneous administration of intravenous solutions and collection of blood samples does much to alleviate the anxiety of the patient and preserve the veins. The nurses, by preparing and administering drugs and performing other duties, free the doctor for his medical duties. The value of intravenous therapy teams has been well documented. In one hospital, despite the fact that the Transfusion Therapy Service maintained 90 percent of the total number of catheters, it was responsible for only 11 percent of the transfusion-related infections [2]. This was attributed mainly to (1) the skill and experience of specially trained personnel in inserting catheters atraumatically and (2) the daily and twice-daily observation and care of catheter sites.

The Center for Disease Control, in its Recommendations for the Prevention of I.V.-Associated Infections [3], reported:

Experience has indicated that proper maintenance of intravenous fluid systems is most efficiently and effectively carried out if intravenous "teams" are responsible for intravenous therapy throughout the hospital. Heterogeneous groups of individuals, such as house officers, staff doctors, and nurses, have been much less successful in methodically and meticulously following the above recommendations.

In a report of the National Coordinating Committee on Large Volume Parenterals, Baker [1] stated:

With regard to nursing personnel, should functional specialization for IV administration be encouraged? An example of this would be the use of IV teams. Should their use be required? Certified? Should special or continuing education be required? There is a feeling that the answer is "yes" to all these questions. Any recommendations will probably stop short of making IV teams a requirement for the smaller hospital.

With the increasing complexity of intravenous therapy and the potential dangers associated with it, hospitals have come to recognize the value of intravenous therapy teams. More and more hospitals are establishing parenteral departments.

Directorship of the Department

Because the functions performed by the Intravenous Department are not generally classified as nursing procedures, the responsibility for this department is often allocated to the head of another department directly involved in the functions of intravenous therapy, such as the Director of the Blood Bank, the Pharmacy, or the Anesthesia Department. The Intravenous Department (1) fulfills an important function of the Blood Bank, administering bloods and blood components, (2) is in close alliance with the Pharmacy, administering infusions of which 50 to 80 percent contain drugs, and (3) executes many of the functions performed by the anesthesiologist. Since some of these procedures may be considered medical functions it is advisable to have a physician share the responsibility or be available for counsel and advice.

Philosophy and Objectives

In organizing a department the first consideration should be given to establishing a philosophy and the objectives necessary to support such a philosophy. An example follows:

Philosophy (purpose): To administer safe and successful intravenous therapy in the best interests of the patient, the hospital, and the nursing profession.
Objectives
1. To develop skills and impart knowledge that will provide a high level of safety in the practice of intravenous therapy (embodies administration of solutions and drugs, administration of blood and blood components, placement of intravenous needles and catheters, and withdrawal of blood samples).
2. To encourage further education and knowledge in the field of intravenous therapy.

3. To assist in keeping the nursing staff educated in the maintenance of intravenous therapy and other nursing needs relevant to intravenous therapy.
4. To collaborate with orientation personnel in the development and implementation of continuing education in intravenous therapy.
5. To develop nursing judgment in intravenous therapy.
6. To keep abreast of the latest scientific and medical advances and their implications in the practice of intravenous therapy.

Functions of an Intravenous Department

In organizing an intravenous department, one must first classify the functions to be performed. They may include the following:

1. Administration of parenteral fluids
2. Preparation and administration of drugs in solution
3. Administration of blood
4. Routine inspection and daily change of all infusion tubings and dressings
5. Bleeding of donors
6. Bleeding of patients under supervision of the physician
7. Administration of hypodermoclysis
8. Collection of venous blood samples for all laboratories: chemistry, bacteriology, hematology, blood bank, and so on. This includes:
   a. Collection of blood samples routinely from all surgical admissions for typing and grouping in the Blood Bank
   b. Knowledge of the requirements of the various laboratory tests, including the proper collection and handling of blood samples
9. Administration of Levin tubes for therapy and for diagnostic tests
10. Computation of blood volumes by means of the Volemetron

Policies and Procedures

Policies and procedures play a basic and vital role in the functioning of a department, serving as a guide to its operations, providing the nurse with adequate instruction, and assuring the patient of a high level of nursing care. They may also provide legal protection in determining whether or not an individual involved in negligent conduct has had adequate instruction in performing the act.

Policies describing the responsibilities of the intravenous nurse vary significantly among hospitals and should be outlined to prevent confusion or misunderstanding. Examples of a few such policies follow:

Administration of Parenteral Fluids

1. Intravenous nurses will, upon written order, initiate all infusions, with the exception of those not approved for administration by the nurse.
2. No more than two attempts at venipuncture will be allowed. If two attempts are unsuccessful, the supervisor must be notified.
3. No venipuncture will be performed on the lower extremities. Veins should be avoided in the affected arm of an axillary dissection.
4. All intravenous lines are to be changed every 24 hours.
5. Solutions are to be labeled indicating the date and time the seal is broken. All intravenous solutions must be used or discarded within 24 hours of the time the container is opened.
6. Double clamps are to be used on all intravenous infusions.

Insertion of Intracatheters and Plastic Needles

1. Catheters are not to be used routinely and are inserted by the nurse upon written order of the physician.
2. All catheters and needles must be labeled indicating the date and time of insertion. All are to be removed after 72 hours.

Preparation and Administration of Intravenous Drugs

1. Nurses will, upon written order, prepare and administer only those solutions, medications, and combination of drugs approved in writing by the Pharmacy and the Therapeutics Committee.
2. Nurses must check the patient's chart and question the patient regarding sensitivity to drugs which may cause anaphylaxis. They must observe the patient following initial administration of such drugs. If a question of sensitivity exists, the drug should be administered by the physician.

Use of Force in Performing Venipuncture

No coercion will ever be used on a rational adult patient. If such a patient refuses an infusion or transfusion, the intravenous nurse will report the fact to the head nurse or physician.

Flushing and Irrigation of Intravenous Needles and Catheters

1. Plugged needles and catheters are not to be irrigated or flushed. Positive pressure, either by the positive pressure chamber of the infusion set or by syringe, shall not be used to remove a stubborn clot.
2. Needles and catheters may be flushed or irrigated for the sole purpose of *maintaining* patency.

Procedures should provide in detail the step-by-step directions for performing each function.

Selection of Personnel

The intravenous nurse is usually a registered nurse who is specially hired and trained since intravenous therapy involves the administration of drugs, blood, and fluids requiring specialized judgment and skill. Because of the highly specialized therapy and the responsibility involved, the success of the department will depend upon the selection of its personnel. Not all nurses are successful as intravenous nurses.

The nurse must be conscientious. She will be drawing blood samples and giving transfusions where carelessness could mean a patient's life. The conscientious nurse will realize the importance of her job, the importance of being accurate, and the importance of careful patient identification. Her duties include mixing and administering drugs which, given intravenously, act rapidly. There is no margin for error.

Cooperation and teamwork are essential to the success of the department. No one individual's job is finished until the entire department has completed its work. If one nurse becomes involved in a time-consuming emergency, the others must show a readiness and willingness to help out and accomplish the remaining work.

Mental and emotional stability play an important part in the nurse's success as an intravenous therapist. Manual dexterity, necessary in administering an intravenous infusion, is greatly affected by the mental and emotional attitude of the nurse. The performance of few procedures is so easily affected by stress as is the execution of a difficult venipuncture.

An understanding and pleasant personality are other assets necessary to the success of the individual and the department. The nurse has unpleasant functions to perform. These unpleasant tasks are better tolerated by the patient if the nurse is understanding and congenial.

She must be tactful. The nurse works in close conjunction with the hospital nursing staff, the blood bank, the various laboratories, and the patient. Her attitude and her personality could do much to impair the harmony of these departments.

The nurse in charge of the Intravenous Department, who must assume responsibility for the teaching, training, and successful functioning of this department, should have a voice in selecting its personnel.

Once the functions of this department are classified, the work load should start at a reasonable level. It may be desirable to start by performing only a few designated functions, such as the administration of blood and fluids. After this program has been successfully organized, other functions may be added. By so doing, the problems that may arise on initiating such a program may be met and remedied, and the success of the department may be guaranteed from the outset.

Before this department can go into operation, the hospital nursing staff must first be educated as to its functions.

Call System

A system for receiving calls must be organized, with special emphasis on emergency calls. Some systems work to better advantage than others under various conditions. The size of the hospital, number of patients, size and location of the department, and the functions to be performed must be taken into consideration in deciding which system would be most adaptable.

REQUISITIONS. Requests for parenteral administrations and other functions may be filled out on requisitions and sent to the department. This system contains drawbacks because of the added paperwork, lost time involved, and the necessity of the intravenous therapist's having to return to the department to pick up the requisitions. It may prove successful in smaller hospitals where calls are not as numerous and where the nurses are stationed in the blood bank or laboratory.

PAGE SYSTEM. The page operator lists the floor extensions as they are received. The intravenous nurse calls in every half hour and picks up her calls. Any emergency call may be put through by means of voice page or by means of a radio pager.

ROUTINE ROUNDS. Routine rounds may be made twice a day by the intravenous therapist. The requests for services are listed on a clipboard with the patient's name and room number. When orders have been filled they are checked off by the intravenous therapist. One nurse in each building is equipped with a radio pager. This is used only for emergency calls or requests that must be performed before the second round, or after rounds are completed.

This system involves less expenditure of time by the nursing staff. It eliminates the necessity for placing calls or sending out requisitions. The intravenous department is freed from unnecessary phone calls. The charge nurse, with a glance at the board, immediately knows what procedures have been performed.

Preparation of Equipment

Setting up the necessary equipment for procedures to be performed must be allotted to either the intravenous department or the nursing staff.

PREPARATION OF EQUIPMENT BY INTRAVENOUS DEPARTMENT. When preparation of equipment becomes the responsibility of the intravenous department, an equipment cart must be provided on each floor. This cart carries all necessary equipment for parenteral administration:

Intravenous solutions	Bandage
Intravenous sets	Adhesive tape
Armboards	Alcohol
Poles	Syringes
Levin tubes	Sterile sponges
Tourniquet	

The nurse checks the orders directly from the doctor's order book. By means of the equipment cart, she sets up the procedures and initiates each order as she continues rounds.

PREPARATION OF EQUIPMENT BY NURSING STAFF. The nurse distributes necessary equipment, solution, set, armboard, and pole for parenteral fluids or a tray containing Levin tube equipment. The intravenous nurse carries a prep tray. This system automatically places a double check on solutions and medications ordered. It saves time. If each nurse is responsible for setting up the necessary equipment for her patient, little time is lost by her, whereas a great deal of time is utilized by the intravenous therapist in preparing all patients. This system eliminates the necessity for an equipment cart on each floor.

Cooperation of Interdepartmental Personnel

Before this department starts to function, a thorough explanation must be made to the staff of doctors, for only with cooperation in every department will success be guaranteed. The doctors should be requested to cooperate by writing intravenous orders early—before 9 A.M. when at all possible. This will assure the physician that his orders are initiated at a reasonable hour. This is particularly important when the Intravenous Department has inaugurated the system of making rounds.

Collection of Blood Samples

The program for collection of blood samples may be initiated and become an added function of the Intravenous Department only after

1. The therapists have been adequately trained in the necessary laboratory procedures.
2. A system has been set up for receiving calls.
3. A method has been arranged for transportation of specimens to the laboratories.
4. The nursing staff and the departments have been made aware of their responsibilities.

Training of Therapist

Before this program is initiated, the intravenous therapist should visit the various laboratories. The nurse should be educated in the proper method of collecting, handling, and transporting blood specimens. She must understand and be educated in the performance of the various laboratory tests.

Requisitions

A system for notifying the Intravenous Department of requests for blood samples must be arranged. (1) Requisitions may be sent directly to the Intravenous Department. (2) Requisitions left at a designated area on each floor may be picked up by the intravenous therapist on rounds. This system saves time and prevents the unnecessary handling and sorting of requisitions from all floors.

Transportation

A safe method of transporting the specimens to the various laboratories must be arranged. This duty may be allotted to (1) Ward helpers on each floor. (2) Intravenous nurse. This is impractical as many bloods must be delivered to laboratories within a limited time. The accuracy of some tests depends upon immediate analysis or proper refrigeration. (3) Messenger service by routine pick up or by call system. (4) By a direct specimen chute to the laboratories.

Operational Activities of the Intravenous Department at the Massachusetts General Hospital

Call System

The Intravenous Department has inaugurated the system of routine rounds and makes use of the radio pager for urgent requests. The department services the wards by means of routine rounds twice a day plus early rounds for fasting blood samples only.

Requests for procedures to be performed are listed with the patient's name and room number on designated blackboards and clipboards. Orders executed are checked off by the therapist. Any orders written after first rounds are added to the board to be carried out on afternoon rounds.

One intravenous nurse in each building is equipped with a radio pager. This page system is used only when (1) emergency procedures are necessary, (2) urgent procedures are required that must be performed before second rounds, or (3) tests involving specific times must be made, e.g., blood samples to be drawn at a specific time after injection of dye. The page system is used full-time after last rounds are made.

A printed card reading INTRAVENOUS NURSE ON THE FLOOR is carried by each intravenous therapist. This card is left at the desk for the duration of time the nurse is on the ward.

ADMINISTRATION OF PARENTERAL FLUIDS. The intravenous nurse initiates all intravenous infusions, with the exception of those prepared by the doctor and containing drugs not on the authorized list. The intravenous nurse does not

1. Administer intravenous infusions in the lower extremities.
2. Apply positive pressure in administering parenteral fluids.
3. Apply force in administering intravenous or other procedures on rational adult patients. Refusal to comply with treatment is reported to the physician.

The intravenous nurse and the nursing service remove catheter needles and intracatheters when infiltration occurs or infusion is terminated, on the order of the doctor.

PREPARATION AND ADMINISTRATION OF DRUGS IN SOLUTION. The intravenous nurse prepares and administers all drugs on the authorized list only, affixing to the solution bottle a label containing the name of the patient, the name of the drug, dosage prepared, and the time and date. The intravenous nurse must realize that she is legally responsible for every medication she administers.

ADMINISTRATION OF TRANSFUSIONS. The Intravenous Department initiates transfusions.

1. All transfusions require filters.
2. Bloods are not delivered to the wards until requested by the intravenous therapist.
3. Bloods are not to be placed in the ward refrigerator.
4. Bloods not used within a half hour are to be returned to the Blood Bank.
5. The intravenous therapist remains and observes the patient for the first 5 minutes after initiating the transfusion.
6. Transfusions are to be terminated at once if reactions occur. *Imperative:* Reaction slips are sent to the Blood Bank with a blood sample.
7. Positive pressure is never applied when administering blood except under the direct supervision of the physician.
8. Staff nurses are not allowed to attach blood to an intravenous infusion. This is the responsibility of the intravenous nurse.

COLLECTION OF VENOUS BLOOD SAMPLES FOR ALL HOSPITAL LABORATORIES. *Program.* Each ward has an allotted area designated for the use of the blood collection program. This area contains

1. Large envelope in which blood requisitions are left for the intravenous nurse.
2. Blood collection equipment, including stock of various Vacutainer tubes and needles.
3. Containers (small wire baskets) to hold blood samples, labeled and painted different colors to designate the various laboratories.

Venous blood samples. All requisitions for venous blood are placed in the requisition envelope until 3 P.M. on weekdays and until noon on Saturdays. After 3 P.M. on weekdays only emergency requisitions and requisitions for the blood bank are honored. Each afternoon the intravenous nurse draws blood samples on all surgical admissions, to be sent to the blood bank for typing.

LEVIN TUBES. The intravenous nurse inserts Levin tubes, except that she does not perform this function on patients (1) with esophageal varices, (2) on aneurysm precautions, or (3) who have had radical neck surgery. She does insert Levin tubes for (1) preoperative cases, (2) feeding, (3) gastric analysis, and (4) acid-fast tests.

ADDITIONAL FUNCTIONS. The intravenous therapist also performs *administration of hypodermoclysis, blood volume computation by means of the Volemetron, phlebotomy* (under the supervision of the physician), and (under the direction of the Anesthesia Department) *insertion of intracatheters and central venous catheters* on patients in the operating room.

Teaching Program

An adequate teaching program and criteria for the evaluation of the intravenous nurse must be established. The criteria will be dependent upon the role of the intravenous nurse as dictated by hospital policies. The competency of the nurse may be substantiated by answering questionnaires on intravenous therapy, transfusion therapy, and drug therapy and a demonstration of involved procedures, such as the administration of parenteral fluids using metal needles and plastic catheters, the administration of blood and its components, the preparation and administration of drug admixtures, and the collection of blood samples. The intravenous nurse receives on-the-job training. The length of time involved in teaching depends upon the individual and may range from 3 to 6 weeks. The following is a suggested outline for teaching intravenous, drug, and transfusion therapy.

I. Legal implications of intravenous therapy
   A. *State policy.* Review state rulings, joint policies related to intravenous therapy
   B. *Hospital policy.* Review health institution's or agency's policy, which has been approved by the medical staff
      1. Responsibilities of nurse in administering intravenous therapy
      2. List of fluids and drugs delineated by the hospital for administration by the nurse
   C. Legal requirements
      1. Qualification by education and experience
      2. Adherence to hospital policy
      3. Thorough knowledge of fluids and drugs: their effects, limitations, and dosage
      4. Order by licensed physician for specific patient
      5. Skilled judgment
   D. Review of policy and procedure books
      1. Policy statements do not provide immunity if the nurse is negligent
      2. The nurse is legally responsible for her own acts
II. Equipment
   A. Review all types of equipment, their characteristics and usage
   B. Review procedures for the proper handling of equipment, changing of in-line administration sets, use of filters, etc.
   C. Adhere to established infection control procedures and guidelines in the use of equipment
      1. Aseptic technique in manipulation of equipment
      2. Inspection of parenteral fluids and containers
      3. Daily change of administration sets
III. Anatomy and physiology as applied to intravenous therapy
   A. Review names and locations of peripheral veins of the upper extremity
   B. Differentiate between arteries and veins. Recognize an inadvertent arterial puncture
   C. Recognize dangers associated with the use of veins of the lower extremities
   D. Understand factors that influence the size and condition of the vein
      1. Trauma
      2. Temperature
      3. Diagnosis of the patient
      4. Psychological outlook of the patient

E. Choose veins suitable for venipuncture
  1. To infuse various fluids and medications, with preservation of veins in mind
  2. To draw blood samples
  3. To administer blood
IV. Intravenous therapy
  A. Methods of infusion
    1. Constant
    2. Intermittent (by "piggyback" or heparin lock)
    3. Infusion by pump
  B. Manner and approach to the patient
    1. Explain the vasovagal reaction (an undesirable autonomic nervous system response)
    2. Alleviate fears
      a. Make patient comfortable
      b. Explain procedure
      c. Reassure patient
      d. Appear confident
  C. Methods of distending veins
    1. Apply a broad tourniquet above selected site
    2. Apply a blood pressure cuff inflated to 50 to 60 mm of mercury or to just below diastolic pressure
    3. Periodic clenching of the fist
    4. Allow arm to hang dependent over the side of the bed
    5. Light tapping slightly distal to the proposed venipuncture site
    6. Moist heat to entire extremity
  D. *Antiseptic and aseptic technique.* Skin flora have been implicated as an important source of organisms responsible for catheter-associated infection. Adherence to aseptic and antiseptic technique is imperative, especially during preparation of the venipuncture site
  E. Choice of cannula (straight metal needle, scalp vein needle, catheter)
    1. Purpose of the infusion
    2. Condition and availability of the vein
    3. Gauge and length of cannula depend upon:
      a. Location of the vein
      b. Fluid employed
      c. Purpose of the infusion
  F. Techniques of venipuncture
    1. Scalp vein needle
    2. Syringe and needle
    3. Vacuum tube and needle holder (commercially supplied)

4. Catheters (over-the-needle, through-the-needle). Complications associated with catheters include mechanical and chemical thrombophlebitis, infection, and catheter embolism

G. Hazards and complications. Observing the patient, reporting reactions, and taking measures to prevent complications are the nurse's legal and professional responsibilities

1. Systemic complications
   a. Infections (septicemia, fungemia)
      Preventive measures
      1) Use aseptic and antiseptic technique
      2) Inspect all fluids and containers before use
      3) Use fluids within 24 hours
      4) Change administration sets daily
      5) Do not irrigate plugged cannulas
      6) Remove nonfunctioning sets and needles
   b. Pulmonary embolism (occurs when a substance, usually a clot, becomes free floating and is propelled by the venous circulation to the right side of the heart and on into the pulmonary artery)
      Preventive measures
      1) Use clot filters for infusing blood and blood components
      2) Use special blood filters of micropore size for infusing several units of stored bank blood
      3) Avoid using veins of the lower extremities
      4) Avoid irrigating plugged cannulas
   c. Air embolism (may be fatal when small bubbles accumulate dangerously and form tenacious bubbles that block the pulmonary capillaries)
      Preventive measures
      1) Vigilance in preventing fluid containers from emptying. Infusions through a central venous catheter carry greater risk of running dry as there is more apt to be a negative venous pressure
      2) Vented Y-type infusions or piggyback infusions allowing solutions to run simultaneously may introduce air into line if container empties. Check valves, safety valves, and micropore filters (wet) reduce this risk
   d. Circulatory overload (a real hazard in patients with impaired renal and cardiac functions)
      Preventive measures
      1) Maintain infusion at prescribed flow rate

2) Never apply positive pressure when infusing fluids and blood
3) Do not administer fluids in excess of quantity ordered to maintain a keep-open infusion
4) Be alert to signs of circulatory overload

e. Speed shock (systemic reaction occurring when a substance foreign to the body is rapidly introduced into the circulation)

Preventive measures

1) Slow injection of drugs
2) Use of controlled volume chambers
3) Use of micropore drip sets
4) Use of double clamps—an extra clamp ensures greater safety should the initial clamp let go
5) Ensure that intravenous fluid is flowing freely before regulating the flow

f. Fluid and medication error

Preventive measures

1) Be familiar with intravenous fluids
2) Know drug, dosage, and rate of administration
3) Clarify orders
4) Substantiate identity of the patient and the admixture

2. Local complications

a. Phlebitis (mechanical, chemical, and septic)

Preventive measures

1) Do not use veins located over an area of joint flexion
2) Anchor cannulas well to prevent motion and reduce the risk of introducing microorganisms into puncture wound
3) Adequately dilute medications
4) Use a needle or catheter relatively smaller than the vein
5) Use aseptic and antiseptic technique
6) Remove needle within 72 hours
7) Remove needle for:
   a) Erythema
   b) Induration
   c) Tenderness by palpation of venous cord
   d) Nonfunctioning needle

b. Infiltration (recognize extravasation)

1) Check questionable extremity against normal extremity
2) Apply a tourniquet tightly enough to restrict venous flow proximal to the injection site. If infusion con-

tinues regardless of this venous obstruction, extravasation is evident

V. Rationale of fluid and electrolyte therapy
  A. Fundamentals of fluid and electrolyte metabolism
    1. Body fluid compartments
    2. Electrolyte composition
    3. Acid–base balance
  B. Principles of fluid therapy
    1. Deficit
    2. Maintenance
    3. Replacement
  C. Intravenous fluids
    1. Classification and effect
      a. Isotonic
      b. Hypotonic
      c. Hypertonic
    2. Parenteral fluids
VI. Drug therapy
  A. Hazards
    1. Incompatibilities
      a. Therapeutic (undesirable reaction from overlapping effect of two drugs)
      b. Physical (interaction which leads to a visible change such as color, precipitate, or gas bubbles)
      c. Chemical (invisible interaction, with degradation of drug and loss of therapeutic activity)
    2. Vascular trauma
    3. Speed shock
    4. Bacterial and fungal contamination
    5. Particulate contamination
    6. Medication errors
  B. Knowledge of the drug
    1. Dose and effect
    2. Recommended rate of infusion
    3. Reactions
    4. Contraindications
  C. Factors controlling stability and compatibility of admixtures
    1. Pharmaceutical agents in drug formation (buffers, preservatives, and stabilizers)
    2. Brand of drug (formulation varies)
    3. pH of drug, pH of intravenous fluid
    4. Concentration (degree of dilution)
    5. Order of mixing
    6. Diluent

7. Period of time solution stands
8. Light
9. Temperature
  D. Preparation of admixture
    1. Procedure for transcribing orders on medication label
    2. Frequency with which medication order should be renewed
    3. Reconstitution of drug using aseptic and antiseptic technique
      a. Correct diluent
      b. Correct volume
      c. Absence of particulate matter
    4. Procedure for adding drug to fluid container
    5. Stability of the admixture
    6. Labeling
  E. Administration of drugs
    1. Substantiate identity of patient and admixture
    2. Check for sensitivities of patient to any drug that may cause anaphylaxis
    3. Observe patient for untoward reactions when administering an initial dose of an antibiotic
    4. Patients known to be sensitive to a drug require the presence of a physician
    5. Inspect admixture each time before administration
    6. Record drug, dosage, and amount of fluid on fluid intake chart and medication sheet
VII. Transfusion therapy
  A. Fundamentals of immunohematology
    1. Factors governing red blood cell distribution
    2. ABO compatibility
    3. Rh compatibility
    4. Handling and storage of blood
  B. Blood and blood components
    1. Uses
    2. Methods of administration
    3. Reactions and protocol to follow
  C. Administration of blood and blood components
    1. Substantiate identity of patient and blood
    2. Inspect blood prior to administration
    3. Follow proper technique in administration
    4. Observe patient

References

1. Baker, K. N. Interim report of National Coordinating Committee on Large Volume Parenterals. *Drug Intelligence and Clinical Pharmacy* 7:477, 1973.
2. Bentley, D. W., and Lepper, M. H. Septicemia related to indwelling venous catheters. *Journal of the American Medical Association* 206: 1749, 1968.
3. Center for Disease Control. *Recommendations for the Prevention of I.V.-Associated Infections* (for training purposes, Hospital Infectious and Microbiological Control Sections, Bacterial Disease Branch, Epidemiology Program). Atlanta, March 1973.

Index

postcatheterization management, 190–191
insertion of, 64–68
  by intravenous nurses, 322
  policies, 316
  sterile technique in, 85
  surgical, 68
Intracellular body fluids, 120, 124
Intramuscular drug administration, 3
Intravenous department, organization of, 313–328
  and blood sample collection, 319–320, 321–322
  and blood transfusion, 321
  call system, 318, 320
  cooperation and, 319
  directorship, 314
  and drug intravenous therapy, 321
  and equipment preparation, 318–319
  and fluid-electrolyte therapy, 321
  history of, 2
  at Massachusetts General Hospital, 320–322
  personnel selection, 317
  philosophy and objectives, 314–315
  policies and procedures, 315
  routine rounds, 318
  teaching program, 322–328
  and value of, 313–314
Intravenous infusion, defined, 155–156
Intravenous push of drugs, 231
Intravenous solution. See Parenteral solutions
Investigational drugs, 13, 14
Iodine in skin preparation, 107
Iron
  intravenous administration, 221
  serum, 290
Iron-binding capacity of serum, 290
Isotonic body fluid contraction, 176, 178
Isotonic body fluid expansion, 174–175, 177, 178
Isotonic multiple electrolyte fluids, 167–168

Jugular vein
  in central venous pressure monitoring, 236
  in parenteral nutrition, 188

Ketone bodies, 144, 151, 152
Kidneys
  acid-base balance and, 125, 128
  bicarbonate concentration and, 125
  diabetic acidosis and, 151–152
  fluid-electrolyte balance and, 128
  fluid-electrolyte therapy and, 137

function tests, 174, 281, 294, 301–302
hydrating fluids and, 165
intravenous flow rate and function of, 75, 76
potassium replacement and, 119–120

Lactated Ringer's soluton, 168
Lactic acid, blood, 290
Lactic dehydrogenase, serum (SLD), 290, 299
Laminar flow hood, 223
Lead, blood, 291
Leg veins
  described, 43
  for intravenous therapy, 43, 53
    complications, 53, 85, 89
    drug therapy, 220
Legal factors, 5–16
  guidelines and definitions, 13–16
  instruction in, 323
  investigational drugs, 13, 14
  Levin tube insertion, 307
  nurse vs. physician responsibility, 5, 12, 13
  professional and government regulations, 5–13
Levarterenol bitartrate infusion, 221
Levin tube, 307–311
  in acid-fast test, 307, 311, 322
  in gastric analysis, 307, 310, 322
  in gastric cytological examination, 307, 311
  indications for use, 307–308
  insertion
    equipment, 308
    by nurses, 307, 322
    technique, 308–310
  use in unconscious patients, 309–310
Liability, rule of personal, defined, 15–16
Light
  for drug solution preparation, 223
  drug stability and, 219
  for venipuncture, 58
Lipase, serum, 291, 298
Lipids, serum, 291
Lipoprotein electrophoresis, 291
Liquid stored plasma, 251
Lithium, serum, 291
Liver function
  gastric replacement and impaired, 120
  tests of, 299–300
Lungs. See also Pulmonary edema; Pulmonary embolism
  fluid-electrolyte balance and, 128, 129

343

Pneumothorax, subclavian catheterization and, 191
Polycythemia vera, phlebotomy for, 263, 264
Porphyria cutania tarda, phlebotomy for, 263, 264
Positive pressure infusion, 29, 30, 31
  responsibility for, 81
  veins for, 54
Postoperative fluid-electrolyte therapy, 140–145
  fluids in, 141, 143
  nutrients in, 144–145
Postprandial blood sugar test, 302
Potassium
  blood stored for transfusion and, 248
  in body fluids, 122, 123, 129–131.
    See also Hyperkalemia; Hypokalemia
  in burns, 146
  chloride loss and, 133
  determination of, 280, 281, 292, 295
  in diabetic acidosis, 152, 153
  exchange with sodium, 131, 143
  glucose metabolism and, 203
  importance of, 129–130, 295
  intravenous administration, 136
    in dehydration, 119–120
    in diabetic acidosis, 153
    flow rate, 145
    postoperative, 145
    precautions and dangers in, 76, 77, 137, 145
  metabolic alkalosis and, 125
  normal level, 295
  packed red cell transfusion and, 249
  regulation of, 128, 129
  sample collection for determining, 292, 295
  shifts in, 123
  transfusion and, 248, 249
Potassium oxalate in blood preservation, 280
Preservation of blood for transfusion, 248
Preservatives, drug stability and, 219
Pressure cuff, 29, 31
Private duty nurses, 13
Protein(s)
  carbohydrates and catabolism of, 144
  intravenous infusion of
    freshness of solutions, 89
    human plasma protein fraction, 254
    infusion rate, 77
    in maintenance therapy, 136
    for parenteral nutrition, 186
    postoperative, 145

serum
  determination of, 174
  total, 292, 299–300
Prothrombin time test, 281, 301
Psychological factors
  complications of intravenous therapy and, 51–52
  in total parenteral nutrition, 205–207
  in infants and children, 210–211
Pulmonary circulation, 42
Pulmonary edema, 83, 93
  circulatory overload and, 175
  hypertonic intravenous saline and, 164–165
  intravenous flow rate and, 76, 93–94
  prevention, 93–94
Pulmonary embolism, 83, 325
  blood clots and, 89
  massive transfusion and, 112
  reducing risk of, 42, 89–90, 325
  thrombosis and, 43, 53, 89
Pulmonary insufficiency, 111
Pulse in evaluation of fluid-electrolyte balance, 171–172
Pumps, infusion, 34, 37–38
Pyrogenic reactions, 83, 101
  to blood transfusions, 257–258
  reducing risk of, 88–89
Pyrogens, defined, 1–2
Pyruvic acid, blood, 293

Quinidine, serum, 293

Radio-opaque material, intra-arterial infusion of, 41
Rate of flow. *See* Flow rate
Red cells
  hemolysis of. *See* Hemolysis
  transfusion of packed, 249–250
Reduction, chemical, 217
Requisitions
  for blood samples, 320, 322
  to intravenous department, 318
Respiratory acidosis, 125
Respiratory alkalosis, 124–125
Respiratory system. *See* Lungs; Pulmonary edema; Pulmonary embolism
Rh factor, 246
  anti-Rh immunoglobulin infusion and, 252–253
  discovery of, 3
  tests for, 303, 328
$Rh_o(D)$ immune-globulin infusion, 254–255
Roller infusion pumps, 34, 37
"Rule of nines" in burn surface area determination, 148